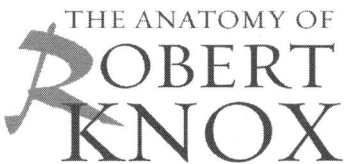

Dr Knox ... is not one of those rote practitioners whose sickening tediousness puts us in mind of the monotonous gyrations of donkeys turning mills. No! Nature is his goddess, and he is her high priest.

Medical Times, 1840; 1: 225

Practical anatomy, at best, is a loathsome, fatiguing, cold, monotonous, and tiresome piece of business.... It is only a select few who, influenced by ... a lofty ambition of professional distinction, bear up against the tedium and disgust of the operation, and continue their dissections after having obtained a license to practise.

The Metropolitan, 1832; 3: 133–4

The greatest absurdity is not less readily conceivable, than the possibility of a good surgeon, or a successful practitioner in medicine, *without anatomy.*

The Hospital Pupil's Guide, 1818

THE ANATOMY OF ROBERT KNOX

Murder, Mad Science
and Medical Regulation
in Nineteenth-Century
Edinburgh

A. W. BATES

sussex
ACADEMIC
PRESS
Brighton • Portland • Toronto

Copyright © A. W. Bates, 2010, 2018

The right of A. W. Bates to be identified as Author of this work has been asserted in accordance with the Copyright, Designs and Patents Act 1988.

2 4 6 8 10 9 7 5 3

First published in 2010 in hardcover, reprinted in paperback 2018, by
SUSSEX ACADEMIC PRESS
PO Box 139
Eastbourne BN24 9BP

Distributed in the United States of America by
SUSSEX ACADEMIC PRESS
ISBS Publisher Services
920 NE 58th Ave   Suite 300
Portland, Oregon 97213-3786

All rights reserved. Except for the quotation of short passages for the purposes of criticism and review, no part of this publication may be reproduced, stored in a retrieval system or transmitted in any form or by any means, electronic, mechanical, photocopying, recording or otherwise, without the prior permission of the publisher.

British Library Cataloguing in Publication Data
A CIP catalogue record for this book is available from the British Library.

Library of Congress Cataloging-in-Publication Data
Bates, A. W. (Alan W.)
  The anatomy of Robert Knox : murder, mad science and medical regulation in nineteenth-century Edinburgh / A. W. Bates.
    p. ; cm.
  Includes bibliographical references and index.
  ISBN 978-1-84519-381-2 (h/c : alk. paper)
  ISBN 978-1-84519-561-8 (p/b : alk. paper)
    1. Knox, Robert, 1791–1862. 2. Anatomists—Scotland—Edinburgh—Biography. 3. Physicians—Scotland—Edinburgh—Biography. 4. Medicine—Scotland—Edinburgh—History—19th century. I. Title.
  [DNLM: 1. Knox, Robert, 1791–1862. 2. Physicians—Scotland—Biography. 3. Anatomists—Scotland—Biography. 4. Dissection— history—Scotland. 5. History, 19th Century—Scotland. WZ 100 B3288a 2010]
  QM16.K6B38 2010
  611.0092—dc22
  [B]   2009031749

Typeset and designed by Sussex Academic Press, Brighton & Eastbourne.
Printed by TJ International, Padstow, Cornwall.

Contents

List of Illustrations, Foreword & Acknowledgements

INTRODUCTION

CHAPTER ONE
The Darling Boy of the Family, 1791–1810
13

CHAPTER TWO
A Beautiful but Seductive Science, 1810–1814
19

CHAPTER THREE
Hospital Assistant, 1815–1820
30

CHAPTER FOUR
Parisian Anatomy, 1821–1822
42

CHAPTER FIVE
Museum Medicine, 1823–1825
51

CHAPTER SIX
Knox *Primus et Incomparabilis*, 1825–1828
57

CHAPTER SEVEN
The West Port Murders, 1828–1829
66

CHAPTER EIGHT
A Nation of Cannibals
78

Contents

CHAPTER NINE
The Most Popular Teacher in Our Metropolis, 1830–1836
85

CHAPTER TEN
A Scandalous Monopoly, 1836–1840
98

CHAPTER ELEVEN
Nature's High Priest, 1840–1844
105

CHAPTER TWELVE
Popular Anatomy, 1845–1848
116

CHAPTER THIRTEEN
The Races of Men, 1848–1851
122

CHAPTER FOURTEEN
A Great Scheme of Nature
130

CHAPTER FIFTEEN
Distrust Your Genius, 1851–1855
139

CHAPTER SIXTEEN
The Hideous Interior
146

CHAPTER SEVENTEEN
Organic Harmonies, 1855–1862
152

CHAPTER EIGHTEEN
Science Run Mad
161

Notes 175
Bibliography 204
Index 221

List of Illustrations

Cover illustrations (from the author's collection): FRONT Dr Knox lecturing, from a contemporary drawing by Professor Edward Forbes; sketch of a Xhosa skull described to the Wernerian society by Dr Knox. BACK Plan of the city of Edinburgh in the early-nineteenth century; Surgeons' Square as it appeared in the 1820s – Knox's school at no. 10, now demolished, lay between Old Surgeons' Hall (left) and the hall of the Royal Medical Society (right).

The following illustrations are placed after page 118.

1. Edinburgh's High School, which Knox attended from 1806 to 1810. The building is now part of Edinburgh University (photograph by the author).
2. Dr Knox lecturing (from the author's collection).
3. Knox's official Edinburgh home at 4 Newington Place (photograph by the author).
4. A display from the Jules Thorn Museum of the Royal College of Surgeons of Edinburgh, showing Knox with his textbook of anatomy (courtesy of the Royal College of Surgeons of Edinburgh).
5. One of the few remaining houses in Edinburgh's Surgeons' Square; No. 1, formerly Handyside's school of anatomy, which Lonsdale joined after leaving Knox (photograph by the author).
6. The Celts in Marylebone, as depicted in Knox's *Races of Men* (from the author's collection).
7. Mary Paterson as Venus in the dissecting room; from a drawing, now lost, by John Oliphant (from the author's collection).
8. Knox, watched by Burke and Hare, receives an anatomical specimen. *Tu doces* suggests both the cause of his celebrity and his fondness for puns ("thou tea-chest") (courtesy of the British Library).

Foreword by the President of the Royal College of Surgeons, Mr John Orr

Robert Knox was the foremost anatomist of his age yet his reputation was irrevocably tainted through his association with Burke and Hare. Dr Bates' work highlights Knox's position as an anatomy teacher of great distinction – the finest British anatomist of his generation. He also provides us with insight into the complex mind of someone who held many of the attributes of genius. Knox was Dux of the High School of Edinburgh, yet he failed his anatomy examinations but later went on to acquire a prodigious knowledge of his subject. He became a Fellow of the Royal Edinburgh College of Surgeons where he was instrumental in establishing the historic Barclay and Bell anatomical collections. He was appointed as the first Conservator of the College Museum, during which time he became the most successful teacher of anatomy in Edinburgh. Unfortunately, following 'the West Port Murders' and Burke's execution, his professional reputation was irreversibly damaged. His relationship with the College rapidly deteriorated and he resigned as the museum Conservator shortly before the opening of the magnificent Playfair building designed to house the collections. In later life, he resisted the introduction of the Anatomy Acts and failed to comply with any form of regulation of the Schools of Anatomy. The refusal of the College to recognise him as a teacher of anatomy effectively ended his academic career.

Throughout his career, he appears to be a man perpetually at odds with the establishment and, inevitably, a victim. This volume not only gives us unique insight into the society of early 19th century Scotland, the professional jealousies which existed at the time, and insight into the horrors of the surgery of warfare, but an insight into anatomy as the most important science supporting surgery just before the anaesthetic and antiseptic revolutions. It is entirely appropriate that more than 150 years after his death, anatomy is being reinvented as a study critically important to this generation of undergraduates and postgraduates. The volume tells us a great deal of his strengths and weaknesses, his refusal to conform when this would undermine his principles, but a recognition that Knox is now being restored as one of the most distinguished surgical anatomists in the history of Edinburgh surgery.

Acknowledgements

This book could not have been written without the matchless facilities of the Wellcome Trust Centre for the History of Medicine at University College London, and of UCL itself, which was so kind as to grant me an honorary appointment. It has been a great pleasure to visit so many institutions associated with Knox: in London, I was particularly fortunate in the assistance of Tina Craig, Deputy Head of Library and Information Services at the Royal College of Surgeons of England, Katharine Higgon and the staff of the Archives of King's College, Sarah Walpole of the Royal Anthropological Institute, and Victoria Rea, Archivist to the Royal Free Hospital. The staff of the Wellcome Library, the London Library, and the Library of the Royal Society of Medicine were, as ever, unfailingly helpful.

Scotland proved, if possible, even more hospitable, and I wish particularly to thank Julie Gardham, Assistant Librarian for Special Collections, and the staff of Glasgow University Library, Sally Pagan and colleagues at Edinburgh University Library, Marianne Smith, Librarian of the Royal College of Surgeons of Edinburgh (where I was extremely glad to be one of the few visitors that day not sitting the notoriously difficult examinations), and Gemma Tougher and the staff of the National Archives of Scotland.

Dr Sam Behjati advised on the German translation.

Introduction

When Oliver Wendell Holmes, whom Robert Knox had once invited to breakfast, came to write of his "hundred days" in Europe, more than fifty years later, he spoke for posterity when he bluntly declared that the "celebrity" of "the monoculous Waterloo surgeon" was due less "to his book [*The Races of Men*] than to the unfortunate connection of his name with the unforgotten Burke and Hare horrors."[1] At the time of his death in 1862, Knox's obituarists tactfully ignored the scandal, but it was soon almost the only thing for which he was remembered: when Dr Robert Lightfoot of Newcastle upon Tyne died in 1908 at the age of ninety-three, *The Times* noted that he had been "a pupil of John [*sic*] Knox, the famous anatomist, who fell into disfavour through the Burke and Hare murders."[2]

The murders themselves were assimilated into the tales of anatomists, graveyards, and body snatchers that had been a source of macabre fascination since the early-nineteenth century, when former medical student Hector Berlioz borrowed the language of the gothic novel to populate the dissecting-room at *l'Hôpital de la Pitié* in Paris, where Knox later trained, with cracked skulls, scattered limbs, grimacing heads, "swarms" of birds and gnawing rats.[3] Such sanguinary accounts of the horrors of the "human charnel-house", it has been argued, gave rise to a popular association between "cannibalism" – represented by the "often grotesque dissolution of the individual" in the dissecting-room – and "godless science", whose rise threatened civilized culture and stirred up fears of the destruction of race, society and nation through "conquest by or reversion to barbarism." Fear of the anatomist – the purchaser of corpses, scientific cannibal and apostle of radical, agnostic, out-of-control science – was the fear of "the mad, the deviant, and the racial Other".[4] In literature and drama, Knox became the anti-hero of a Faustian morality play in which his noble, scientific ideals were perverted by an immoderate passion for knowledge that drew him into the company of the most repulsive of criminals. When their crimes came to light, he was professionally ruined and, with his reputation "irrevocably tarnished", was driven from Scotland and reduced to working as a barker for a travelling "Indian" show, before dying "in poverty".[5]

It makes a good story, though it is substantially untrue: Knox continued as an anatomy teacher in Edinburgh for more than ten years after the murders, much in demand with students, and he played a leading rôle in organizing the resistance of the city's anatomy teachers to the 1832 Anatomy Act. Murder for dissection was not even the most damaging episode in a career punctuated by scandals any one of which would have ruined a less tenacious protagonist: calumniating a fellow officer in the Cape, evading the provisions of the Anatomy Act, academic plagiarism, unlicensed teaching, and signing false certificates. In the face of so many unfortunate episodes it is difficult to disagree with the conclusion of Knox's detractors, that he could be utterly unscrupulous.[6] He was also more successful than many would have liked. After leaving the army at a time when many Scottish doctors were emigrating for want of opportunity, he continuously earned his living from teaching, writing about and practicing anatomy (with the addition of a little journalism and surgery) for the rest of his life. In his later years he held a unique post as pathological anatomist in a London hospital, and while he may have been cramped by the exiguousness of his salary, he was not living in penury.

One hundred and fifty years after his death, Knox is finally being restored to the pantheon of distinguished sons of his native Edinburgh: the university that repeatedly refused him a professorial appointment has accorded him posthumous recognition amongst its "famous members of staff",[7] and the Royal College of Surgeons, which once ended his hopes of an academic career by refusing to recognize him as a teacher of anatomy, has granted his waxwork a prominent place in its historical museum, next door to the museum of pathology that he helped establish. Ironies such as these seem appropriate to a life and career filled with paradox. Regarded by his contemporaries as a leading scientific anatomist, in a fifty-year career of sustained and sometimes frenetic activity Knox discovered little of lasting value, excepting anatomical *minutiae*, and lived to see his elaborate philosophical speculations on the formation of new species undermined and, though he never accepted it, superseded, by Darwin's theory of evolution. Acclaimed as the finest British anatomy teacher of his generation, he never held an academic appointment, and taught no medical students at all for the last eighteen years of his life, fulfilling instead "the office which he has imposed upon himself – that of becoming an anatomical teacher through the medium of the Press", and finding fresh audiences as a popular lecturer, journalist, artistic anatomist, curator of a museum of anatomical models, and director of a troupe of dancing "Bushmen".[8]

The incongruities of Knox's career are matched by those of his writings. Evelleen Richards, the most perceptive of recent commentators on his work, characterized him as an "unviable hybrid", whose anatomical theories, at once materialistic and non-progressive, fitted no stereotype, and satisfied no political dogma.[9] He was an abolitionist and anti-colonialist whose idiosyncratic work on race was pressed into service by

Introduction

pro-slavers and the imperialist Anthropological Society of London, and though he proudly proclaimed his descent from the "Radical Reformer" John Knox, he never attended Kirk and was dubbed an atheist: "We doubt", wrote one critic, "whether old John would rejoice much over him".[10] He built up the celebrated museum of the Royal College of Surgeons of Edinburgh from primitive foundations, and dismissed the result as "of no value whatever"; he spent innumerable hours in the "charnel-house" of the dissecting-room, and found it "always horrible"; he taught anatomy to artists, and repudiated dissection as "frightful, hideous, shocking to behold"; he was an outsider and a constant critic of the medical establishment who came to personify the profession's arrogance.[11]

When Knox yielded to the temptation of blaming his professional troubles on the machinations of jealous detractors, he had a point. The celebrated Edinburgh medical faculty was the largest in Britain, anatomy was the basis of medical teaching, and he was its most successful teacher, but he won no official position. The city was governed by an unelected council, a Member of Parliament for whom he could not vote, and a church of which he was not a member; the Councils of the medical Royal Colleges were unelected and unaccountable, and the university professors and inspectors of anatomy were political appointees. Yet many others successfully made the transition from private teacher to university professor. Knox's "peculiar characteristics" stymied his progress: his wilful obstinacy and defensive intellectual pride prevented him from toadying to the establishment, and his "hangings, drawings, and quarterings" of "all such dabblers in science who maintained the contrary opinion to his own" alienated him from the learned societies that were his natural home.[12]

His views were notorious: he championed freedom of thought and action, anathematized "kingcraft" and "priestcraft", praised "Napoleon the Great" to the skies, opposed colonialism, slavery and vivisection, and lauded the French Revolution. Students and colleagues knew him as a "savage radical", and his "private conversation" was that of an "atheist" or an "infidel", but there were rumours this was something of a pose; that he was "as orthodox or Trinitarian as the best of them" and, after the Reform Bill, voted Tory.[13] Knox, it seems, was less a political agitator than a chronic malcontent, always "agin the government". He relished twisting the tails of those in authority, but there is no evidence he was ever active in, or even a member of, any political group, and if he read Paine, Burke, Coleridge, or Marx, he left no record of what he thought. He kept a bible by his bed, complained about papists, and boasted of his friendships with the aristocracy. He tried too hard to enter Edinburgh society, talking up his supposed family connections, overdressing in lectures, and keeping a separate establishment for his lowborn wife for fear his rivals would discover he had married beneath him.

Introduction

Interest in Knox's life and work has always extended well beyond those custodians of anatomical tradition, the medical schools and Royal Colleges, which promote "great men" histories of a subject they no longer teach. He is public property, and through retellings of his story successive generations have engaged with the achievements, the dangers, and the strange fascination of the science of anatomy. In explaining his approach to the biography of the French pathological anatomist Xavier Bichat, Knox, who was as fulsome in praise of the few he admired as he was trenchantly critical of the many he despised, sketched out a method that might have been written with his own biographer in mind: "To appreciate justly the vast merits of this profound genius, we must consider first – What is anatomy and what is its object? How stood it before the times of Bichat, and how since? What were and what are the views which the public, as well as the professional mind, had adopted in respect of it?"[14]

At present, the average person is probably, and the average medical student certainly, less knowledgeable about anatomy than were their counterparts in the early-nineteenth century, when it was a controversial subject with a claim on the attention of all persons of learning. When Knox was first introduced to it, anatomy was a revolutionary science that at the "higher", philosophical, or transcendental level promised biological laws, comparable to those of chemistry or physics, that would explain the organization of life without recourse to a divine plan. German transcendental anatomists explored the significance of "unity of type" among diverse species, and their French followers, also struck by the apparent serial affinity of all living things, caused a sensation by abandoning the dogma of fixity of species since the Creation and postulating transmutation of some forms and extinction of others. Napoleon promoted anatomical museums, models and lectures, and General Lafayette regretted not having studied the subject in his youth.[15]

It is small wonder then that, when Knox was a young man, anatomy fired the imagination of medical students; it was the highlight of an otherwise dreary syllabus of chemistry, botany and *materia medica*, in contrast to which it appeared both forward-looking and tantalisingly unorthodox. When students made their nocturnal visits to the churchyard with a dark-lantern and spade to resurrect the dead, there was more at stake than their final examinations: dissection, it was anticipated, would shed light on the origins and interrelationships of animals and man, while post-mortem examinations performed according to the innovative principles of Bichat would reveal "the effects of disease on organs", without which knowledge "medicine must ever remain a mere empiricism".[16]

The dissident, avant-garde continental ideas that Knox and others

Introduction

introduced into Britain, the doctrines of unity of plan and species change that established his early reputation and made Edinburgh the cradle of biological evolution,[17] did not outlast him, but fell swiftly into obscurity along with the work of all those historically unhonoured transcendental anatomists who failed to acknowledge the pre-eminence of natural selection as set out in the *Origin of Species*. If "philosophical" anatomy, which at its most luxuriant purported to explain not only homologies between species but also aesthetics, human history and politics, was congruent with Darwinism, it had merely prefigured it, if not, it had been superseded by it, but either way it had become intellectually redundant.

It was more than a hundred years before philosophical anatomy was restored to the intellectual map of nineteenth-century science: in America, Philip F. Rehbock's *The Philosophical Naturalists* (1983) raised the transcendentalists from obscurity as false prophets or at best forerunners of Darwin, while Adrian Desmond's *The Politics of Evolution* (1989) examined the hitherto undervalued contribution of radical science and private anatomy schools to the introduction and promotion of evolutionary ideas in Britain. These and other significant reappraisals of British transcendentalism, especially the work of L.S. Jacyna and Evelleen Richards, have left the biographer of Knox better placed to assess his contributions to transcendental biology.[18] If the Scylla of claiming Knox's work to be a blind alley and the Charybdis of presuming him to have assembled a cogent hypothesis of evolution are easily avoided, the precise evaluation of his higher anatomy, in the context of many interrelated contemporaneous theories, remains problematic. Though it is possible to wrest from his voluminous and sometimes self-contradictory oeuvre a plausible theory of species change, his philosophy was never evolutionistic in a conventional sense, for evolution was "the child of the hopes of Progress" and Knox's overriding anti-progressive views militated against such a world view.[19] Nonetheless, Richards' reading of his mature hypothesis as a form of saltatory evolution – evolution by jumps – is an attractive proposition, not least because saltationism is a characteristically Knoxian idea: quirky, heterodox, and regarded by some mainstream biologists as bad science, if not positively heretical.

As a teacher of medical students, a career followed out of necessity as the most practical route by which a man without private means or patronage could fund researches in anatomy, Knox found a receptive audience for speculations on his "favourite and engrossing" subjects: "comparative anatomy, embryology, and the transcendental".[20] In his lectures he fleshed out dry anatomical descriptions with innovatory Parisian teachings and texts, some of which he translated, which traced the interrelated forms of the animal kingdom to an ideal body plan supposedly common to all, and he taught a generation of medical students that the formation of new species and races, and their survival, were products of biological laws, independent of design or providence. Edinburgh supplied the science that nineteenth-century medicine took as its intellectual foundation, and as its popularity burgeoned, anatomy became the focus of medical power struggles in Scotland and London as young, radical private teachers challenged the authority of the universities and royal colleges by deploying continental ideas of extinction, inter-species homology and progressive change against the conservative view of nature and society as static and divinely ordered.[21]

Anatomy underpinned the "great cultural authority" of early-nineteenth century medicine as it shifted its focus from health and the bodily economy to the pathology of disease, and from the whole patient to isolated tissues and organs.[22] Practical experience in dissection was increasingly sought after as rising numbers of traumatic injuries (in an age of wars, machinery and mechanical transportation) and better anaesthesia increased the need for surgeons, and the medical licensing bodies' demands that pupils attend anatomy lectures and dissection classes confirmed the subject's hegemony. As training became increasingly standardized and regulated, anatomy emerged as the ideal medical knowledge – detailed, complex, testable, and unlikely to be acquired outside recognised schools – and the skeleton and diploma in the consulting room replaced the bob-wig and gold-headed cane as symbols of the learned medical practitioner, whose scientific authority was founded on privileged access to the secrets of the dissecting-room.

The raw materials for these studies were increasingly hard to come by: the legal status of body-snatching was ambiguous (coffins and shrouds were property but bodies were not) but, in Knox's words, anatomists could obtain "subjects" only by "violations of the law, without which anatomy can scarcely now be practised."[23] Edinburgh did well out of this anatomical free-for-all, and since the income generated by the medical school helped the town to thrive while the rest of Scotland was struggling, the city's anatomists were justly celebrated, and the manoeuvres necessary to supply them with subjects were generally ignored.

Given the rising demand for corpses as the school's popularity grew, the wholly inadequate legal supply, and the appalling conditions in Edinburgh's slums, it can be argued that murder for dissection was almost inevitable. The depredations wrought by Burke and Hare in Edinburgh's West Port district during 1828 were a national scandal, but it took further murders in London before legislation was passed by parliament and even then the 1832 Anatomy Act, intended to eliminate the need for body snatching by making available sufficient numbers of pauper cadavers, was poorly conceived and implemented. Its failings have been comprehensively described in Ruth Richardson's *Death, Dissection and the Destitute*, a seminal work on the social history of human dissection in the nineteenth century[24] that recounts how, after 1832, anatomy became subject to specific legal controls rather than the general law of the land, and who taught anatomy, who learned it, and how, became matters for the state. Anatomy was the gateway to medicine, and the Anatomy Act metaphorically, if not literally, set "a Police man at the door of each Dissecting Room".[25]

The West Port murders made Knox the best-known anatomist in Britain: his class was of record size, and he used his influence, most notably as chair of the Association of Teachers of Anatomy, to oppose the provisions of the Anatomy Act which, by legalizing the supply of bodies without increasing it, had replaced a free market, in which successful teachers could afford to pay more, with a quota system that favoured university and hospital schools to the detriment of private teachers. Students abandoned Edinburgh for Paris or London, and those that remained found the best opportunities for dissection in Professor Monro's mandatory classes at the University. State control of medical education, which Knox and his contemporaries had so admired in radical France, had started an inexorable decline in Britain's private anatomy schools.[26]

Though all extramural lecturers suffered under the Anatomy Act, Knox's privations were extreme, for while most complied with the regulations most of the time, he was wilfully obdurate: he flouted the rules and refused to pay his dues when it did not suit him, until the intervention of the anatomy inspectorate forced him out of business. There is little evidence to support his claims that his colleagues set out to ruin him, but after the death of his wife his professional and personal isolation grew and he spoke his mind regardless, seeming no longer to care. It would be tempting, especially for a medical writer, to diagnose his misanthropy, hubris and mistrust as the fruits of an abnormal personality, were it not that he had much to be bitter about: Edinburgh society had (he fancied) shunned his wife and family, while second-rate colleagues and former pupils who gained cherished positions failed to repay his kindnesses when in a position to do so.

Knox's response to the failure of his school was to reinvent himself as a public anatomy teacher through popular lectures, shows, books and articles in which he confidently asserted that anatomy, descriptive and transcendental, was the key to understanding the organization of life. Ironically, it was only after the West Port murders had drawn unprecedented public attention to the subject that it "suddenly turned to gold": anatomical models were dusted off for public display, and public lectures were given, usually by those outside the medical profession, which was, in general, unwilling to share its hard-won specialist knowledge with audiences of "gaping fools".[27] Knox, however, seems to have enjoyed lecturing to the much maligned public, and the audiences at his ethnological shows, eager to be informed and entertained, were probably closer in spirit to his enthusiastic classes of the 1820s and 1830s, when medical men had travelled from England to hear him lecture, than were the conscripted audiences of drinking, smoking, brawling, wrestling, rat-hunting medical

Introduction

students who filled (or failed to fill) the hospital dissecting-rooms of the 1850s.

Under the auspices of the General Medical Council (created by the Medical Act 1858), anatomy became the dragon that guarded the gate of orthodox medicine, and with hospital dissecting-rooms effectively closed to all but ticketed medical students pursuing state-recognized courses for registrable qualifications, the subject was touted as both the foundation of scientific medicine and a formative influence on the pupil's mind: a shared, tabooed and privileged experience that excluded patients and, more especially, self-taught practitioners who, if they lacked anatomical training or learned from books and waxworks, could be dismissed as mountebanks and charlatans.

By the 1860s, little remained of the previous generation's anatomical zeal: no longer a subject to engage enthusiasms, anatomy was at best an exercise in mental discipline (learning its minutiae was to medicine what Latin grammar was to academe) and at worst a mass of useless facts. Universities and professional associations tolerated dissection as a grim necessity that distinguished the properly trained practitioner from the quack: the certificates of attendance that examination candidates were required to present were notoriously unreliable, but it was easy enough for an experienced examiner to detect, and fail, a candidate who had never dissected.[28] Some medical men objected on principle to students being compelled to dissect, a practice they thought beneath the dignity of aspiring physicians, while others complained it was a savage and brutalising undertaking that eroded the finer feelings and encouraged coarse appetites, like those of the "savage" races, for "strange flesh".[29]

In his latter years, Knox turned from the horrors of the dissecting-room to the heights of philosophical anatomy, and strove, through his studies of race, art, and comparative anatomy, to achieve a theoretical breakthrough comparable to those of the continental anatomists who had inspired him. Though an admirer of these "great anatomists", he was never a wholehearted follower, and having ultimately rejected, among other ideas, Cuvier's creationism, Lamarck's ladder of progress, Geoffroy's transmutation of species, and Darwin's natural selection, he continued to plough his own furrow, despite his failures, with unwavering devotion to his transcendental cause. "So you see", he declared towards the end of his life, "I am still the same as when you first saw me, full of life, mad after the discovery of the unknown in science . . . ".[30]

"Posterity will put all right", wrote Knox at the conclusion of his own attempt to burnish the posthumous reputation of Cuvier, who hardly needed it.[31] Knox was fortunate in his first biographer, his former pupil, colleague and fellow "philosophical radical" Henry Lonsdale, who

Introduction

treated his reputation sympathetically and gave due prominence to his work on comparative anatomy and anthropology. Lonsdale was aware that he lacked the expertise in these fields necessary fully to evaluate Knox's contribution, and had intended to collaborate with the anatomist John Goodsir, who was to have written chapters on Knox's science and the "import of his teachings", but Goodsir made no progress with the work before he died in 1867.[32] Notwithstanding its deficiencies, Lonsdale's biography provides much valuable information and should be the first port of call for any serious enquirer into Knox's life. It was clearly intended as a tribute that would be read by former pupils and admirers, and it would be vain to criticize Lonsdale, as the gossipy Sir John Struthers did in 1895, for having "suppressed" some aspects of Knox's career.[33]

Lonsdale had access to some of Knox's letters and possessions, such as the High School gold medal whose inscription he transcribed, but Knox had destroyed most of his manuscripts shortly before his death, and Lonsdale was obliged to rely on recollected conversations with a man who, despite a passionate devotion to scientific truth and a fondness for talking about himself, could be notoriously misleading when he wished. Under the circumstances, Lonsdale evidently did his best, and even Struthers, who disliked the "vulgar" Lonsdale, considered the book "reliable as to facts".[34] Lonsdale is sometimes assumed to have passed over Knox's failings, but if he did it was probably just the medical profession defending its own; his personal friendship with Knox seems to have come to an end around 1842, after he joined Peter Handyside's school when Knox was in difficulties, and on a subsequent occasion when he could have defended Knox, who stood accused of falsely signing a certificate of attendance, Lonsdale went out of his way to discredit him by checking the register of Knox's school and informing the *Lancet* that on the date when he had supposedly signed the certificate Knox had not been in Edinburgh.[35]

The only other full length biography of Knox is Isobel Rae's *Knox the Anatomist* (1964) which focuses primarily on Knox's life rather than his academic work and contains valuable background information on the West Port murders and nineteenth-century Edinburgh. More recent contributions to Knoxian scholarship are Kathy Stephen's pamphlet in the "Scottish men of medicine" series, which includes additional material on Knox's exploits in the Cape colony, and articles by the Edinburgh anatomist and medical historian M.H. Kaufman, whose books on military surgery and nineteenth-century anatomy schools are important sources for students of Knox's career.[36]

The loss of Knox's personal letters and papers – the records of his anatomy schools also failed to survive, the usual situation for these ephemeral institutions – renders it unlikely that there will be many more significant additions to his personal biography. This book is concerned primarily with his professional life, and therefore includes ancillary material that sets his work as a scientist and teacher in context without, I hope, unduly disrupting the narrative. Three areas that seemed to call for more extended comment – the association of anatomy with cannibalism, Knox's transcendental theories, and the links between anatomy and aesthetics – have been relegated to separate chapters outside the chronological sequence. In view of these digressions, it might seem perverse that the West Port murders are described only in such detail as is necessary to follow the story; however, the tale of Burke and Hare has been very well told elsewhere, and readers who wish to explore their crimes further will find ample material in the accounts of Burke's trial by John Macnee and William Roughead, and in the more recent works of Hugh Douglas, John Mackay, and Owen Dudley Edwards.[37] I have particularly avoided any speculation on whether Knox knew or believed the bodies he purchased were those of murder victims. We cannot know what he believed, or whether he, his students, his rivals, the wretched inhabitants of West Port or the burghers of Edinburgh entertained any suspicions. If they did, they kept them to themselves.

One reason that Knox remains a better-known figure than his more illustrious contemporaries is that his career, especially in its fictionalized form, has proved of particular relevance to subsequent moral and ethical debates in medicine. There were other teachers of transcendental anatomy, other scandals that ushered in the Anatomy Act, and other critics of state regulation, but it was Knox's name that became linked with anatomy dispassionately pursued as a subject in its own right, rather than as an adjunct to surgery (he despised the unmethodical teaching of "practical" anatomy): a quest for knowledge in which the end justified the means.

The intellectual and moral justification of dissection was important to the nascent medical profession in the mid-nineteenth century, which defined itself by its grounding in anatomical pathology, without which, "the art of medicine would lose its best claim to be ranked as a profession".[38] Until recently, the one experience that all orthodox medical practitioners shared, and that distinguished them from other healers, was that they had, early in their career, dissected the human body. Anatomy was the *sine qua non* of scientific medicine, and since Knox represented anatomy, he came, by a process of synecdoche, to stand for the medical profession as a whole.

Recent social histories of nineteenth-century anatomy have focussed on its rôle in establishing medical authority over patients' bodies, especially the bodies of women and the poor,[39] which it reduces to the status of "subjects". For medicine's critics, Knox still represents such abuses of power: recent autopsy "scandals" have been compared to "a modern-day Burke and Hare story", in which organs were "stolen" from cadavers by the successors of the "infamous" Knox, "the surgeon who knowingly received murdered and resurrected bodies" and who is "seen in some

Introduction

quarters as being as much a butcher as Burke and Hare".[40] But power, according to Michel Foucault, is located not in individuals, institutions or ideas, but within complex situations in society, in the "daily jostlings for status and position" within the medical profession and among practitioners, government and the public.[41] Taken in context, Knox's actions were far removed from the autocratic exercise of authority imputed to the formidable anatomists of nineteenth-century sensational fiction: his career path was shaped by the constraints of Edinburgh's academic and civil authorities, and his vicissitudes owed at least as much to legal and professional pressures and to the changing currents of public opinion as they did to the impulses of his mercurial personality.

Since he failed to make the great discovery he hankered after, it is easy to dismiss him as a figure in permanent opposition, testing and challenging theories but contributing nothing new. His unceasing self-advertisement and references to his "vast experience", his penchant for describing every distinguished acquaintance as "my friend" and his "unseemly displays of vanity and ignorance" left some of his contemporaries with the impression that his performance was mere braggadocio: "Who is Dr. Knox, and what has he done", asked one exasperated reviewer.[42] A glance at his bibliography would have shown that in terms of quantity at least – he published over a hundred papers and five books – Knox's output would have shamed many university professors, though he spread his theories so widely, in popular works on race and art as well as in medical journals, that during his lifetime they were not fully understood; indeed, so chaotic was their presentation that it was sometimes difficult to know "what Dr Knox would really be at". While he did not elaborate a fully-fledged theory of species change, his claim that sudden alterations in embryonic development gave rise to new species foreshadowed the "hopeful monsters" of Richard Goldschmidt's "macro-evolution",[43] making Knox perhaps the earliest contender for the much-disputed title of "father of evo-devo". It would have pleased him to be named in connection with so controversial a field.

For his contemporaries, it was as Britain's most successful teacher of anatomy, whose lectures to medical pupils and lay audiences ranged widely over race and art, comparative anatomy and natural philosophy, sometimes shirking the dry details but always seeking to engage his audience's enthusiasm, that Knox made his outstanding contribution. From a present day perspective, as the importance of anatomy in the medical curriculum dwindles, university museums fall into desuetude, and the medical profession, through its *soi-disant* "leaders", dismisses attempts to engage with the public as trivial, macabre, or even grotesque,[44] the nineteenth-century vogue for anatomy may seem of interest to no-one except medical historians and the morbidly curious; yet despite, or perhaps because of, the moral ambiguities of this most relevant of subjects, public interest in anatomy, in museums and demonstrations, artworks and

Introduction

autopsies, remains high. There is interest, too, in Robert Knox: not just morbid curiosity for his failings, but genuine interest in his work. As a character in popular fiction, where he appears more often than any other British doctor, he is, as the review of his fictional career in the final chapter will show, more subtly drawn, and more persuasive in his arguments, than might initially be supposed: the audience is invited to sympathize with him as his desire to educate medical students, to understand the body's workings and to supplant the authority of received wisdom with that of direct observation is frustrated by regulations, narrow mindedness, and professional jealousy. When, inevitably, he oversteps the mark, his downfall atones for the moral cost to his profession, and to society, of a supposedly dispassionate but ultimately destructive penchant for scientific rationalism. We, the beneficiaries of this science, are relieved of responsibility for the human tragedies of the dissecting-room because Knox, and the profession he stands for, has accepted the guilt on our behalf.

CHAPTER ONE

The Darling Boy of the Family, 1791–1810

The Scotland into which Robert Knox was born on 4 September 1791, at the height of the French Revolution, was closer historically and culturally to France, its oldest ally, than to England. The '45 uprising, when Jacobite clan chiefs and lairds had rallied to the French-backed Prince Charles Edward Stuart, was within living memory, and it had only been twenty years since the last of the rebels' heads had finally fallen from its spike on London's Temple Bar. By the 1790s, the Scottish aristocracy had mostly been won over by the economic benefits of the union, but the Revolution unsettled the ruling class and emboldened the lower orders, who looked to France as a paradigm for the future: "trees of liberty", a French revolutionary symbol, sprang up in many Scottish towns, and the middle classes ostentatiously adopted the republican language of the Jacobins.[1]

Not that one needed to be a red-hot radical to crave reform in a country where there was so little representation of the people: Henry Dundas, the Tory MP for Edinburghshire and "uncrowned King of Scotland", had arrogated to himself control over Scottish affairs following his appointment as Lord Advocate in 1775, and Edinburgh, a city of some 85,000 inhabitants with an electorate of thirty-three, was run by a town Council that was largely self-appointed.[2] When mob rioting broke out during George III's fifty-fourth birthday celebrations in 1792, effigies of Dundas were burned, the Lord Provost's house was attacked, and one of the city's best-known surgeons, Alexander Wood, was almost killed after being mistaken for that unpopular dignitary.[3] There were fears of an uprising, and in the following months groups of "daring miscreants" organized themselves into radical clubs to lobby for parliamentary reform, or even a republic.[4]

One such was Knox's father, also named Robert, a teacher of mathematics at George Heriot's School, who joined the Society of the Friends of the People.[5] Founded in July 1792, the Friends included aristocrats and politicians, though the majority of members were tradesmen, professionals and skilled artisans (an annual subscription of one and a half guineas excluded the lower classes),[6] who looked enviously at France and the new-found wealth and status of the bourgeoisie. The Friends organized three increasingly radical annual conventions, at the last of which, held in Edinburgh in October 1793, they demanded universal male suffrage and expressed support in principle for the French Revolution. In an excess of enthusiasm, they rashly adopted a revolutionary calendar, naming 1793 as the "first year", though "thank God", wrote William Cobbett, who had experienced the Revolution at first hand, "it was also the last".[7]

Britain and France had been at war since February 1793, and Prime Minister William Pitt the Younger acted decisively against potential appeasers and supporters of the enemy. "[D]isorganizing clubs that threatened the dissolution of society",[8] were suppressed, and the leaders of the Friends of the People were convicted of sedition and transported as part of Pitt's own "reign of terror", ruthlessly implemented in Scotland by Dundas – who claimed there were plans for revolutionaries to seize Edinburgh by force[9] – and "hanging judge" Lord Braxfield, who, on being told by one prisoner that Jesus had been a reformer, was said to have chuckled "Muckle he made o'that; he was hanged".[10]

There is no record of Robert Knox senior taking any active part in public demonstrations, and it seems that either his revolutionary ardour was lukewarm or discretion prevailed and he kept his radical views within the family. While he was still a student in Edinburgh in 1775 (he never graduated), he had married Mary Scherer (the family name was sometimes anglicized to Shearer), the orphaned daughter of German-born farmer Archibald Scherer, and their first child, John, was born the following year in Mary's home town of Ayr.[11] Two sons, William and Archibald, and a daughter Mary were born in 1777, 1779 and 1781 in the Stewartry of Kirkcudbright in south-western Scotland, where Robert worked as a "writing master", before the family finally settled in Edinburgh, where two more daughters, Elouisa and Janet (known as Jessie), followed in 1787 and 1789.[12] Robert, the subject of this biography, was the eighth of nine children, the youngest being Frederick John, who was born on 3 April 1794.[13] The "missing" child probably died in infancy, an unrecorded tragedy at a time when infant mortality was high due to infectious diseases, of which smallpox alone killed one child in ten.[14]

The family house in Edinburgh was in North Richmond Street, close to Surgeons' Square and about ten minutes' walk from Heriot's school, an impressive French gothic building, more like a castle than a school, founded in 1628 to provide for the education of Edinburgh's "puire fatherless bairnes". Robert senior's duties there were not exacting: he was expected to devote his "whole time" to teaching, but in practice this amounted to an hour's daily instruction on Euclid, algebra, logarithms and trigonometry to each of the four senior "sections" of the school.[15] He customarily described his calling as "mathematician" or "accomptant" rather than teacher, and had a series of business addresses in the Old Town – Baxter's close, Toderick's Wynd and finally, until his death in

The Darling Boy of the Family, 1791–1810

1812, Cant's close – where he presumably carried on his accountancy practice.[16]

Robert Knox senior was an active freemason, and was present when the brethren of the Edinburgh lodges, in order of seniority, marched through the city with the professors and students of the university, the Lord Provost and the town council to witness the laying of the foundation stone of the new university buildings by the Grand Master Mason of Scotland, Lord Napier, on 16 November 1789.[17] Edinburgh had a strong Masonic tradition, perhaps the oldest in Britain, and for the liberally minded, such as Robert Burns, the lodges offered an alternative social framework that paralleled that of the Kirk. The Craft's freedom from religious dogma and its ideals of fraternal support and moral responsibility appealed to supporters of "liberty, fraternity, and equality", and though, unlike their French counterparts, Scottish Masonic lodges were never overtly politicized, the British government was sufficiently concerned that they might become hotbeds of revolution to threaten them with charges of "traitorous conspiracy" under the 1799 Secret Societies Act.[18]

While we do not know how radical Robert senior's views actually were, he was certainly less outspoken than Robert junior, who grew up to be an ardent Francophile, a passionate admirer of Napoleon, and an enemy of priestcraft, privilege, nepotism and the outmoded social distinctions that he felt made professional advancement in Britain as capricious as it had been in France under the Bourbons: "a filthy dynasty, seeking merely place and patronage for their flunkey partisans".[19] Though he was his father's son politically and intellectually, in later life Robert Knox spoke little of his parents. If his reticence stemmed from a desire to conceal his comparatively humble origins, it was apparently successful, since Henry Lonsdale's *Life of Robert Knox*, published in 1870, stated that "scarcely anything is known" about his family.[20]

Lonsdale, a former friend and pupil, seems to have relied on Knox's own anecdotes for information about his early life. One story placed his parents at the home of Helen, Countess of Selkirk as guests on the historic night of 23 April 1778, when sailors from the American ship *Ranger* under the command of John Paul Jones broke into the house in an attempt to kidnap the Earl for ransom. Finding him absent, the Rangers stole some of the family silver, which Jones eventually returned. Although this "comic opera" of a raid did Jones little credit, it caused consternation in Scotland and England, accustomed as they were to the security of the Royal Navy's wooden walls.[21] The event was widely reported in the press, but not one account mentioned the Knoxes, who were "favourably received at the Hall of the Earl of Selkirk" only in their son's imagination.[22] Knox would not be the only medical man to embellish his family background in order to meet society's unreasonable expectation that doctors, however humbly employed and poorly remunerated, should be gentlemen by birth as well as manners, and he later claimed that his family would have been lairds of Ranfurly, had the place and title not been occupied by his "Irish kinsman", Thomas Knox, Earl of Ranfurly, an argument remarkable both as a *non sequitur* and as the anti-Celtic Knox's sole acknowledgement of his Irish kinship.[23]

Young Robert was said, most likely by himself in later life, to have been "the darling boy of the family", a good-looking child with soft, blonde hair and big blue eyes. Others remembered him as "an imp of mischief, even from his cradle".[24] As an infant, only a few years before Edward Jenner introduced an effective inoculation with cowpox virus, he contracted smallpox, the most devastating complication of which was blindness due to secondary bacterial infection of an ulcerated cornea. Robert's left eye was destroyed and his face disfigured by pockmarks (the story later current that he lost his eye in a trout fishing accident was probably another of his tall tales).[25] Though physically still quite robust, his early instruction was carried on at home, where along with a liberal education he imbibed his father's radical opinions. Napoleon Bonaparte was his boyhood hero, an adulation that continued throughout his life, untainted by his customary scepticism, perhaps because it owed more to romanticism than to practical politics. Unlike many radicals, including Thomas Paine, whose *Rights of Man*, an appeal for the overthrow of the British monarchy, sold a staggering twenty thousand copies, and who saw revolution as progress towards a "more perfect civilization" that would alleviate the wretched "savagery" of the masses,[26] Knox entertained no hopes of collective progress and never became disenchanted with Napoleon's rule as the Emperor grew increasingly autocratic. His own response to the savage masses would be predominantly one of scientific curiosity, and though revolutionary change, under the guise of periodic extinctions and sudden transformations in the natural world, was to become central to his scientific thinking, he remained unmoved by ideals of social or biological progress: "progress towards what?", he enquired sarcastically.[27] As a child, he could not have been unaware of the appalling poverty endured by the "very dregs" of society in Edinburgh's densely packed, disease-ridden wynds and closes,[28] but these wretched folk, who lived in Britain's cultural capital but played no intellectual part in it, must have seemed as remote from him as a foreign race.

If we assume he spent the customary five years there, Knox must have matriculated at Edinburgh's Royal High School in 1806, at the age of 14 or 15, considerably older than most of the boys in the class and with the additional advantage of having been tutored by his father.[29] The "Tounis School" as it was known, one of the oldest grammar schools in Britain, was located in a classical building at the end of Infirmary Street (which currently houses the University of Edinburgh department of archaeology), where in 1806 it was flourishing under the rectorship of Dr Alexander Adam (1741–1809), who had just confidently raised the fees from 5s to 10s 6d a quarter.[30] Adam was a "benevolent" and rather eccentric looking

The Darling Boy of the Family, 1791–1810

old man who still wore his hair in a queue, and whose old fashioned knee breeches, buckled shoes, and threadbare coat struck one visitor as a sign of "economical habits" (all the more so since his income, mostly from fees, was over £400 a year), though others were more impressed by the "order, readiness, and accuracy" of his class of a hundred boys.[31]

Knox joined the class of James Gray, a Greek scholar and the son of a shoemaker, who set the older boys to teach Latin to the younger, a practicality with large classes. Despite, or perhaps because of, his humble origins, Gray had no illusions that all could be "*equally* successful": "Nature", he wrote, "has made strong and marked distinctions in the extent of capacity; but I will venture to assert that every one may be made to turn his talents to the best account."[32] The younger boys were taught for just four hours a day (two on Saturday), their time being divided roughly equally between classics and other subjects. Of the latter, English and divinity were the most important, and a mere ninety minutes a week were devoted to "elementary science".[33] One visiting English clergyman reported that the High School was the best in Scotland, and as good as any in England, for producing classical scholars. Unfortunately, the street leading up to it, Blackfriars' Wynd, was "inhabited by some of the most abandoned of both sexes":[34] its "twenty-seven houses of bad fame" left many pupils' morals "so corrupted, that they became scarcely good for any thing", and the more enterprising boys could boast of "gallantries and intrigues (and in a line too) which their parents little think of."[35]

Classes began at nine every morning (a daunting prospect in winter, when the sun rose at a quarter to nine and temperatures were barely above freezing) with prayers, Latin verse translation and an examination on grammar, with promotions in class order for detecting blunders and demotions for committing them. As the boys progressed through the school, French, arithmetic and "book-keeping" were added to the curriculum, though natural history and chemistry were not taught until 1849.[36] In the end of year examinations, which were taken in the presence of the magistrates, professors and ministers of the city, the boys' classical knowledge was tested by such exercises as the translation of the *Iliad* into Latin verse, and they were required to work out arithmetic problems on a slate under the watchful gaze of the examiners.[37] While these early studies may not have been very exciting, after four years the boys were literate in three or four languages, numerate, and ready to pass on to the Rector's class for their final year.

Dr Adam taught them Latin, history, antiquities and "mythology". He was fond of travelling, and in his lighter moments he talked of Paris, constitutional freedom, and his successful pupils from the past. "The Doctor", a farmer's son, was an energetic teacher who never sat down in class; he questioned his students constantly and flourished a leather strap that he used for theatrical effect rather than chastisement. Instead of punishing the boys at the bottom of the class, he preferred to encourage

The Darling Boy of the Family, 1791–1810

their "honest ambition" by questioning them first, and promoting them if they answered correctly.[38] Knox responded well to what was for its time a liberal mode of education, and Adam's engaging style of instruction may well have inspired his pupil's subsequent performances in the lecture theatre. The Rector's class was the largest in the school and it was demanding work for a man of sixty-eight: in the winter of 1809 Adam became too ill to teach, and he died soon afterwards. In Knox's final months at the school the Rector's class was taken by James Pillans, another progressive liberal who went on to become professor of humanity and laws at Edinburgh University.

Knox was later remembered as the boisterous "bully" of the school, "thrashing" his contemporaries "mentally and corporeally";[39] he won a string of prizes, rose to the top of every class, and was *dux* (head boy in the final examination) when he left in 1810. Though he later told Lonsdale that he achieved this success "without effort", anyone who has tried it knows that learning is never effortless, and his mastery of Latin and Greek, subjects for which he showed little enthusiasm in later life, indicates that he applied himself diligently to his studies. When, at the final prize giving, in front of the magistracy of the city in their robes, he received from the Lord Provost a gold medal inscribed *Roberto Knox puero optimo merito condiscipulorum DUCI*, and a folio of the works of Virgil,[40] he must have anticipated a career in which his talents and industry would earn him even more gratifying rewards.

CHAPTER TWO

A Beautiful but Seductive Science, 1810–1814

Medicine was the obvious career for an Edinburgh man from a modest professional background with a grammar school education and no strong religious convictions. Thomas Charlton Speer, an Edinburgh MD who graduated in 1812, estimated that three-quarters of the university's two thousand students were medics, though a more conservative estimate was five hundred out of a total of fourteen hundred, "only a small proportion" of whom went on to take a degree.[1] A doubling of the number of medical students graduating, from some fifty a year in the first decade of the nineteenth century (ten times more than Oxford and Cambridge) to around a hundred a year after 1820, suggests that student numbers were rising, though it seems the examinations were also getting easier.[2] This "great resort of medical students", the largest medical school in Britain, was less exclusive than Oxbridge, as it did not require students to subscribe to the articles of the Anglican faith (one Oxford professor dismissed Edinburgh's students as "rabble"), and cheaper than training in London's private medical schools.[3]

The combination of academic medical education and practical studies, the latter having fallen into abeyance in the English universities, attracted students from "almost every civilized country". In Edinburgh, "idle, care-for-nothing" Irish mixed with "indefatigable" Germans, wealthy West Indians, "Good Genevese", "supercilious" Englishmen and "combustible Americans",[4] though the early-nineteenth century rise in student numbers was probably due to more Scotsmen embarking on a medical career, a prudent choice at a time when trade was restricted by the war with France. In these economically hard times, the influx of young men with money to spend was of considerable financial benefit to the town, which could afford to carry out civic "embellishments" in "the spirit of improvement" at a time when the rest of the country was "stagnant".[5]

Although Knox was the first in the family to study medicine, he must have had a good idea of what was involved. His home, the university, and the Royal Infirmary were all within a few hundred yards of each other, and the High School lay directly between the Infirmary and Surgeons' Square. He could have seen Old Surgeons' Hall and the adjacent anatomy schools from the school windows, and had he been at all curious about what went on in these institutions it would have been easy enough to get into conversation with the students. Knox entered Edinburgh University as a "med" in November 1810, three months after leaving school, and along with the other students signed the matriculation album in the university library in the presence of the Principal, the Reverend George Husband Baird, Moderator of the General Assembly of the Church of Scotland and son-in-law of a former Lord Provost.[6] This little ceremony was the only formality: there were no entry requirements and anyone could matriculate who paid half a crown, which went to the library to boost its poor stock of medical books.[7] Clearly, it was only worth a young man's while matriculating if he knew enough Latin to get through the final *viva voce* examination and write a short thesis, but this ordeal was three years off and there were crammers to help those, particularly the English, Irish and Americans, whose Latin was mediocre.[8] Lectures were in English, and at the beginning of term the students bought tickets for those they wished, or were required, to attend. Many professors relied on lecture fees for the bulk of their income[9] and so hoped for large classes, which might include "occasional auditors" who did not intend to sit for a degree.

Edinburgh had a higher proportion of students than any other British town, but unlike Oxford and Cambridge the university was not collegiate and neither provided accommodation nor attempted to regulate students' conduct. Hundreds of young men, many away from home for the first time, were left to their own devices, "unguardianed and unguarded" in the cosmopolitan city, where it did not require much money to cut a dash in "large blue cloaks" and "long brass spurs" (even if they had no horse to use them on), or to indulge in "free" behaviour: many a young man with "more money than brains" developed a "partiality for the bottle" and for "racy jokes and anecdotes" that relied on "punning", a form of humour that Knox subsequently favoured.[10] "This negligent mode of education," wrote one critic, "in which no sort of authority or discipline is exerted by the professors over their students, and in which every student is allowed to live as he finds convenient while attending the university, without incurring farther expense than the professor's fees . . . is well suited to the character and situation of the Scottish nation."[11] There were, however, concerns that Edinburgh men acquired less "moral feeling" and "a less clear perception either of intellectual or of moral truth" than their English counterparts, and that consequently, "they are not very pre-eminent for sagacity as counsellors, or trust-worthiness as friends": in short, it was felt that student life "tends to debauch their morals".[12] The popular notion was that medical students indulged in the "lowest debauchery" and consequently "even" the town's tradesmen regarded them as "contemptible".[13]

Those, like Knox, who lived at home, had fewer opportunities for misbehaviour, but all faced a particular moral challenge at the start of

A Beautiful but Seductive Science, 1810–1814

their medical training, when they began to study anatomy and encountered, in the dissecting-room and operating theatre, sights that could shock and demoralize them. Laurence Holker Potts, a young surgeon and inventor of, amongst other things, a suspended railway, a velocipede, and a manual paddle-boat, wrote a *Hospital Pupil's Guide*, under the bumptious pseudonym of Aesculapius, in which he counselled:

> A medical practitioner should be a man of just feeling; and as this will depend greatly on his possessing habits of just thinking, I shall here add a few observations on the influence of the study of anatomy (a beautiful but seductive science) on the moral perceptions. A man who is gifted with the right exercise of reason, almost believes it impossible that the study of the profession should lead its disciples *to entertain inferior ideas of the Deity*.[14]

Anatomists were notorious unbelievers, and while they might be forgiven for failing to find proofs of the "theological doctrine of the soul ... amid the blood and filth of the dissecting room", they had a "highly unreasonable" tendency to employ their discoveries "to overturn *that proof*, by invalidating the truth of those sacred records, which form the venerable basis on which alone the 'sublime dogmas' in question are built."[15] According to the radical-turned-conservative Samuel Taylor Coleridge, when Voltaire and others had tempted men away from the spiritual they "openly joined the banners of the Antichrist, at once the pander and the prostitute of sensuality, and whether in the cabinet, laboratory, the dissecting room, or the brothel, [were] alike busy in the schemes of vice and irreligion."[16] "Flippancy and slang, beer-drinking, and heartlessness, brutality and debauchery" followed from the "awful revelations of morbid anatomy", as "materialism chases the philosophy of God from the heart and from the lips."[17] Anatomy, it was feared, would draw its devotees into "the vortex of Atheism": when a Scottish visitor to Turkey in 1828 found students handling "human flesh" in the dissecting-room "as if it had been mutton or lamb" he asked whether this was contrary to Islam and was told the students were all followers of Voltaire.[18]

Medical men made much of the horrors of the dissecting-room to stress that their knowledge of anatomy was all the more valuable for being hard-won. The "heroic" anatomist, as Simon Chaplin termed him, made a virtue of his stoicism, and his work, as Knox testified, was undertaken dispassionately: "By dissection, the dead are analysed or reduced to certain assemblages of organs, holding relations, often mechanical, to each other."[19] However, the student's very indifference during these "searches in death for the explanation of life" might cost him his humanity: "[d]oes he become unfeeling, as, day after day, he looks upon that accumulating heap – that horrible tower of Babel, composed of the fragments of human bodies of all languages and nations?"[20] "Aesculapius", mindful that anatomy was regarded with "odium" for treating the body as a mechanism, rehearsed the well-worn counter-argument that it substantiated the case for intelligent design: "It is impossible to survey ... this complicated machine ... without discovering the traces of obvious design in every part of nature's work, and consequently acknowledging the hand of an Intelligent Being."[21]

Quite apart from religious and moral arguments against dissection, many simply found it distasteful. As one medical man wrote:

> How well do I remember the sickening feelings of degradation I had when living in hospital, where our examinations of the dead bodies, far from being sympathized in by the heartfelt interest of the patients and their friends, were viewed with loathing and horror; ourselves regarded at times as butchers, and every attempt made to baffle our laudable endeavours. The patients were afraid of dying in hospital, and would sometimes cause themselves to be carried off, when nearly at the last gasp, to escape those whom they regarded as the sworn foes to the decency of death. No provision had been made to allow of the examination of the dead, and therefore it was done clandestinely by the physicians and students; and at every death there was a series of stratagems between the doctors on the one hand, and the friends of the deceased on the other, to effect or prevent the examination. At these most indecent and degrading scenes the deep glow of sorrow and indignation entered my heart.[22]

The dead body was perhaps a more emotive and tabooed object even than it is today, for though men and women often had to cope with the deaths of family and friends, there were elaborate mourning rituals to sanitize death and conceal the corpse. Dissection rudely exposed that which was not meant to be seen: for the celebrated utilitarian theologian William Paley, the very fact that bones, bowels, muscles and the whole "disgusting materials of a dissecting room" were covered by an attractive integument of skin was itself "a strong indication of design".[23]

More worrying, for some, than anatomy's squalid nature was its latent sensuality: it was the anatomist's duty to examine "all the parts of the body without distinction or reserve", but he must "use caution, in order to preserve his mind uncorrupted, to keep at a distance from vicious disorder and irregular desire [because] to act as an anatomist in the common scenes of life, would render him obnoxious to punishment for corruption and seduction."[24] Anatomy was a dangerous subject for young men: it was "calculated to awaken the passions ... *already inflamed by study*", and required them to "set an additional guard upon the conduct", lest their unwholesome studies "usurp the government of reason".[25]

Yet, in the opinion of the Royal College of Surgeons of Edinburgh, which oversaw the training of surgeons in the city, the unprecedented interest in anatomy in the early-nineteenth century proceeded from the students themselves.[26] Anatomy was the last major science for which general laws had yet to be established, and as living things seemed to call for dauntingly complex regulatory processes compared with those governing, say, chemistry or physics, it was fertile ground for intellectual enquiry. New approaches derived from German *Naturphilosophie* had raised comparative anatomy from dry description to a search for common forms that could reveal nature's essential organization. The proponents of this new, "philosophical" anatomy, also known as "transcendental" or "higher" anatomy, whose origin Knox would later trace to the works of Goethe and Oken, assumed the interrelatedness of all living things and dissected their myriad forms in search of unifying principals: "*laws*, not *details*".[27]

Though difficult to define succinctly, transcendentalism's essential premise was that structural resemblances between species (homologues) were an expression of an ideal form or archetype. These interspecies correspondences were known as unity of type, which Darwin later defined as "that fundamental agreement in structure, which we see in organic beings of the same class, and which is quite independent of their habits of life".[28] According to Goethe, the common plan or archetype from which all living things were contrived was like the theme of "a vast musical symposium" (architecture as frozen music) whose variations were endlessly recapitulated and transformed.[29] Philosophical anatomy did not require the action of a Creator, but its emphasis on the grandeur and unity of Nature tended to appeal to those with a religious, or at least a mystical, view of the world.

Goethe's claim that "[a]ll the parts of an animal, taken together or separately, ought to be found in all animals" and his theory that the skull was formed from modified vertebrae – two of the tenets of philosophical anatomy – were based not on comparative anatomical studies (though he had studied anatomy in the 1780s) but on *a priori* reasoning and an "instinctive conviction".[30] The embryologist, romantic and radical, Lorenz Oken, whom Goethe selected for the post of professor of medical sciences at Jena in 1807, reached the same conclusion on the vertebral origins of the skull as his distinguished patron, apparently independently. As Germany's leading transcendental naturalist, Oken took up the quest for structural elements common to different parts of the body and to different classes of the vast array of creatures that constituted Nature's "multifariously-constructed temple, with its nave, choir, chapels and towers". This search for a common plan was inspired by well-worn systems such as alchemy and numerology rather than by any presumption of evolutionary change: for Oken, different classes of animals were not "gradually evolved metamorphoses of one system, but sudden productions 'en avant' with new tissues, forms, and functions."[31]

In Knox's undergraduate days, transcendental anatomy was scarcely taught in Britain. He recalled first reading of "the doctrine" in 1811, in a paper given by "M. Dunevil" (André Duméril, professor of anatomy and physiology at *l'école de santé*) to the French Academy of Sciences: Duméril's reference to the theory that "the cranial bones were only vertebrae, cranial vertebrae" led Knox to the works of Goethe and Oken, which kindled his interest in comparative anatomy, and he soon began his own studies on unity of type, claiming, like Goethe, an intuitive perception of the structural homologies between animals of different classes.[32] A comparison of the bones of the forefoot of the horse with those of the hand of man provided a practical demonstration of the priority of form over function, since the horse had "rudimentary fingers" even though its foot served a very different purpose than the human hand. During his next two years as an undergraduate, Knox went on to study the comparative anatomy of the eye, satisfying himself that here too "one great plan regulated all".[33]

Oken's quasi-mystical influence is apparent both in Knox's lifelong pursuit of "knowledge for the sake of knowledge" and his ambition "to discover in the interior the secrets of the organization, the mysterious laws of transcendentalism and the theory of life". For the transcendental anatomist, "the book of Nature is always patent to those who know how to read it", and so "in Nature's manifestations you must learn to read her intentions, learning to trace her great scheme of perfect form; that form so often aimed at and so seldom attained."[34] It was like the initiation into a secret society: to most anatomists, the vertebra was merely "a portion of the skeleton", but to Knox, it had become "the type of all vertebrate animals, of the entire skeleton . . . of the organic world. . . . It possesses the form of the primitive cell; of the sphere; of the universe."[35] On a more practical level, he was also inspired by the work of Xavier Bichat, the French pathological anatomist and microscopist who regarded tissues rather than organs as the basic components of life and performed hundreds of autopsies to investigate how tissues were changed by disease. When he discovered Bichat's work "early in 1811–12", Knox "felt that a man had appeared whose destiny it was to bring a close to the era of his youth and of mine, substituting for it other thoughts, other terms, and other views."[36]

Knox's interest in the latest scientific developments far exceeded that of the average medical student, and he was twice elected president of the Royal Physical Society, an undergraduate club that met in an "elegant" hall near the Knoxes' house in North Richmond Street to hear essays on topics as varied as "The Migration of Animals", "Love", "Haemorrhagy", "Satellites of Jupiter" and "Strictures of the Urethra". Two lectures of which Knox may have taken particular notice concerned Xavier Bichat and the physiognomic basis of beauty. His own contributions were more prosaic: he read two essays, on "Hydrophobia or Rabid Erethismus" and on "the Conversion of Diseases".[37] The former was a simple summary of the literature, but the latter, a speculative piece on "changes of one disease to another" suggests he was (like Bichat) contemplating "a natural arrangement of diseases . . . to which we can only hope to contribute a few materials", presumably, since he expressed concern

A Beautiful but Seductive Science, 1810–1814

that medical science was becoming overcrowded, with a view to an academic career.[38] Though he was yet to fix on anatomy as the subject on which, also like Bichat, he would endeavour to "bestow an intelligible, systematic form",[39] his radical views ("letters can only flourish as a republic: the very shadow of that royal authority . . . by crushing free discussion proves pernicious") and combative style are already very much in evidence in these early essays: "[p]erhaps", he wrote scathingly of an egregious contribution to the literature by one Dr Ferrier, "there never was a case so foolishly related by any medical man whatever".[40]

These precocious extracurricular studies took up time that might more profitably have been spent learning basic anatomy. Many able students are prone to stray from the syllabus, but Knox's total neglect of the fundamentals of anatomy for the flights of transcendentalism was to prove his undoing. He was a diligent student when his interest was caught – twenty-six years later, he still had his notes from the first pathological dissection he had seen in Edinburgh, a case of "soft pulpy tubercle of the lungs"[41] – but in Alexander Monro *tertius* (1773–1859), the last of a dynasty that held the chair of anatomy at Edinburgh for a total of 126 years, he had an uninspiring teacher.

Monro's distinguished grandfather, Alexander Monro *primus*, had been appointed to the chair in 1720 and lectured at Surgeons Hall, until it was besieged by a mob who had discovered that Greyfriars Kirkyard provided some of the bodies for dissection.[42] Soon after, the university built a "theatre for dissections" inside the College buildings, where he taught to great acclaim until succeeded by his son Monro *secundus* in 1758. In 1800, Monro *tertius*, who was, like many Edinburgh MDs, completing his education in Paris, was appointed to the chair conjointly with his sixty-seven year old father, and eight years later he took over completely, though he had neither the ability nor the character to make a good teacher. Darwin wrote that he "made his lectures on human anatomy as dull as he was himself" and his scholarship was similarly uninspired: in the second volume of his *Outlines of Anatomy* (1825) he pedantically substituted "curvum" for "rectum", a terminological innovation of which he was rather proud.[43] The often-told story of Monro *tertius* reading out his grandfather's lecture notes makes the point not only that he was a poor teacher – only about a third of his students attended the compulsory lectures for which they had paid in advance[44] – but also that anatomy under Monro was seen as an unchanging canon of topographical details to be delivered verbatim.

In October 1812, Knox was placed under additional pressure to succeed when the death of his father left him, in effect, as the head of the family. Robert Knox senior did not leave a will, but for the time being his family were adequately provided for, and his son was able to continue his education. After three years of study, the minimum time permitted, he sat the MD examinations but received a humiliating setback when he failed the *viva voce* in anatomy.[45] Previous biographers have been unanimous in blaming Monro's lacklustre teaching, which Knox thought "haphazard", "fragmentary", and "at times coarse and contemptible", though these cavils were not specific to Monro, and he subsequently found others no better.[46] As some men with poor Latin managed to "blunder" through the *viva* by memorising the answers to common questions, a practise known as "grinding",[47] Knox, who had been a prizewinning Latin scholar at school, must have had a very limited knowledge of anatomy indeed, which suggests that he had as yet no plans to become an anatomy teacher. His failure may have been due to lack of experience in the dissecting-room, as it is very difficult to learn topographical anatomy – the names and relations of the body's bones, muscles, nerves and blood vessels – from books alone. Monro *tertius* gave demonstrations of practical anatomy between 1 and 3 p.m. when the light was best, but these were too rare to learn much from, however good the view; the surgeon John Bell, (Sir) Charles Bell's older brother, complained in 1810 that "In Dr Monro's class, unless there be a fortunate succession of bloody murders, not three subjects are dissected in the year."[48] It was of course the murderers, rather than their victims, who were dissected.

To make good his deficiencies, Knox needed to join the class of one of the town's extramural anatomy lecturers, independent teachers not employed by the university, and undertake dissections for himself. Prior to the 1832 Anatomy Act, the only lawful sources of corpses for anatomists were voluntary donations and the gallows. The ritual mutilation of the bodies of murderers in the secularized hell of the dissecting-room that the Murder Act 1752 permitted as an additional punishment, literally a fate worse than death, made dissection so widely feared and socially unacceptable that voluntarily to submit to it was an extreme rarity: to be dissected was an ignominious fate, and the anatomist seemed, and sometimes was, no better than an executioner, for when the body of a hanged man was cut down there might be a fight between medical students, who wanted the corpse for dissection, and the man's friends waiting to revive him, a real possibility following hanging without a drop. It was rumoured that a hanged man revived in a dissecting-room at Newcastle upon Tyne only to be killed by a surgeon unwilling to be "disappointed" of his dissection.[49]

If these punitive associations were not deterrent enough, fears of being dissected alive by an over hasty anatomist were fuelled by folk tales of cataleptics, sleeping beauties and moribund cardinals.[50] The story was told of a farmer from the Edinburgh area who, finding the corpse of his recently dead wife by the roadside, assumed that she had dug her way out of the grave, until he was persuaded that an interrupted grave robbery was a more likely explanation. Even medical students, who were able to find a callous humour in body snatching, were afraid of the corpse coming back to life,[51] and new researches only increased their fears: in Glasgow, the body of murderer Matthew Clydesdale had breathed and grimaced after the application of a galvanic battery, and in the dissecting-room of the Royal College of Surgeons in London electricity had produced "such wonderous [sic] exhibitions on dead bodies" that re-animation seemed in prospect.[52]

The scant legitimate supply of bodies did little to hinder the extramural anatomy schools, whose wants were supplied by the resurrection men. Knox enrolled at the best known of these schools, that of John Barclay (1758–1826) at 10 Surgeons' Square, thus beginning a long association that was to end in his taking over the school after Barclay's death. When Monro *secundus* finally retired, Barclay's roll of pupils rose to over three hundred: a combination of enthusiastic teaching, well-supplied practical classes and up to date lectures on comparative anatomy attracted some of Edinburgh's most promising students, including the future surgeons (Sir) George Ballingall and James Syme, and the veterinary surgeon William Dick, who in later life would send Knox animal specimens for his research.[53] Between 1810 and 1815 Barclay's assistant was a young man named Robert Liston (1794–1847), who would later become a successful anatomy teacher in his own right, and Knox's most acrimonious rival.

Barclay, who had been schooled in theology and licensed as a minister before switching to medicine, had started his anatomy school in 1797, but continued as an Elder of the Kirk, with a seat on the General Assembly.[54] On the face of it, his views would not have appealed to Knox: "All seem agreed", he wrote in 1822, that souls "with new bodies, are to exist in a future state, and in that state to be more or less happy, according to the deeds of the present life", and he saw the huge variety of animal species as evidence for an intelligent Creator – how else could diversity be explained when "[p]lants and animals propagate only after their kind"? Though Knox would find very different answers to such questions, he shared Barclay's enthusiasm for comparative anatomy and dislike of vivisection. Barclay was a humane man, who abhorred the Cartesian view of animals as "automatous", which he saw as justification for unnecessary cruelty.[55] Liberal, hearty and convivial, he had a marvellous store of anecdotes and a sly wit, less obvious than Knox's but just as mischievous: he once commenced an evening lecture on the sexual organs with the words "for what we are about to receive, the Lord make us thankful".[56]

The relationship between the out-lecturers and the University was a mutually beneficial one: the Napoleonic wars created a demand for doctors, and as the number of students taking degrees rose, the extramural lecturers became increasingly important in delivering high quality teaching. The "out lecturers" were recognized as "the chief source of all the knowledge requisite for obtaining a Physician's Diploma in Edinburgh", but since, unlike the university faculty, they had no guaranteed audience, they could not afford to become complacent.[57] Barclay's twice-daily performances in the lecture room were "all fire and zeal",[58] and at other times he was constantly in the dissecting-room to supervise and answer questions. Extramural lecturers were essential to Edinburgh's pre-eminence as a medical school, but the faculty ensured they were kept in their place: Barclay was a Fellow of the Royal Society of Edinburgh, and well known as one of the city's most "learned men", but a move to create a well-merited chair of comparative anatomy for him in 1817 was blocked by the professors, who were shown in a contemporary cartoon barring his way as he attempted to ride into the university on the skeleton of an elephant.[59]

Having passed his anatomy examination at the second attempt in 1814, Knox successfully defended his doctoral thesis, a twenty-nine-page Latin dissertation on the effects of stimulants and narcotics on the body, which was published in English the following year in the *Edinburgh Medical and Surgical Journal*. In reporting the results of his observations on variations in his own heart rate, Knox included the following description of himself:

> The subject of the experiments is about 22 years of age, of a moderate height, and somewhat muscular; his constitution may be called irritable,– by which is meant only, that it is easily excited by stimulants of almost every kind. He has not laboured under a serious indisposition for a great number of years, nor is he conscious of any hereditary or acquired tendency to disease in any organ.[60]

Though never, apparently, a games player, he was remarkably fit and active:

> August 30th 1813, the day being moderately warm, I walked, between 1 and 11 P.M. a distance of nearly 40 miles. Not having much appetite, retired to rest about 1 A.M. after drinking a little coffee, but slept none, perhaps owing to over-fatigue. Next morning (31st) . . . performed a journey that day of 27 miles, at a tolerable pace.[61]

As a student, he displayed the same energy and abstemious habits that would characterize his maturity. A breakfast of coffee, bread and eggs sustained him until dinner ("of animal food principally, and a small quantity of vegetables; to which was added a little spirits or porter"), taken a little before 5 p.m. After a light supper, with a "small quantity" of spirits, "much diluted", he usually retired to bed by midnight.[62]

At his graduation, the 24-year-old Knox was one of eighty-eight young men who signed the oath in the library where they had first matriculated and, with a tap on the head from the Principal with a cap said to have belonged to George Buchanan, were granted "the title and privileges" of Doctor of Physic, with full leave to practise and teach, "*ubique gentium* – all over the world".[63] In reality, however, Edinburgh graduates had to be re-licensed or serve an apprenticeship before they could practise in

A Beautiful but Seductive Science, 1810–1814

England, where it was seen as presumptuous that a "Scotch physician so easily gets the degree of Doctor", a qualification reserved in England for a scholarly few. The Edinburgh men might have answered that their training left them far better prepared for practice, but the English were concerned that many Scottish MDs took up surgery, a manual activity that required less "exertion of mind" than medicine. For one English physician, the suggestion that medicine and surgery were on the same level was so revolutionary as to be "fitted for the Marat Club of Paris".[64]

Though the Scottish medical schools seemed radical to the English, their curricula retained many elements of the time-honoured classical training of gentleman physicians. The ability to write a thesis in Latin and discuss Hippocratic aphorisms may have distinguished university men from jobbing surgeons and apothecaries, and impressed those patients who thought classical knowledge "indispensable",[65] but this largely theoretical training left them ill prepared for day to day work as medical practitioners. They may have started out with high expectations, but in Scotland, as in England, plum hospital and university appointments were scarce, and required the right social connections. As one "Student of 1815" commented: "Tell me the name of the successful individual, and I will tell you who his uncle was."[66]

After a holiday in the highlands, where the "opportunity of observing the Caledonian Celt" was as great a lure as the scenery,[67] Knox, apparently concerned that his training left him poorly equipped for the demands of practice, decided to spend some months studying under the celebrated John Abernethy (1764–1831) at St Bartholomew's Hospital. Many Edinburgh graduates made the trip to London (so many that young ladies were deterred from sailing on the same boat), and many, like Knox, were destined to be disappointed.[68] Abernethy was an "interesting, instructive, clear, and amusing" lecturer, who often sent his audience into convulsions of laughter, and Knox had much in common with this "man of high genius", who preferred observation over experiment and abhorred vivisection. Abernethy's confident, even brusque, public manner, quite unlike his natural personality, probably cost him thousands of pounds a year in private practice and may well have inspired Knox's own robust professional persona, but his deliberate disregard of topographical anatomy proved exasperating: he "talked of the abdominal muscles", complained Knox, "as so many steaks, which he buffoon-like tossed over each other, when dissected, counting them as steak first, steak second, steak third, muscles and tendons which the first of descriptive anatomists have failed clearly to describe."[69]

CHAPTER THREE

Hospital Assistant, 1815–1820

So successful were Scotland's "cheap universities" in turning out doctors of medicine that there were concerns a "general inflation" in qualifications had devalued the degree and obscured the traditional distinctions between physicians, surgeons, and apothecaries (the equivalent of general practitioners). Edinburgh MDs still enjoyed local privileges – they could, for example, become fellows of the Royal College of Physicians of Edinburgh without sitting a further examination – but after the 1815 Apothecaries Act they could not practise in England without serving a five-year apprenticeship, and many were obliged to seek employment further afield.[1] A surplus of Scottish graduates was seen in some quarters as "necessary" to provide physicians for the British Empire, where there were said to be ten Scots doctors for every English one, for what English-trained physician would settle for being "frozen in Newfoundland, Hudson's Bay, or the Orkneys; or broiled for a pittance in the West Indies", or "waste his health, his vigour, and his talents, among the outcasts and convicts of New Holland"? Nor, for that matter, would he wish to end up "starved" in a "dirty" Scottish borough.[2]

If Knox, who returned to Edinburgh in 1815 to attend some surgical cases, probably as an observer or assistant, had not already considered working overseas, the news that Napoleon had escaped from Elba and raised an army in France may have decided him.[3] Many Edinburgh medical graduates began their careers in the armed forces, and almost one in ten joined the army,[4] usually as Hospital Assistants, a commissioned rank newly created in 1813 to replace the less professional sounding "Hospital Mates". Advertisements in London and Edinburgh medical journals promised "advancement" in the Army Medical Department for "well-educated persons" of "liberal education", but promotion was often slow, and regular officers treated their medical colleagues with scant respect.[5] The army, however, offered a guaranteed income for a comparatively small outlay – Knox had to provide his own uniform and surgical instruments – and the prospect of service overseas was attractive to any natural philosopher, especially the travel-struck Knox, who had recently been "lost in wonder" at the sight of the "Chinese bridges, pagodas, and heathen deities" of Hyde Park.[6]

There was an urgent need for surgeons to tend those wounded at Waterloo. The casualties on the 18th of June had been exceptionally heavy in proportion to the numbers of men involved, and some of the injuries were appalling: over twenty thousand coalition troops and a similar number of French died, most from wounds or infection in the days and weeks following the battle. Each regiment, comprising some four to six hundred cavalry, or between five hundred and two thousand infantry, had one surgeon and an assistant, and they struggled to cope. Knox was commissioned Hospital Assistant on the 24 June 1815, and was sent immediately to Belgium.[7] In later years he spoke of his military service as professionally valuable, and many would-be surgeons gained their first experience on the battlefield, but his arrival in Belgium, days after the battle, when the hospitals were full of wounded pleading for medical attention, must have been a daunting experience.[8] Georgina Capel described the scene in Brussels, eleven miles from Waterloo, in a letter to her grandmother, the Dowager Countess of Uxbridge: the streets were crowded with wounded and with "wagons filled with dead and dying", and three thousand dead bodies lay exposed on the ramparts, "there not being room to bury them", with wounded men "heaped" upon the dead. The rotting carcasses of horses in the streets added to the risk of contagion, and many civilians fled for their own safety.[9]

After two weeks, Knox was sent to Ostend to join the first British hospital ship to sail for Portsmouth. There were some ninety patients aboard, and he had only a sergeant as his assistant: his duties were "urgent, most pressing, and harassing", and he got no more than six hours sleep during a voyage of six or seven days, but he was pleased to record that he did not lose a single life. Abernethy's training proved invaluable, particularly his axiom that one must do everything of importance oneself, and Knox successfully treated a young soldier with a neck wound by adopting his technique of leaving the wound open to the air.[10] His patients were mostly uncomplaining, and he later recalled that men whose bodies had been transfixed by musket balls or sword thrusts had been most anxious to tell him they had received their wounds facing the enemy and not running away. Not all wounds acquired on the continent were so honourable: Knox saw some "striking" cases of venereal disease among the hospitalized British troops.[11]

Having delivered the wounded to the Navy hospital at Haslar in Gosport, Knox was ordered back to Brussels "without delay" to take charge of the wards of the first division of the *hôpital de la gendarmerie*, a converted barracks filled with French wounded.[12] One memorable patient, sufficiently recovered to work as an orderly, was a *chasseur* of the Imperial Guard, who had received a musket ball in the temple and had lain unconscious for three days. When he was discharged he thanked his attendants for their humanity, adding that he felt so little pain that he would willingly be shot on the other side too, if it would benefit the Emperor.[13] Many of his compatriots with limb wounds were less fortunate: they developed gangrene or infections, and when "secondary" amputations of the mortifying limbs, performed as a last resort, failed to prevent death from septicaemia, the Belgians blamed the British surgeons, some of whom were unable to explain their actions as they spoke no French. Knox, however, had learned the language at school, and he enjoyed discussing the battle with the French officers, who professed themselves unable to understand the reason for their defeat. They could count on his sympathy, for he regarded Napoleon as "the greatest of men", "betrayed" by the continental Celts.[14]

Knox continued in his post until Christmas, when he was ordered to close the wards and accompany the remaining wounded home to France.[15] Back in England, he was placed in charge of the depot hospital at Hilsea near Portsmouth, which received wounded men and invalids returning from service overseas.[16] Conditions there were poor: a few years earlier, Lady Grey had been so shocked by the sorry state of the patients that she sent them two cartloads of warm clothing.[17] There were many deaths, especially among those men whose health had been broken by service in India and Ceylon, and Knox performed between forty and sixty "dissections" to look for evidence of "hepatic dysentery", though only two or three turned out to have obvious disease of the liver.[18] He also experimented with non-mercurial treatments for syphilis, which he claimed healed the majority of primary chancres (they are often self healing) and he made home visits to convalescing officers, some of whom endured constant pain from unhealed and infected wounds, particularly the stumps of hastily amputated limbs.[19] In 1816, for example, "Captain B_____ residing in the south of England" sought his advice "regarding a discharge of purulent matter from the thigh, which had been amputated about two years before." There was little he could do to treat these chronic infections, though he saw many examples:

> W.S. of the hussars was wounded on the 18th June 1815, by a cannon shot, which destroyed the knee joint. He suffered amputation on the 20th; the bone was sawn through about four inches above the knee; the stump remained open. In the beginning of 1817, a long exfoliation or sequestrum came away from the face of the stump, which still remained open, with a discharge of purulent matter. Such cases are very common.[20]

Many medical men left the army after the peace and took their chance in civilian practice, if they were eligible to practise under the 1815 Apothecaries Act, but Knox, who was comparatively well qualified for the rank he held, stayed on, and in April 1817 he was posted to the Cape of Good Hope: "I went out to Africa", he would tell his students in later years, "with the spirit of philosophic research strong within me, and in this I ever indulged."[21] On the outward voyage, the sailors amused themselves catching dolphins, sharks, and other fish, which Knox dissected to study the anatomy of their hearts. Though light, his shipboard duties

Hospital Assistant, 1815–1820

carried considerable responsibility for a young man. Writing in 1856, he recalled the experience of a surgeon in charge of troops heading for a distant colony, who was called upon to treat a cabin boy seriously ill with a fever after having wounded his thigh by falling onto a boathook. The surgeon instructed his orderly sergeant to give the boy a dose of calomel but the sergeant mistakenly gave corrosive sublimate and the boy died "in frightful agony". It is quite possible that Knox himself was the surgeon whose catastrophic error he remembered nearly forty years later.[22]

∞

The Cape Colony was the oldest European colony in South Africa: established by the Dutch, invaded by the British in 1806 and ceded to the British Crown in 1814, its population numbered some sixty thousand, about half of whom were Europeans; the rest comprised roughly equal numbers of native South Africans and imported African or Malay slaves. In 1816, the British publicly hanged five ringleaders of a Dutch rebellion at Slachters Nek, which stirred up considerable ill feeling between Dutch and English settlers, though they were united in a common cause against the indigenous Xhosa, who constantly crossed the Great Fish River, which the Europeans recognized as the Eastern border of their Colony, into the territory occupied by Boer settlers. Usually, little notice was taken of incursions into this "forsaken" frontier,[23] but a fresh wave of English immigrants who arrived in 1817 were settled along the border to provide a barrier against the Xhosa. The military reinforcements that accompanied them from England were mostly deserters and criminals, who in the opinion of the historian of the Cape Colony G.E. Cory were "almost useless",[24] and even after their arrival the British military presence in the Cape, a region of some 230,000 square miles, numbered a mere 2,700 regulars. In addition there was the Cape Corps, composed mostly of "Hottentots" – seventy-eight cavalry and 169 infantry – under the command of "that most excellent officer and man"[25] Major G.S. Fraser and six other European officers.

Though African service might have seemed a daunting prospect for a recently qualified medical man, Knox's duties were lighter, and his patients healthier, than he could reasonably have expected in Edinburgh. The Cape, he later wrote, was the healthiest of countries, whose salubrious climate was responsible for the "immunity from the host of diseases" that its colonists enjoyed.[26] He was the only surgeon for some 140 miles along the Great Fish River, and if an accident occurred it took many hours of riding, if not a day and a night, before he reached his patient. Apart from accidents, however, calls were few, as the soldiers, "in the prime of life", were "the healthiest body of men I have ever seen".[27]

For most of the time, life was comparatively easy: a typical Boer family kept perhaps twenty or thirty "Hottentot" servants, who had little work to do, while their masters "never labour at all. . . . I presume they act like other men; there being no necessity for labour they very naturally avoid it."[28] Knox learned to ride and shoot, and occupied his time exploring the country, recording the weather, collecting and dissecting specimens, and studying the local people. Mounted on his "famous Arabian mare", he surveyed the geography of the districts he visited, possibly with some official encouragement, as he was able to amend British maps, and he hunted wild animals for their skins and skeletons. According to Lonsdale, who presumably heard it from Knox himself, he also practised swordsmanship, a skill he was later to employ in unfortunate circumstances.[29]

Between May 1818 and April 1819, Knox continuously kept meteorological observations at Graaf Reinet, a small Karoo town two thousand feet above sea level in the Eastern Cape. To the South and South East of this remote spot was open semi-desert, and to the West the Great Karoo extended over three hundred miles to the Atlantic Ocean, while the Snow Mountains lay to the North. The town itself was well watered by a canal from the Sunday River, and with streets lined by lemon and orange trees it resembled a green oasis in the desert.[30] There was little work for a medical man: "bilious fevers" were sometimes induced by the summer heat, and piercing North winds occasioned "considerable mortality amongst infants", but overall the climate was, wrote Knox, "one of the *healthiest* in the world".

Most of Graaf Reinet's inhabitants were Boer farmers; the English presence consisted merely of a small garrison and the Auxiliary Missionary Society. Knox found the Boers boorish, the English vulgar (he blamed their "Saxon nature") and both uninteresting: "From London to Graafkeynet [*sic*] . . . it is all the same."[31] His companions did not inspire him but the landscape did. As a child, he had read "the five enchanting volumes" of François Le Vaillant's (1753–1824) *Travels Into the Interior Parts of Africa*,[32] and now he was free to explore the land of his youthful daydreams:

> As I wandered by the banks of the Rio d'Infante, and climbed the heights separating the valley of the river from those beauteous grassy and umbrageous plains, through which wind their way the clear and crystal streams of the Koonap, gaining a view of the vast plains of '*het land den Caffre*,' themselves shelving towards the Indian Ocean, in the distance reposed in solemn grandeur the Winter Bergen and Anatolo Mountains, through whose wooded and deeply-tangled ravines once roamed freely the dreaded Caffre, I could not fail to recollect that on the spot where I then stood Le Vaillant gazed on that identical landscape! Simple and unaffected lover of the simple and beautiful in nature.
>
> But how was it that the landscape before me transported me with pleasure? No castle rose to view, nor churches nor spires, turrets nor palaces; man nor man's hands had touched this field. Nature prevailed everywhere: antelope and ostrich, zebra and quagga, bustards of all hues, birds of every plumage, deco-

rated this glorious landscape; dark forests clothed the steep slope of the Winter Bergen nearly to that summit whose grassy and shelving rocky crown reached far into the heavens.[33]

This response to a landscape so "beautiful and perfect" that it "speaks directly to the soul" foreshadowed Knox's future emphasis on aesthetics in understanding the works of nature. For a man not yet thirty, it was a personal awakening, and it was "whilst gazing on such a landscape" that "the would-be civilized man – cribbed, trammelled, and confined; the thing in harness – the state flunkey; the biped in harness; the clock-regulated animal" realized that "his soul perhaps for the first time feels independent":[34]

> There is a feeling in the human mind, that is, in the mind correctly formed, which no artificial condition, no conventionalities, no civilization can overcome; it is the feeling which connects it with the earth, its parent – its mother earth teeming with life. In her winter garb, man feels the desolation around him; in her black robes of winter, his instinctive sense sees the emblems of death, although his experience and his judgement and his reasoning mind tell him that Nature will revive. But spring returns, and all that lives rejoices. This is the connecting link between him and the decorated earth, the parent from which he came, unto which he returns. The landscape . . . calls forth feelings and passions he has no language to describe; a chord in his brain, which civilization had masked and thrown into abeyance, but could not destroy; the chord which makes him independent of artificial things, reminding him that he was made to walk and hunt on that landscape unfettered, unrestrained. With this landscape he cannot but choose to sympathize; it is the field on which Nature first placed him; his whole existence harmonizes with it; his physiological destiny proclaims it as his own; from it he sprung – to it he must return.[35]

According to his own account, Knox enhanced his reputation as a surgeon by his willingness to undertake procedures that others would not, such as the removal of "half of the lower jaw of a sergeant", and the Boers offered him the post of chief surgeon to the Dutch Free States. This was probably just rodomontade, and in any case Knox did not intend to spend his life in the colonies. Freedom for the spirit came at the price of professional and personal isolation, and on 10 September 1818 he wrote to his younger brother Frederick complaining of the boredom of his African "banishment". Despite mixing only with the "first society" in the Cape, he lacked "promotion", and the "amusements of the chase" were growing "irksome", although, he told Frederick "without vanity", he could "generally acquire friends" wherever he went.[36]

Knox's contact with the indigenous peoples of the Cape, who "differed in an extraordinary manner" from Europeans, stirred up his interest in race, which became a "favourite pursuit". He described the "Hottentot"

(Khoi) and "Bushmen" (San) as "yellow races" (they are now usually referred to as a single race, the Khoisan) quite different from the "warlike, bold and active" "Caffres" (Xhosa) and "Amakosos" (Zulu).[37] He was particularly impressed that the San knew the names of all the animals, and could distinguish different antelope by their slightest movements, an illustration of the principle that accurate observation of nature was a prerequisite for its classification.[38]

Though he initially ridiculed the Khoi's fear of serpents after seeing a corps of them "routed by a snake eight i[n]ches long", he soon came to respect their caution as "the accumulated experience of ages". While travelling in the desert with a young Khoi servant, Knox was obliged to turn their horses loose to graze on the scanty scrub, and in searching for them next morning he almost trod on a puff adder. His servant shouted a warning and Knox shot the snake with his fowling piece, aiming at its neck so as to preserve the head for dissection. The poison fangs, "of great size" were still in his private museum twenty years later. On another occasion, he carelessly handled a wounded yellow snake, which he assumed from its appearance was not poisonous, but some Khoi who were present expressed alarm, and after the snake died he examined it and found poison fangs. He became experienced at dealing with snake bites, which he treated by cutting out the surrounding tissues: when a Boer farmer was bitten on the toe by a Berg adder, Knox gave him two minutes to decide whether to have the wound cut out. Fortunately, the farmer was too ill even to speak before the two minutes were up, so Knox "cut down to the tendon" and washed the area in alcohol, and after four days the patient had recovered.[39]

The native peoples of the Cape were known in early-nineteenth century Europe only through exhibitions such as the "Hottentot Venus" (Saartjie Baartman or Sarah Bartmann), which were not far removed from freak shows (Baartman's "abnormalities" were commented on), and which emphasized supposed anatomical differences between Africans and Europeans. Though Saartjie was baptized and earned enough money to make her desirable, in the opinion of *The Times*, to "some of our minor fortune-hunters", "Hottentots" were commonly supposed by Europeans to be "the most savage of mankind".[40] "As wild as a Hottentot" was a common figure of speech, though one missionary protested that they were no more dirty or savage than the English "peasantry".[41] Nonetheless, the unfortunate Khoisan came to exemplify "all that is most debasing to humane nature", and travellers returning from the Cape brought back lurid tales of "Hottentots" who lived in a state of "brutalized ignorance": "atheists", "savages" and devotees of witchcraft, they supposedly gave birth in the open like a "brute beast" and "perform[ed] their ablutions with cow-dung". As with all "savages", the "spirit of cruelty" was "innate" in them: they were aggressive and merciless warriors, and when slaughtering animals they disembowelled them alive, "lapping, like wolves or jackalls – without the loss of a drop – the warm and reeking life-blood of their victim whilst the smoking and still quivering entrails were torn asunder, greedily devoured, and naught escaped their ghoul-like voracity, save the contents of the latter, together with the animal's hide."[42]

Knox formed his own opinion, and noted with disapproval the Boers' "contempt and inward dislike to the Hottentot, the Negro, the Caffre", whom in his view they had robbed and enslaved. He admired the love of independence and liberty that drove the Boer to colonize South Africa, but thought his behaviour there that of the "vulgar barbarian", the "cruel oppressor of the native dark races", in which task, he wrote ironically, "[t]he Anglo-Saxon assisted him bravely". The Boers, however, were "honest and straightforward" in comparison with the European statesmen who justified the plunder of Africa and Asia with their sanctimonious rhetoric.[43] Knox's plea for common humanity did not presume equality: he accepted the widely-held notion of a "scale of humanity", in which he assigned the lowest place to the "Basoos" of the North, who were "still smaller than the colonial Bushmen" and who made "little hollows in the ground in which they burrow at night, sleeping with their feet outside the caross or cloak made of the skins of some animal taken in the chase", but he reproached the "Christian Dutch" settlers for treating the native peoples as subhuman, and for having "practically denied the first canon of scripture in a body, as the United States men do now; there is no denying it."[44]

In 1819, an army of ten thousand Xhosa under the command of Chief Ndlambe, emboldened by a prophecy of the "witch-doctor" Nxele, or Makanda, that the British bullets would be turned to water, defiantly sent a message informing Colonel Willshire in Graham's Town that they would breakfast with him next morning. When morning came, however, they were no match for the garrison's musketry and grapeshot. Reprisals against this unprecedented assault were swiftly organized under the "commando" system, which allowed the civil authorities to organize armed raids into Xhosa territory. Over a thousand settlers left their families and homes, joined the "great commando", and accompanied British forces under Colonel Willshire across the Great Fish River. A separate commando from Graaf Reinet, commanded by the town's *landrost* (chief magistrate) Andries Stockenström, a future Lieutenant Governor of the Eastern Province, was charged with clearing the impenetrable bush along the river, and Knox joined these Graaf Reinet cavalry on their foray beyond the Winterbergen, across the Bontebok plains and back to the Anatola mountains, which they re-crossed at the source of the Kat River to join the main force.[45]

Stockenström had previously made the acquaintance of an Edinburgh-trained British Army Hospital Assistant in the person of Knox's predecessor, James Barry,[46] who went on to become a highly successful army doctor and administrator, though only after her death was she discovered to be a woman, the first British woman to qualify as a doctor of medicine.[47] Barry could be argumentative and opinionated, and if Stockenström had formed the opinion that these were characteristic Edinburgh traits, Knox certainly did not disabuse him of it, though, even after their eventual falling out, Stockenström magnanimously recorded that he had found Knox, the only British soldier in his division, to be a man of "great abilities, not only in his medical capacity, but as a man of general knowledge and science, [who] rendered great service, especially in tracing the nature of the horse distemper, by the dissection of the many subjects which unfortunately daily presented themselves, and his enlightened political and ethnological views were deeply interesting to me during the many months he remained under my command."[48] Knox had been a frequent visitor to the *landrost's* house, where he had seen his first "bushman", a little servant who had amused the ladies by imitating Knox's "peculiar" gait, and Stockenström, an outspoken critic of British rule noted for his "principle of justice for all men of whatever race",[49] had taken a liking to Knox's liberal advocacy of the rights of man and condemnation of slavery.[50]

In retrospect, the apparent complicity of Knox in the burning of native villages, trampling of crops, carrying off of cattle and cold blooded slaughter that the commando wrought seems all the more reprehensible given his ostensibly liberal attitudes, but as a soldier he had little choice but to do his duty. It was not an experience he cared to recall, and not until 1850 did he mention it in print:

> Thirty years ago a military *rhazia*, composed of English soldiers, Dutch boors, and native Hottentots, devastated the beautiful territory of the Amakoso Kaffirs. We reached the banks of the Kei, and the country of the noble Hinsa, where wandered the 'wilde' of Nature's creation. All must disappear shortly before the rude civilization of the Saxon boor – antelope and hippopotamus, giraffe and Kaffir.[51]

He later used a piece of anonymous journalism to describe the settlers' victory over the Xhosa: "The men were hunted and shot down like beasts; the women who escaped, dispersed; and the children were brought into the colony as booty."[52] To end the carnage, Nxele surrendered himself to Stockenström[53] and the Graaf Reinetters returned home.

Stockenström's reward for his part in the campaign was promotion to Captain, but his relations with Knox became strained after he heard "several reports" detrimental to his brother O.G. Stockenström's character, "one of which had originated with Dr K". According to Andries Stockenström's autobiography, O.G.'s promotion to senior lieutenant in the Cape Corps had riled his fellow officers, many of whom had been placed on half pay, and a group of them "concocted" a charge against

Hospital Assistant, 1815–1820

him of "stealing a copper coin not worth sixpence" so that he could be "got rid of".[54] The matter came to a head when Knox met Andries in the street and "anxiously" asked for his mail. Andries handed him his letters in silence and walked away, but Knox hurriedly tore one open and went after him, exclaiming "What does Major Frazer [sic] mean? – He has written me an official letter . . . as if he were my Commanding Officer, had it not been for the sake of your Brother's Character I would not have accused him, but I have accused him in such terms as will enable your brother to put a stop to that vagabond plot." Knox implied that he too was the victim of a conspiracy, and named several officers who "would be glad to destroy me by the same blow because your brother and myself were always together; but I hope . . . *I may have an opportunity of exposing the villains which have brought my name into the business.*"[55]

As it turned out, a court martial dropped all charges against O.G. Stockenström: Knox's testimony apparently failed to convince, and the Governor, Lord Charles Henry Somerset (1767–1831), stopped the proceedings after another officer, James Fleeson, withdrew his accusation. According to Andries, the whole business had been trumped up by the "blackest treachery" of Knox, and "those very individuals he had declared it his determination to expose, as the vilest conspirators, had been pressed against the unfortunate subject of his slander by himself only . . . his prevarications became palpable, when a conviction of guilt made him tumble before the court like a Criminal . . . ".[56] In a letter to Somerset written from Graaf Reinet on 19 November 1819, Andries complained that he had arrived in Graham's Town after the court martial to find his brother still under arrest, and no-one except those who had been present in court aware that the charges had been dropped; furthermore, the officers who had accused his brother were still serving, and Knox was taking "the opportunity of giving whatever colour to his shameful conduct the most refined and plausible cunning could suggest".[57]

Not surprisingly, Andries's friendship with Knox came to an end. He expected Knox to challenge him (to judge from his surviving letters, he had openly accused Knox of slander), but Knox passed him by in silence in front of a crowd of other officers. In the following months, each accused the other of not wanting to fight. At the end of December, Andries received a letter "in the well known hand writing of Dr Knox" but he let Knox know that he had not opened it. He consulted a friend, Captain Andrews, who wrote to Knox offering to act as a "mediator" – the illegality of duelling necessitated this ambiguous term for "second" – and Knox duly replied on 22 January 1820 that if he "rightly comprehended" Andrews's letter, "the only offer I can possibly return is that my present residence is at Roodwaal, where I am to be found . . . at such time as may best suit your convenience." Andrews did not call on Knox, but replied the same day by letter, asking Knox to "meditate on the Manner you treated Mr Stockenström under the Cloak of Friendship & to reconcile it to your self if you can."[58] Andries called this a "decided insult" intended to force Knox into a "meeting",[59] but Knox blamed Andries for holding back, claiming that even after he had publicly "affronted" him, Andries did not respond, except to have him bound over to keep the peace.[60]

The Stockenströms demanded, and got, a court of enquiry, which sat at Graham's Town on 23 June 1820 and exonerated O.G., calling his conduct "highly creditable". The court records have not survived, but, according to Andries, Knox's behaviour on the occasion was that of "the most wretched of Beggars" and "such as to astonish the whole court".[61] The official opinion was no less damning: "With regard to Dr Knox the court look upon his conduct in such a light that they hope they may be excused from giving an opinion, and refer the Commandant to the above proceedings, relative to the calumnies issuing from him."[62] Captain Henry Somerset, who Andries felt had, like his father Lord Charles, stepped into a senior position ahead of longer-serving officers,[63] apologized for O.G.'s treatment, but Andries thought "the contrition was as mean as the attack was dastardly".[64]

A key witness at the enquiry, and a supporter of the Stockenströms, was Bishop Burnett, a former lieutenant in the Royal Navy who had arrived in the Cape as a civilian settler in 1820.[65] Unlike most settlers, the hot-headed Burnett had paid for his own passage, and expected to have his say. He disliked the self-important Lord Charles Somerset, against whom he waged a campaign over many years, and quickly sided with the Stockenströms against the British administration. His testimony, he claimed, had been enough to "rescue the character of Captn Stockenström the Landroite of Graaf Reinet from eternal infamy" and bring about "the complete transfer of public odium and contempt to one Doctor Knox his Calumniator." According to Burnett, Knox tried to discredit him with an *ad hominem* attack and he called Knox out, but after initially agreeing to fight, Knox backed down. Burnett then "posted" Knox, *i.e.* he made public his calumnies and refusal to fight, which led to Knox's "expulsion from all society". It was then that Knox called Burnett a blackguard. Burnett's is the only account of the events that followed: "I soundly horse whipped him on the parade before every Officer of the Garrison. Would you believe that the Coward rushed into a house for a sabre and like an assassin attacked me unarmed my foot unfortunately tripped and I lay at his mercy, in this state he was too arrant a poltroon to run me thro', and I escaped with only a slight cut on the arm, & a dislocated finger."[66] While Burnett's account of this incident is obviously partial (what was "every Officer of the Garrison" doing while Knox rushed off for a sword?), it is at least substantially true ("I refer you to any officer returning from the Frontier", wrote Burnett), and Knox's silence is incriminating. In his autobiography, Andries recorded that in addition to being "publicly horsewhipped and placarded" Knox had his promotion to assistant surgeon cancelled.[67]

Hospital Assistant, 1815–1820

In the absence of the original records of the court martial, the motives for Knox's slanders against his former friend O.G. Stockenström remain obscure.[68] Andries blamed professional jealousies and ill feeling in the Cape Corps between Boer and British officers, referring to the latter as "malicious conspirators" who had been reluctant to answer questions in court, perhaps because of intimidation by Captain Somerset. Knox, who did not hold a regular commission, could not have profited professionally from O.G. Stockenström's disgrace, and he may have been acting out of misplaced loyalty to his brother officers: apart from Fleeson, who, having withdrawn his charges, agreed to go on half-pay, Andries mentioned an unnamed third person whose promotion had been facilitated by O.G.'s removal.[69]

With his reputation ruined, it was impossible for Knox to remain in the Cape, and having seen how its civilized and uncivilized inhabitants behaved, he was probably not sorry to leave. As long ago as September 1818 he had mentioned, in his letter to Frederick, that he intended to take "steps" towards returning home. He sailed aboard the brig *Brilliant* on 22 October 1820. During the homeward voyage he continued to pursue his meteorological interests, and made "Observations on the Temperature of the North Atlantic Ocean and the Superincumbent atmosphere", beginning at 6 a.m. every day. On 21 November, at lat 6°4'N, long 20°31'W, the ship encountered a "sublime" storm, his account of which, published in the *Edinburgh Philosophical Journal*, demonstrates a singular aptitude for incorporating a passionate emotional response into a scientific report:

> After the most perfect calm, heavy, dense, and gloomy clouds are seen collecting at every point of the horizon; they form themselves into vast arches, having their abutments in the ocean; suddenly at one point they blacken to an inky hue; the sails are furled; the crew stand in mute attention, each at his station, and every eye is directed towards that vast and hideous mass of clouds, which, resting on the surface of the deep, and reaching heaven with its top, advances upon the devoted vessel. Now, sweeping the ocean, it pours a deluge on the ship; the storm rages, and, by the terrific force of the blast, the masts seem ready to start from the decks. When these squalls happen at night, and are attended with much rain, a ball of meteoric fire is seen at the mast-head, tending to increase the horrors of the storm.[70]

Brilliant arrived safely in England on Christmas day.

CHAPTER FOUR

Parisian Anatomy, 1821–1822

Knox advertised his return from the Cape with a generous distribution of souvenirs: the University museum received two rare antelope, a leopard, and some native weapons and clothes, and there were personal gifts for Professors Jameson and Monro of what Knox claimed were the first "Kaffir crania" ever seen in Europe. Knox kept a third skull for himself, maintaining thereafter that he was the first to describe "this fine race" to science.[1] Robert Jameson (1774–1854), geologist and Regius Professor of natural history (in which capacity he had blocked the proposed chair for Barclay), was an enthusiast for Abraham Werner's theory of Neptunism, according to which all rocks had crystallized from a primeval ocean. Jameson was president and founder of the Wernerian Natural History Society, whose members were mostly Edinburgh medical men, and which met in his rooms at the university; he invited Knox to join, and on 10 March 1821 Knox read his first paper to the Society, on a "Caffre albino".[2] His foray into Edinburgh scientific society was, however, short-lived, for after reporting to Sir James McGrigor (1771–1858), the director-general of the Army Medical Department (and an Edinburgh MD), who praised his chart of the Eastern Frontier and either did not know or did not care about the Stockenström scandal, he was immediately given leave of absence from the army on half-pay to study in Paris.[3]

Since the Peace, Parisian training had become the goal of many medical students and recently qualified doctors: subjects for dissection cost three shillings compared with twenty pounds in Britain; lectures, colleges, museums and libraries were freely open to visiting medical men; realistic wax anatomical models were available; books were a quarter of the price they were in England; food was cheaper, and the cafés were filled with "noblemen, gentry, loose women, rogues, all in the same place, all in high glee, with newspapers, laughter, and lots of converse."[4] Though Knox thought it just possible that civilization might "proceed higher even than in Paris" it was incomparably better than the Cape, or "[b]eer-drinking, smoky London".[5]

Knox later claimed that "France owes everything, as regards science, literature, and art, to the revolutionary assembly of 1793", when "aristocracy, priest, king were destroyed", thus ending the "slavish terror of free enquiry" that had held back anatomists labouring under the "odious incubus" of the *ancient regime:*[6]

On the English side we had no Revolution setting free the human mind from the bondage of ages, and producing such intellects as those of Arago and Cuvier, Laplace and Fourier, Geoffroy and Savigny, Malus and Gay Lussac. With us, on the favoured side of the Channel, Sot George succeeded Idiot George; the English mandarins, with whom, of course, was the English Parti-prêtre, successfully resisted the claims of men to be free; the progress of Science, especially of zoological Science, was successfully resisted; the labours of the Count de Buffon continued to be scandalously mutilated by English compilers to suit the taste of the English public; Paley's well-written, but superficial, erroneous and piratical compilation was the zoological text-book at the Universities. . . . In the meantime, what did the great bulk of people read on zoology? Goldsmith's "Animated Nature" and "A History of the Three Hundred Animals," that being the limit as to what was "useful to be known," and to which the English mind was permitted to aspire.[7]

These sweeping, romantic claims do not stand up to scrutiny. Anatomy had not lacked students under the Bourbons, and among the amateurs who studied this impious science at the *Collège de France* were several aristocrats, including, controversially, women:

> Many of them use the lancet and even the scalpel; the Marquise de Voyer attends at dissections, and the young Comtesse de Coigny dissects with her own hands. The current infidelity finds fresh support on this foundation, which is that of the prevailing philosophy. Towards the end of the century "we see young persons who have been in society six or seven years openly pluming themselves on their irreligion, thinking that impiety makes up for wit, and that to be an atheist is to be a philosopher."[8]

These were no mere dilettantes; the Comtesse de Coigny's passion for this "horrible study" apparently led to her death from breathing the "foul air" of the dissecting-room.[9] In retrospect, Knox's words on the "terror of free enquiry" seem more pertinent to Britain, where students were unable to obtain bodies without breaking the law.

While the French Revolution did not start a revolution in anatomical science in the way Knox supposed, it created positions for ambitions young republican scientists, for example on the staff of the reorganized *Jardin des Plantes* (as the revolutionaries renamed the *Jardin du Roi*) and on Napoleon's Egyptian expedition. There was also a new emphasis on anatomy as a process rather than as a description of static nature, a conceptual change that had begun in the late-eighteenth century – when, for example, embryological preformation, which hypothesized the presence of a complete animal in miniature in the egg or sperm, was superseded by epigenesis, in which the embryo progressed through a series of increasingly complex forms *in utero*[10] – but which accelerated as the Revolution popularized comparisons between change in the natural world and progress in human history.

Parisian Anatomy, 1821–1822

The first of the triumvirate of Parisian comparative anatomists who shaped Knox's thinking was Étienne Geoffroy Saint Hilaire (1772–1844), a political radical for whom the Revolution had provided a timely opportunity. Only nineteen years older than Knox, he had prepared for the priesthood (becoming a tonsured clerk) before taking up medicine, a career more in keeping with his revolutionary ideals. When the *Muséum National d'Histoire Naturelle* was founded in the *Jardin des Plantes* in 1793, Geoffroy was appointed professor of vertebrate zoology (Jean-Baptiste Lamarck held the corresponding post for invertebrates), notwithstanding his youth and hitherto modest achievements.[11] In preparation for his academic rôle, he studied *Naturphilosophie*, and, impressed by Goethe's attempt "to sing the grandeur of the universe" (Goethe later supported Geoffroy against Cuvier), Geoffroy took up the idea that lay at the heart of all transcendental anatomy: "that nature is confined within certain limits and has formed all living things on only one single plan."[12] A keen traveller in the pursuit of science, he joined the commission that accompanied Bonaparte to Egypt in 1798, and after three years he returned with valuable natural history specimens to Paris, where he was elected to the *Académie des sciences*. In 1808, after a successful mission to Portugal, he was appointed professor of zoology and physiology in the *Université de France*.

Geoffroy's career was linked with that of Georges Cuvier (1769–1832), who started out as first assistant at the *Muséum* in 1795 on Geoffroy's recommendation. While Geoffroy travelled, Cuvier exercised his indefatigable intellectual energy and astute political skills at home, becoming professor of animal anatomy, a founder member of the *Institut de France* in 1795 and permanent secretary of the Physical Sciences division of the *Académie des sciences* in 1803. By 1821 he was the most successful anatomist, in worldly terms, that Europe had ever known: councillor of state, chancellor of the university, and inspector-general of public education, his prestige reflected the importance of comparative anatomy in France and made a sharp contrast to Scotland and England where professors of anatomy were primarily teachers of medical students. Cuvier's *Tableau elementaire de l'histoire naturelle des animaux* (1798) was regarded as a landmark work on comparative anatomy, and his *Règne animal* (1817) became the standard text on zoological classification.

Knox may have exaggerated when he wrote that few British anatomists were familiar with Cuvier's work (he was fêted during a visit to Britain in 1818), but its acceptance was certainly slower in Britain than in France. According to Knox, fewer than twenty people in Britain took note of Cuvier's *Leçons d'anatomie comparée* (1800), and it was only after the publication of *Recherches sur les ossemens fossiles des quadrupèdes* [*Research on the Fossil Bones of Quadrupeds*] in 1812 that his reputation there was established.[13] Edinburgh students were more likely than most to be aware of his writings, since Jameson had contributed to a translation of the *Discours préliminaire* of the *Recherches* in 1813, though ironically the arch Neptunist employed Cuvier's challenge to existing chronologies of the world, with its fossil evidence for "the true antiquity of the earth", to argue for the historicity of the Biblical Deluge.[14]

Knox later claimed that his own researches in comparative anatomy were sufficient introduction to Geoffroy and Cuvier, though as he had published nothing on the subject they could have been forgiven for not having heard of him.[15] He was ever "fond of flinging about celebrated names with an air of easy familiarity", and it is likely he exaggerated the closeness of his relations with the great Parisian anatomists.[16] Fortunately, it was not necessary to be invited to Cuvier's soirées to see the great man: anyone who attended his lectures, which were always crowded, might enter the cabinet where he worked.[17] One visitor to the *Muséum d'Histoire naturelle* was as amazed by the variety of people, wealthy and humble, urbane and provincial, learned and unlettered, who attended Cuvier's lectures as he was by the stuffed snakes, crocodiles, and other specimens of the animal world crammed into the Museum. Knox judged Cuvier a "clear and methodical" lecturer, but not a great orator, though his appearance was suitably impressive: his "enormous" head (his "voluminous" brain weighed, post-mortem, 3lbs 13½ oz,[18]) atop a neck as thick as a "well-grown tree", was a striking sight as he worked at his high, black-painted desk while his "acolytes" dissected and a servant stoked a huge wood-burning stove, for he felt the cold acutely, despite having grown "enormously fat" since the restoration.[19]

The Museum was not an examining body (though certificates of attendance at lectures could be obtained as proof of assiduity) and entry was cheap and unrestricted. Medical students, amateurs and sightseers all came along: women could, and did, attend, and in all there were some two thousand visitors a year.[20] According to Cuvier's biographer Dorinda Outram it was a kind of utopia to which the public resorted in order to exchange the tensions of Parisian life for the pleasures of nature, and the large, mixed audiences encouraged professors to adopt the crowd-pleasing simplicity of a grand plan.[21] Cuvier's functionalist anatomy – the form of an organ was determined by the function it was to fulfil – lent itself to the "design" argument that complex structures were created for a purpose, and his commitment to fixity of species, which he supposed remained unchanged over time, was reassuring to those who saw the diversity of animal forms as evidence of a Creator.[22] His most revolutionary claim, based on his study of fossil skeletons and described by Knox as "the greatest discovery ever made in science", was that extinct species and genera differed from those now living.[23] As he was adamant that one species could not transform into another, Cuvier proposed that there had been several zoological creations at successive points in geological time. This seemed to Knox, and to many others, over reliant on the "miraculous", and he doubted that Cuvier was fully satisfied with this explanation.[24] The political significance of mass extinctions was, however, inescapable: Cuvier called them "Earth's revolutions".[25]

In 1821 there were already tensions between Cuvier and Geoffroy: "our friend Geoffroy is not an anatomist", Cuvier allegedly told Knox, and while Knox thought the criticism legitimate, he realized that Geoffroy possessed "original powers of thought" that went beyond Cuvier's "logical mind".[26] Geoffroy's doctrine of "unity of composition", which came to prominence in 1818 with the publication of the first volume of his *Philosophie anatomique* – a work which, with characteristic immodesty, he claimed marked the beginning of "a new epoch" – followed Goethe's premise that vertebrae were the building blocks of all animals, a hypothesis Geoffroy extended in 1820 to include insects as well as vertebrates, thereby uniting two of the four great "embranchments" into which Cuvier had divided the animal kingdom.[27]

Geoffroy adopted a conciliatory approach to Cuvier, whose ideas, he wrote, differed from his own "only in expression". Cuvier had, after all, acknowledged "a kind of general plan . . . of which we can find some traces in those [beings] that we thought most abnormal", though he was notoriously so averse to transcendentalism that he would not have it discussed in his presence.[28] Though interpretations of the seriousness and depth of the disagreement between Cuvier and Geoffroy have varied, there can be no doubt that the "overbearing" opposition of the most celebrated anatomist in Europe hampered the acceptance of Geoffroy's theory of transmutation – change of one species into another – because "[t]o attack Cuvier was to assail the dignity of France."[29]

When he came to write the history of transcendental anatomy, Knox distinguished great ideas from great men, and concluded that Cuvier and Geoffroy were not "great or first-rate men in themselves". He claimed to have discussed the doctrine of unity "at great length" with both men early in 1821, and to have foreseen the rift between these two "personal friends" whose "innermost thoughts on the nature of science and of scientific research were known to me."[30] According to Knox's account, his studies had provided him with sufficient knowledge to dispute both Geoffroy's views on unity of organization and species change, and Cuvier's claim that there had been four creations – "three at least must be superfluous" he wrote many years later.[31] Despite his lifelong Geoffroyan sympathies, Knox allied himself more closely with Cuvier, whom he regarded as "the greatest anatomist – *Descriptive Anatomist* – of any age", and "[a]fter the most deliberate reflection" he accepted Cuvier's doctrine of fixity of species, convinced that no "physical laws now in operation" could convert one species into another and that hybrids were, outside artificial situations such as domestication, impossible to sustain.[32] He was to remain loyal to this dogma throughout his career.

The third of Knox's "illustrious trio" of teachers was Cuvier's protégé

Parisian Anatomy, 1821–1822

Henri Marie Ducrotay de Blainville (1777–1850), who would succeed to Lamarck's and Cuvier's chairs after their deaths.[33] Blainville's acceptance of *naturphilosophisch* homologies between vertebrate skeletons distanced him from Cuvier (fortunately he had other patrons), as did his conclusion, based on meticulous studies of "the relation between the natural families of the extinct and living", that extinct forms "fill up the gaps in the scale" so that "out of the living and the extinct, the present and the past, is formed one great chain of beings."[34] This static series, an updated version of the Aristotelian "chain of being", in which all animals were arranged in sequence so that "they follow each other like the links of a vast chain" had, in Cuvier's opinion, "proved more detrimental to the progress of natural history in modern times, than it is easy to imagine", but Knox, who "carefully attended" Blainville's lectures in the winter of 1821, found the all-embracing grandeur of "one great self-created chain connecting the living and the extinct world" intellectually and aesthetically appealing, and judged Blainville to be Cuvier's equal.[35]

One notable Parisian anatomist whom Knox did not seek out, despite Blainville's admiration for him, was Lamarck. We know from the lists of auditors at Lamarck's lectures that Knox did not attend them, though his friend and fellow student Thomas Hodgkin did.[36] During Knox's time in Paris, Lamarck's evolutionary theory of environmentally-driven change from monad (the most primitive animal form) to man enjoyed scant professional support, and Cuvier, who saw him as a rival, ridiculed his transformist views and accused him of plagiarism. Though opinion is divided as to whether Cuvier (ab)used his position as Permanent Secretary of the Academy of Sciences to silence Lamarck during life, when he died, in poverty, in 1829, Cuvier disparaged his work in a bitter eulogy.[37] While Knox may have been influenced by Cuvier's opinions, he was not so easily led as to reject Lamarck's work without reasons of his own. Lamarck's theories were too speculative for some critics, though this would hardly have posed a problem for Knox, whose objections were most probably to transmutation of adult species and biological progress – Lamarck's "march of nature" from simple animals to more "perfect" ones[38] – both of which ideas he consistently rejected.

Geoffroy did not publish his theory that species present in the fossil record had transmuted into different, modern forms until 1825, but in 1821 he apparently discussed it with Knox, who claimed to have challenged his proposal that gills were transformed into lungs during embryonic development. Knox maintained that organs were not convertible and that rudimentary gills and lungs coexisted in the embryo "with a view to the future". This was in line with Goethe's conjecture that "the germ of any animal" was, potentially, "the germ of every other", and would form the basis of Knox's mature theory of species formation.[39] Though Knox appreciated that Geoffroy and Blainville had left Cuvier's doctrine of separate creations "rudely shaken", he was not prepared to commit himself to environmentally driven transmutation of one species into another. In his Edinburgh anatomy classes he would teach Geoffroy's theory that "there can be no new species, strictly speaking" since the apparently new "may simply be the extinct, altered in form by the then existing circumstances", but he still agreed with Cuvier that species change could not be caused by the action of physical forces.[40] Much of his subsequent work on race and comparative anatomy would be directed towards reconciling these apparently contradictory positions.

Paris not only awakened Knox's interest in the big questions of higher anatomy – how species were formed and how they related to one another – to which he would devote his scientific career, but also provided him with a personal ideal of how such research could be sustained by lecturing: Cuvier was a popular teacher who derived a significant proportion of his income from public lectures.[41] Both Knox and Cuvier were of part German ancestry, and Knox's comments that Cuvier was "not a Celtic man" but "the antithesis of their race" and that "how he assorted and consorted with them it is difficult to say" recalled his own Saxon background and experiences: it was Knox, rather than Cuvier, who found his countrymen difficult to consort with. In the winter of 1821–2, in his private library in the Museum of Comparative Anatomy, Cuvier told Knox there were fewer than forty unprejudiced men in France. "How different", mused Knox, "must have been the lot of Cuvier had fate cast his nativity in Britain", where he would have been "frowned down" and "sneered at" until forced either to leave or to turn his "vast intellect" to teaching "mathematics to boys" or "the anatomy of the parts of the body, concerned in surgical operations, to medical students."[42] In short, a British Cuvier would have been Knox, condemned like his father to pedagogic drudgery.

In later years, Knox tried, not always successfully, to convince his readers that he had moved, during his Parisian years, in the highest intellectual circles. In fact, though it would have been surprising if he had not seized every opportunity to attend the lectures of the anatomists whose work he admired, there is nothing to indicate that his relationship with them was any closer than that of an enthusiastic pupil to a lecturer. The main purpose of his spell in Paris, and the reason the Army had allowed him to go there on half pay, was to learn practical anatomy and pathology. It was probably the best place in Europe to do this, since the two state dissecting-rooms at *l'Ecole de médecine* and *l'Hôpital de la Pitié* were so well supplied with bodies for students' use that privately-run schools were unnecessary. His companion in study was the industrious young Quaker, Thomas Hodgkin (1798–1866), an Edinburgh medical student later known as the discoverer of an eponymous disease of the lymph glands, whom Knox invited to share his "private" dissecting-room at *la Pitié*, which he had obtained, he told the genuinely well-connected Hodgkin, through his "powerful interest" with some of the physicians and lecturers.[43] In fact, anyone could obtain a private room by paying a fee, a wise move, as the floor of the great, galleried "dissecting pavilion", in which most students worked, was strewn with "portions of viscera, detached limbs, pieces of dissected muscle, fat, and cellular membranes", and the stench was "almost insupportable". The mephitic atmosphere was alleviated somewhat by the windows being kept constantly open, but the students, who removed their hats and coats while dissecting, were prone to catch pneumonia.[44]

Knox and Hodgkin spent four to six hours a day at *la Pitié*, either in their private room making more detailed dissections than had been possible in Edinburgh – more than twenty years later Knox could still recall seeing the cutaneous branch of the vagus nerve for the first time – or studying specimens in the museum.[45] They got on well, forming themselves into "a little physiological society", which Hodgkin thought would help him with his thesis, and discovering a common interest in race.[46] Hodgkin, an abolitionist who would later become a leading light in the Aborigines Protection Society and the Ethnological Society of London, was struck by Knox's account of atrocities committed against the Xhosa in the Cape Colony, which confirmed "all that has been said of the amiable and excellent qualities of that deeply-injured race".[47] When Knox wished to have some portraits of himself printed by the new technique of lithography, Hodgkin introduced him to the proprietor of one of the presses, Comte Charles-Philbert de Lasteyrie (1759–1849), who was "pretty civil" to them, though no portraits were made.[48] In the Spring of 1821, Knox also met Le Vaillant, the celebrated traveller, friend of Cuvier, and fellow member of the *Société des Observateurs de l'Homme*, in whose books he had first read of the glorious landscapes of the Cape.[49] He also joined a Masonic lodge, where he could enjoy congenial society, philosophical speculation, radical politics, and rituals intended to make known, through symbols, the Great Architect of the Universe.[50]

In addition to his dissections with Hodgkin, Knox studied morbid anatomy at *l'Hôpital de la Charité* under his "friends" the physicians Auguste-François Chomel, an early enthusiast for anatomical pathology, and F.J. l'Herminier. He also followed the practice of the royal (formerly imperial) surgeon Alexis Boyer (1757–1833) and his son-in-law, the surgeon and professor of pathology Joseph-Philibert Roux (1780–1854), though he was not impressed by the operations he saw: Boyer "clumsily" punctured a small cyst on the face of an "extremely beautiful" young woman, who died of typhoid, and Roux's operation on a perianal fistula was "a ludicrous failure".[51]

Knox later maintained that he left the Parisian Faculty of Medicine never to return in 1821, after an unfortunate meeting with the professor of anatomy and surgeon-in-chief Pierre Béclard (1785–1825) under a bust or painting of Bichat, whose *Anatomie générale* Béclard was revising. Béclard pointed to Bichat and remarked "that man never performed the experiments given under his name", which left Knox "shocked and deeply grieved" by this slur on "[t]he idol I worshipped".[52] However, though he greatly admired Bichat as the "founder and discoverer of true descriptive anatomy", and later claimed to have introduced his system of pathological anatomy to Britain,[53] Knox considered Bichat's work inferior to Cuvier's because it was concerned only with the "practical" sciences of medicine and surgery. Descriptive and pathological anatomy were necessary for the surgeon, but the anatomist's greatest goal was to discover the secrets of animal organization, and this required insight rather than just observation. "The springs of the action constituting life cannot be displayed by the scalpel and forceps", wrote Knox in his tribute to Bichat; "by this means we discover the effects of disease only, not diseases themselves."[54] He returned home intent on the study of philosophical anatomy, compared with which the work of surgery seemed mere "mechanical routine".[55]

CHAPTER FIVE

Museum Medicine, 1823–1825

On 31 December 1822, a week or so after arriving back at the family home in Edinburgh's Nicolson Square, Knox wrote asking for the two years of army half pay owed to him and resumed his researches with the support of Professor Jameson, who gave him access to the university museum. There he made "beautiful anatomical preparations" of the eyes of reptiles for a study of the retina, dissected a duck-billed platypus, a present to the University from the Governor General of New South Wales, and provided editorial assistance for Jameson's *Edinburgh Philosophical Journal*.[1] Between 1822 and 1824 Knox was very active in the Wernerian Society, at which he read papers on the beaver, the cassowary, the poison fangs of serpents, the red-throated diver and the platypus, the latter illustrated with "excellent drawings" and a "perfect skeleton".[2] Whales, which could be obtained from the Scottish coasts, were another interest (perhaps stemming from his time with Abernethy, a keen cetologist), and he spent many days tracing their lymphatics as they decomposed in the "sultry" dissecting-room.[3]

In an address to the Wernerian Society on the "savage races" of South Africa, in April 1823, Knox presented his observations from the Cape along with comparative measurements of skulls of different racial types from the museums of Jameson, Monro and Barclay.[4] It was already widely accepted that the shape of the skull differed between races: Johann Friedrich Blumenbach, the anatomist often regarded as the founder of physical anthropology, had published findings based on his own "unrivalled collection of the crania of different nations from all parts of the globe", and physiognomy and phrenology (though not disciplines that Knox recognized as sciences) had popularized cranial morphology to the extent that no anatomy museum was complete without its "sundry comparative crania".[5] Knox did not attempt to distinguish races on the basis of skull measurements, but instead measured "known" racial types: perhaps his service in the Cape, where all non-Europeans were "blacks" regardless of skin colour or appearance, had accustomed him to prejudge race rather than rely on physical characteristics.[6]

Skull collecting has latterly come to be seen as the ethnological equivalent of body snatching, and some early anthropologists literally stole body parts and traded in human skulls, though there is no evidence that Knox, despite his lifelong interest in cranial morphology, was among them.[7] In recent years it has been suggested that he extensively collected human bones in the Cape: for example, Zine Magubane writes that "[Knox's] interest in the anatomy of the indigenous peoples of South Africa . . . provided him with the skulls and skeletons that would form the basis for his research", but it is possible that the three skulls mentioned previously were all he collected, for he was a prolific author and would not have failed to write up further specimens had he gone to the trouble of obtaining them.[8] Nor is there any evidence to support the allegation that he performed human dissections in the Cape: the "many subjects" Stockenström recorded his having dissected were horses, during an outbreak of distemper.[9] A more unpleasant misunderstanding arose from Knox's black humour: he was supposedly asked how he came to have "so many Caffre skulls in his museum", and replied that in the Cape he had been permitted to "shoot as many Caffres as I wanted". If he did make such a remark, it would have been to satirize European brutality in the Cape, but his "enemies" repeated it as a fact.[10]

In the early-nineteenth century, limited collecting of human remains for scientific purposes was widely accepted; human skeletons were exhibited in many European museums, and were considered appropriate for public viewing. Edinburgh's University Museum displayed the skull of the scholar George Buchanan next to that of a "fool", to facilitate comparison; that the Buchanan skull was probably not authentic does not alter the fact that its exhibition was not considered improper.[11] Racial differences in the acceptable use of human material were most apparent in attitudes to the collection and display of human skins: removing the skins of Europeans was considered disrespectful to the dead and brutalizing to the perpetrators – tanning human skin for bootmaking was one of many accusations of savagery directed at the French revolutionaries[12] – but the skins of "savage" races were collected like any other "natural curiosities". Even scholars who were advocates of monogenism, the common kinship of all human races, tolerated skin collecting from non-Europeans: the monogenist, anti-slavery Bishop Henri Grégoire referred to the work of Andreas Bonn of Amsterdam, "qui a la plus belle collection connue de peaux humaines [who has the finest known collection of human skins]" without expressing any disapproval.[13] Knox was in a minority of anthropologists who neither collected human skins nor approved of their display, and he curtly dismissed an exhibition of the stuffed skins of "Hottentots" in London and Paris as "a great curiosity, no doubt".[14]

Inevitably, Knox's account of the Cape was influenced by imperialism: the virgin landscape passively awaited European colonists, and the indigenous people were material to be studied, classified in European terms and described to science, but while it may be a valid criticism of nineteenth-century science that it imposed European systems on everything it encountered, it is hardly a significant criticism of an individual scientist. Knox the anatomist treated the African races in the same way he did

Europeans, as subjects for study. His remarks in a lecture to the Wernerian Society that the Dutch had already "partly exterminated" the "Hottentots" were an early expression of a lifelong, though initially guarded, anti-colonialism,[15] and from the time of his earliest writings on race, in 1823, his position was consistently monogenetic, that is to say he recognized a common origin for the races of men ("we may view the human race as derived originally from one stock") and accepted that races could be "modified by intermarriage". Yet when, on a visit to London to see Belzoni's exhibition of paintings and casts from the tomb of "Psammuthis, King of Thebes" in winter 1821–2, he discussed the question of race with his friends Hodgkin and W. F. Edwards, he argued that races were unalterable by either time or climate.[16] Reconciling this view with monogenism, by explaining how different races arose "from one stock" without being altered over time or by "external means", a task that promised to throw light on the wider question of how new species could be formed without environmentally-induced change from one to another, was a challenge to which Knox was to devote most of his academic career.[17]

Knox's papers to the Wernerian Society, though accomplished, are unlikely to have been read outside Edinburgh, and he had earned nothing from his anatomical studies since his return from the Cape. He may have been content to go on living on his army half pay, indulging his interests and occasionally taking on surgical cases, had he not decided to marry. Little is known about his wife, Susan, who was about twenty-one when they married in 1828. There was no formal ceremony – Scottish law did not require one – and the date of the marriage rests on the testimony of W. Syme Wilsone, the husband of Knox's eldest daughter Mary, who wrote to the *Lancet* after Knox's death to correct the date given in the journal's obituary and thereby establish his wife's legitimacy.[18] According to Lonsdale, Susan was "a person of inferior rank" and the marriage was kept secret, but some rumour must have got out, because the marriage "put shackles" on Knox's "social progress".[19] It may also have inspired him to advance his career by applying for the position of curator of the pathology museum at the Edinburgh College of Surgeons.

Anatomical museums had their origins in the polite science of the enlightenment, when the virtuoso's cabinet displayed his wealth and learning (women rarely collected). The most celebrated museum, John Hunter's (1728–93) collection of more than 10,500 specimens, was bought by the government in 1799 for £15,000 and given to the Company (from 1800 the Royal College) of Surgeons in London, who idealized Hunter as the type of a gentlemanly, scientific and learned surgeon, guided in his work by a profound knowledge of anatomy and science. Hunter was one of the few British anatomists whom Knox unreservedly admired, though he thought Everard Home's arrangement of the Hunterian collection had turned "a more remarkable work than the wall of China" into "a sealed book" no better than "a Dutch collection".[20] Compared with Cuvier's Museum of Comparative Anatomy in Paris, with its fifteen hundred specimens of mammals of five hundred different species, six thousand birds, eighteen hundred reptiles and five thousand fishes, all arranged according to Cuvier's system and "ticketed with the greatest exactness", all other museums were, in Knox's eyes, merely collections: only Cuvier had set Nature properly in order.[21]

On 1 December 1823, in recognition of his scientific work, Knox was elected to the Royal Society of Edinburgh,[22] where he joined Monro *tertius* and Barclay, who was at the time the only extramural anatomical lecturer among the distinguished Fellowship. The following April, Knox wrote to Dr Russell, the "oldest member" of the Royal College of Surgeons of Edinburgh, who had expressed an interest in his work, and offered to devote his "whole labour and time" to "the formation of a museum of comparative anatomy", a task to which he would bring "that energy which the cultivation of a favourite pursuit naturally gives", on condition that he could have the use of the museum throughout his lifetime.[23] He was apparently hoping that, under the auspices of the College of Surgeons, which was an "incorporation" (like the butchers and bonnet makers) rather than an academic body, and correspondingly wealthier, he could build a collection at no cost to himself which, though it would remain the College's property, he could use, like Cuvier, for teaching and private research. He began to work informally on the collection at Surgeons' Hall and in the winter of 1824–5 he revisited Paris, where he saw Cuvier for the last time and presumably sought inspiration for his new project.[24] Any misgivings over the suitability of "trading corporations" as custodians of museums were put aside when on 13 January 1825 the College appointed him curator with a salary of £100, in order to secure his services "on a more permanent and efficient footing".[25]

By the standards of English collections with which Knox was familiar, from the Hunterian museum to those at Alfort Veterinary School and Chatham hospital, the museum at Surgeons' Hall, which comprised between two and three hundred preparations dating back to the "collection of curiosities" held by the Guild of Barber Surgeons in the eighteenth century, seemed "antiquated and useless".[26] He would probably have known, however, that Barclay planned to bequeath his own collection to the College as a gift, and that in November 1824 Charles Bell, who was said to be the only person with whom Knox never quarrelled,[27] had offered to sell the College a large part of his Great Windmill Street museum. One of Knox's first tasks as curator was to visit London and inspect Bell's collection, which he did in February 1825 along with one of the keepers of the College museum, Alexander Watson. They recommended that the College should pay up to £3,000; the purchase was completed on 22 July, and at the beginning of August Knox returned to London to supervise the packing of more than three thousand items for transportation by boat to

Leith.[28] He refused to accept the College's offer of £21 to cover his expenses for the trip, saying that he "conceived it a duty".[29]

As there was no room for the collection in Surgeons' Hall it was temporarily housed next door in Barclay's school, where it would have been a welcome addition. The Parisian-inspired vogue for correlating clinical findings with pathology, coupled with the difficulty in obtaining fresh human material, had increased the value (scientific and monetary) of preserved specimens: few medical pupils could attend enough autopsies and dissections to familiarize themselves with the range of normal and diseased appearances, and they needed well ordered, representative collections. In June 1826, the *Senatus Academicus* of Edinburgh University, aware of medical students' needs, resolved to charge them a guinea for the use of the museum assembled by Monros *primus* and *secundus*.[30] From now on, no school or teacher would be taken seriously without a museum: the London teaching hospitals set about acquiring collections for their pupils' use, and possession of an anatomy museum worth more than five hundred pounds was proposed as a condition for a private teacher to be recognized by the London College of Surgeons.[31] Museum work became an accepted route to an academic career for medical graduates: in 1825 Thomas Hodgkin, who had qualified two years earlier, was appointed curator of the pathology museum at Guy's Hospital, where he catalogued some three thousand specimens, including a cast of one of Knox's Xhosa crania.[32]

In 1825 Barclay, then aged 65, offered Knox a partnership in his anatomy school: Knox was to undertake the "whole labour" of the school, excepting any work Barclay chose to do himself. This unfavourable split was necessitated by Barclay's failing health, and both men must have known that, in offering a partnership, Barclay was in effect appointing his successor. Knox's contract made provision for the eventuality of his obtaining a university professorship, a realistic ambition at a time when out lecturing was an accepted route to a university chair (a total of thirty-six extra-mural teachers became Edinburgh professors in various branches of medicine), though he would have known that the attempt to create a chair for Barclay had been frustrated by, amongst others, Professors Hope, Jameson, and Monro. Despite the animus that existed between some university professors and out lecturers, Edinburgh's private anatomy teachers, who included James Syme and Barclay's former assistant Robert Liston, tended to compete amongst themselves rather than with the university, on which they relied to attract students to Edinburgh.[33] The students dutifully signed up for the professorial lectures of Monro *tertius*, but they went to the private lecturers to learn anatomy: it was well known that "students pay their fees and enter their names at the college, not with any view of attending the classes there, but because the fees and entries are necessary for the ceremony of graduation."[34]

In order for Knox's lectures on "Descriptive Anatomy" to be recognized by the College of Surgeons, he had to be admitted to its Fellowship, and in April 1825 he duly presented a thesis, *On the causes and treatment of lateral curvature of the human spine*, which he dedicated to the eminent oculist and Surgeon in Ordinary to the King, John Henry Wishart (1781–1834). The dissertation was in English rather than Latin, but the requirements were otherwise similar to those of an Edinburgh MD, and the process was a formality, albeit, with an admission fee of £250, an expensive one.[35] Having obtained his diploma, Knox paid another short visit to Paris in the winter of 1825–6. The College apparently anticipated no conflict of interest between his private teaching and museum work, and on 15 May 1826 its Council elected him Conservator of the pathology museum, with a salary of £150 a year, by thirty-four votes to Robert Grant's eight.[36]

One of the last cohort of students to attend Barclay's classes was Richard Owen (1804–1892), a bright twenty-year-old just starting out on a career in medicine, who would later make a name for himself as the "English Cuvier". Owen remembered Knox's lectures as "the most brilliant ever delivered on anatomy", and they earned the school over £250 in fees, of which Knox received £190 and Barclay, £60.[37] The introductory lecture of the 1825–6 session was the last that Barclay ever gave: soon afterwards a "palsy" affected his speech, and as the term progressed he had difficulty breathing. He died on 21 August 1826, leaving Knox in sole charge of the school, and bequeathed his museum, "a monument of zeal and energy" that contained some 2,500 preparations, to the Edinburgh College of Surgeons, on conditions that "the College will build a Hall to receive it", that it be known as the Barcleian Museum, and that Knox be made a trustee and appointed Conservator for life.[38] This appointment was distinct from his curatorship of the pathology museum, though according to the official history the two posts were merged in 1828.[39]

In the course of his teaching career Knox became an enthusiastic collector in his own right, spending hundreds of pounds on animal specimens. Lonsdale recalled him paying fourteen shillings for a brace of grouse (in Scotland!) and local fishermen sold him seals "in the freshest condition", but he rarely contributed anything to the College museum: only four out of over three thousand specimens in the 1836 catalogue were attributed to him, and two of those were pieces of tapeworm.[40] His achievements at the College were largely administrative, but they were still considerable for a young man with no curatorial experience: he furnished them with a collection comparable to or better than those of other Scottish medical institutions, and catalogued it methodically. Ultimately, however, he came to regard his labours there as a failure: the "ample" collection he had assembled was, he claimed, "of no value whatsoever" to the surgeon and "equally useless" to the "scientific anatomist", and the museum, though the finest in Edinburgh and open "in the most liberal way" to the medical profession, was "never visited by them."[41]

CHAPTER SIX

Knox Primus et Incomparabilis, 1825–1828

Knox excelled as a teacher in Barclay's "academical" tradition: his lectures were "free" and "expressive", with an "aesthetic colouring" as idiosyncratic as it was effective, and he quickly established a rapport with his students, towards whom he showed none of the acerbity that characterized his dealings with officialdom.[1] The Newcastle surgical apprentice Thomas Giordani Wright remembered Knox inviting him to dinner during his early days in unfamiliar Edinburgh, and recorded in his diary that when he was ill during the winter of 1825–6 Knox "was so good as to visit me four or five times a day during the most critical period".[2] Another enthusiastic pupil was John Reid, later to become Knox's assistant, who attended his lectures morning and evening, and sometimes invited friends along to enjoy Knox's "literary elegance" and "flashes of wit".[3] Knox did not confine himself to practical anatomy: his talk ranged widely over comparative anatomy and zoology, and in 1826 he joined forces with the geologist Samuel Hibbert-Ware (1782–1848) and the botanist Robert Kaye Greville (1794–1866) to form a short-lived "School of Natural History."[4]

In the small world of Edinburgh, Knox was quickly acknowledged as a leading anatomist: he published eleven papers in 1823 alone, and in 1826 the Plinian Society, an Edinburgh University natural history society of which Robert Grant was secretary, resolved to offer him honorary membership, along with Cuvier, David Brewster, and Barclay. Alas, the proposal was thwarted by an officious committeeman, who quibbled over the correct procedure until Barclay died, and the plan was shelved.[5] Knox, perhaps offended by this apparent snub, never joined or attended the Plinian, though two papers were presented there on his behalf in 1826.[6] His name was probably known in London too, and he provided a testimonial when Hodgkin applied, successfully, for a post as physician to the London Dispensary in 1825: "if you do not like it let me know", he wrote in the accompanying letter, "I will with pleasure write a dozen for you."[7]

Hodgkin, however, had another favour to ask, and wrote requesting support for his efforts to publicize the plight of the aboriginal peoples of the Cape. As his letters to Knox have not survived we do not know exactly what he proposed, perhaps a public statement from Knox or even legal action, but Knox thought it a step too far: "it would be very dangerous to move in it, as I then was and still am an Officer in the Army – After all perhaps it [the commando system] may justifiable [*sic*] according to our notions of the *lex talionis* [law of retribution] which you know is scriptural."[8] Knox appeared to be making light of a serious wrong, and the principled Hodgkin was not minded to let the matter drop. Knox had injudiciously fuelled his zeal with stories of "atrocities" in the Cape, but now Hodgkin wanted to make the facts public, Knox demurred, writing disingenuously: "I shall be very glad if the Caffres can be secured for the future from any further atrocities, but feel so averse to the ripping up of old sores that I must positively request it of you as a favour, never to mention my name in any shape whatsoever as connected with Caffraria – I have already destroyed all the papers I had relation [*sic*] to that country." Pusillanimous as his rebuff was, Knox had a point: newly married and with a career to build, he could not risk losing his army half pay and starting a scandal in the vain hope of changing British policy in the Cape.[9]

When Knox took over from Barclay, anatomy was "universally acknowledged" to be the "foundation of medical science", and it occupied most of the neophyte medical student's time.[10] Nine hours of dissection a day, five days a week, for nine months was considered the minimum necessary, and aspiring surgeons often sought additional experience, as Knox had, to prepare them to operate unsupervised, for it was accepted wisdom that "he who dissects most assiduously will be the most expert operator".[11] Physicians, on the other hand, had little practical need for anatomy, though it was thought, like the classics, to improve the mind, and it enabled them to converse on an equal footing with educated patients. Frederick Tyrell, keen to promote his newly-opened Aldersgate Street anatomy school in London, told his audience that, while there were many who practised medicine "apparently with success" despite an "entire ignorance" of anatomy, a thorough knowledge of the subject would win them the "respect" of patients and colleagues as well as providing "a never-failing source of internal satisfaction ... a source of pleasure, which increases at an age when all other powers of enjoyment begin to decline." Such was the high regard of patients for the subject that some medical men set themselves up as teachers just so they could use "the title of anatomist", which was "of infinite advantage" to their practice.[12]

Edinburgh's population of medical students was already so large that demand for bodies far exceeded the legal supply. While Knox was in the Cape, a pamphlet war had been going on between those appalled by the activities of the body snatchers and those who argued that dissection was a no more ignominious fate than to be eaten by worms.[13] The traffic of dead bodies to Surgeons' Square was an open secret: they were carried "through the public streets in open day, (in baskets, in gigs, in hackney coaches, in boxes, and in various other shapes) by some of the most respectable inhabitants of Edinburgh", as "hundreds" of people living near the lecture rooms could testify. But the resurrection trade still failed to meet students' needs, and some headed for Paris or Dublin "in disgust", while others took advantage of the London schools, which obtained bodies from Paris, a practice to which customs turned a blind eye except for having a few opened at random by a surgeon in case contraband goods were hidden inside.[14] The London surgeon William Lawrence, who acknowledged that "the Scotch schools cannot be surpassed" for teaching anatomy, could afford to be sanguine, and argued that the shortage of subjects for dissection would encourage the Scots to "make opportunities for themselves, if they do not find them".[15]

According to Alexander Leighton's *The Court of Cacus*, a fictionalized account written long after the event, Barclay had obtained bodies from the infirmary and the workhouse: the former, if unclaimed, came straight to the dissecting-room, while the latter were buried in a plot conveniently close, almost immediately exhumed, and carried into the school under cover of darkness.[16] When he took over, Knox increasingly relied on resurrection men to exhume fresh corpses from churchyards and transport them to the school, where they were received by a doorkeeper or assistant who accompanied the grave robbers to "a known house near [Knox's] residence" to collect payment. Knox would have known when bodies were delivered and by whom, but would not have seen them until the next morning by which time they would have been "stripped and laid out" ready for dissection. They presented a gruesome sight: having been dragged from the grave by a rope around the neck, and, if still in *rigor mortis*, "tied with ropes and beat[en] into shape" so they could be crammed into a small box for inconspicuous carriage, they were then "disfigured about the face to prevent recognition" and had their teeth "broken out" for sale to dentists.[17]

So prevalent was the violation of graves that it became a public nuisance, and the watchtowers, guards and mort-safes required to protect the sanctity of the tomb were expensive and ever-present reminders of the hated resurrection trade. Since body snatchers risked being shot by those guarding the burial grounds, it was safer for them to appropriate bodies before inhumation if possible: they purchased or stole corpses awaiting burial, they picked up the bodies of "persons of the lower orders" who had "dropped down dead from hard drinking" in the streets and delivered them directly to Surgeons' Square, and on one occasion they even stole a body from Lizars's dissecting-room and sold it to Knox.[18]

Anatomists had obtained bodies clandestinely since the time of Galen,[19] but in early-nineteenth century Britain growing public concern about body snatching was bringing discredit on their work. John Lizars complained bitterly and eloquently of scaremongering by the popular press:

> In place of living in a civilized and enlightened period, we appear as if we had

been thrown back some centuries into the dark ages of ignorance, bigotry, and superstition. Prejudices worthy only of the multitude have been conjured up and appealed to, in order to call forth popular indignation against those whose business it is to exhibit demonstratively the structure of the human body, and the functions of its different organs; the public journals, from a vicious propensity to pander to the vulgar appetite for excitement, have raked up and industriously circulated stories of the exhumation of dead bodies, tending to exasperate and inflame the passions of the mob; and persons who, by their own showing, are friendly to the interests of science, have, in their excess of zeal, that bodies should remain undisturbed in their progress to decomposition, laboured to destroy in this country, that art, whose province it is to free living bodies from the consequences inseparable from accident and disease.[20]

Such polemical accounts of human dissection, whether by supporters or detractors, can give an exaggerated impression of strong passions; Edinburgh's well known anatomy schools carried on their work without hindrance from the public, and the truth may have been closer to the surgeon George Guthrie's comment on the London schools: "no-one knows or cares what is going on, unless he is interested in it."[21] Lizars blamed the courts, for punishing resurrection men ("the unhappy persons necessarily employed, in the present state of the law, in procuring subjects for the dissecting-room") as felons and so preventing students from obtaining the necessary experience of dissection, without which their early efforts at surgery would be little better than "cruelty and murder".[22]

The educated public sympathized with the students' efforts to learn their trade. In 1825, a correspondent to the *Mechanic's Magazine* wrote that on the few occasions he had visited a dissecting-room "much of the disgust and horror which the scene is calculated to produce, was subdued and overpowered by a stronger feeling of commiseration at the sight of so many young men poring over the putrid objects of their study, at the imminent risk of imbibing disease at every pore, and of inhaling the pestilence of death at every breath they drew."[23] They worked in their ordinary clothes, though some wore cheap "dissecting-trousers", and handled the viscera with ungloved hands, which they anointed with lard as a preventative against blood poisoning and which, however well washed, retained "a peculiarly fetid cadaveric odour" for hours afterwards.[24] Forced to spend much of the day in an insanitary atmosphere "loaded with noxious emanations, which more or less poisoned the blood of those who continuously inhaled it, and caused nausea, sickness, diarrhoea, a bad taste in the mouth, and other symptoms", anatomists was sometimes seen as martyrs to science, so "utterly dangerous" were the "poisons" exhaled by putrefying bodies, and concerns were voiced in parliament over the risks faced by "medical students . . . spending much of their time amid the putrid effluvia of a dissecting room."[25]

Apart from its practical utility to the surgeon, training in anatomy was a requirement of many of the United Kingdom's nineteen medical licensing bodies. In England, the 1815 Apothecaries Act made attendance at anatomy classes a prerequisite for sitting the Society of Apothecaries' examinations, the usual portal of entry to what would now be termed general practice. In 1826, the Royal College of Surgeons of Edinburgh made dissection compulsory for its diploma candidates, who had to produce "a Certificate from a Professor or Teacher of Anatomy" that they had "actually engaged in the dissection of a human body . . . ", and the following year Edinburgh University followed suit and imposed the same requirement on candidates for the MD.[26] These changes reflected a nation-wide trend towards greater regulation of medical training, under which "every corporate body of the profession rigorously exacts a well-grounded knowledge of anatomy from all, to whom the legal authority to exercise any branch of medicine or surgery is granted."[27]

Between 1826 and 1834 the average number of students in Knox's class was 335, and the maximum was over five hundred.[28] As the lecture room could not hold more than about two hundred he was obliged to give each lecture two or three times, yet so engaging a speaker was he that some people, including the writer and MP Sir George Sinclair (1790–1868), attended the same lecture morning and evening. Classes were open to all who paid – anatomical studies were traditionally carried on in public, which helped avoid accusations that dissection was a self-indulgent study – but the majority of the audience were medical students, who in their hurry for good seats at the eleven o'clock lecture would run the short distance from the university to Old Surgeons' Hall. Notwithstanding the popularity of his classes, Knox generously gave free tickets to students from the veterinary school run by his old pupil William Dick.[29]

Knox's course in "anatomy and physiology", which included "a full Demonstration on fresh Anatomical Subjects", cost £5 9s, and "practical anatomy and operative surgery", with two demonstrations daily, was the same price. An additional three guineas guaranteed "subjects" for the student to dissect: "Arrangements have been made", promised the flyer, "to secure as usual an ample supply of Anatomical Subjects."[30] Other private anatomy schools in Edinburgh included those of Liston, who was noted for his proficiency in arranging for bodies to be resurrected, James Syme, Lizars and McIntosh. Syme was forced to retire at the beginning of the 1828–9 session for want of *materiel*, and competition for bodies among the remaining teachers drove up prices: an adult "subject" could cost upwards of sixteen guineas, twenty-four times the price in Paris,[31] and Lonsdale claimed that Knox spent, in one session, between £700 and £800 on bodies at anything from £10 to 25 guineas each. In an attempt to obtain a "supply of Subjects from London" he once wrote to Hodgkin enclosing £20 and offering £50 more "if you require it".[32]

Knox carefully rehearsed his lectures and their accompanying gestures, spoke without notes, and spiced his discourse with radical opinions, quotations from Shakespeare, Horace and *Tristram Shandy*, and humour that bordered on the improper: some wordplay on *cul de sac* amused a knowing few.[33] Jokes, asides and controversial opinions are the parts of a lecturer's repertoire that students remember best, but their purpose was to hold the attention of classes over many weeks of teaching the basics, and the minutiae, of topographical anatomy. C. Carter Blake, a former student, thought Knox "perhaps, the most simple-minded and thorough teacher of anatomy that the Edinburgh school ever produced...". Blake's reminiscences tally with other accounts of Knox as candid, possibly even guileless, before his audience: "Knox had an unfortunate habit of letting out all he thought to his students; a habit we cannot commend to all those who prefer the profits to the verities of science."[34]

At the appointed hour, his domed head and smiling countenance would be seen peeping round the half-open door of the lecture room; when he was satisfied his audience was in place he walked smartly across to the desk and took out his watch, with its bunch of dangling seals. He wore a dark puce or black coat, a purple embroidered waistcoat, a frilled shirt with an immensely high collar and a huge striped cravat, the folds of which passed through a diamond ring. Jewellery "redolent of a duchess's boudoir" – diamond rings and festoons of gold chains – completed his costume. He spoke in measured, mellifluous tones, and concluded the lecture with a suave "tomorrow, gentlemen", accompanied by a graceful bow.[35] A lecturer is there to be seen, but Knox's finery also made the point that the anatomist, though labouring among "decaying mortalities", could be a person of refined and elegant manners. The London anatomist Richard Partridge, while a demonstrator at King's, adopted a similar approach, dressing immaculately and livening up his lectures with barbed remarks about colleagues and mildly improper jokes ("That skeleton is one of the prettiest girls I ever saw").[36] Lecturers, however talented, who appeared dirty and unkempt, as had Joshua Brookes, Knox's English counterpart, risked making a poor impression.[37]

Despite being only 5'6" ("the intellectual height", he called it), badly scarred from "confluent small-pox", prone to "involuntary twitchings" and lip smacking, and possessing "not one single good feature", Knox's debonair appearance, helped by his "fine intellectual head" and "smooth liquid voice", won him admirers professionally and socially, and ladies "(who he especially worships)", found him a welcome companion.[38] His performance in practical classes was as polished as in the drawing room, and as he stood before the dissecting table, "like a necromancer about to perform some mystical operation", his audience was struck by "the ineffable feeling of scepticism which seemed to thrill through his very scalpel".[39] He was quite a contrast to Monro, who "skulk[ed]" into the lecture room, with "[h]is head sunk betwixt his shoulders", wearing a threadbare coat and his father's hat.[40] Even a correspondent who wrote to the *Lancet* in defence of the University's teachers admitted that Monro was "a little tame and rather insipid".[41] Knox, on the other hand, could seem too anxious to please, and some found his expression while lecturing "something between a leer and overdone sincerity".[42]

Knox had inherited Barclay's fiery enthusiasm, and was critical of those surgeons who, like Abernethy, taught anatomy without interest in or respect for the subject: "There are many persons, indeed, some of them, I regret to say, teachers of anatomy, who seem to think that anatomy is in itself the most tiresome, disgusting, and uninteresting of all studies; and ... have taught it as a mere appendage to surgery ... as if anatomy were a nauseous draught requiring to be masked by some palatable, overpowering ingredient."[43] Not surprisingly, given the compulsory requirement to study it, many medical students tried to get away with learning the minimum anatomy necessary and performing "the smallest possible quantity" of the "disgusting process" of dissection: just enough to satisfy the examiners.[44] Teaching medical students can be frustrating for an educated man, and Knox complained that many Scottish medics "cannot write, cannot spell, and can scarcely read", but he never resorted to "parrot" learning, nor did he confine himself to teaching the bare minimum required for the aspiring surgeon, which would in his opinion have been to "reduce anatomy to mere empiricism, and the operator to the level of the common mechanic."[45]

As well as daily classes for medical students, Knox also gave Saturday lectures on general and comparative anatomy and ethnology, tickets for which were sold separately, and which attracted large audiences. His introductory lectures were particularly celebrated, and medical practitioners travelled miles to hear him.[46] According to his own account he lectured on transcendental anatomy from 1825 onwards, presumably not as a separate course but as part of his general lectures. He taught the theory of a common vertebrate plan, but not transmutation: "that [Geoffroyan] doctrine which maintained that . . . organs might be converted into each other; that the hyoid bones were ribs &c." In the 1820s he did, however, teach a limited form of Geoffroy's doctrine of *formation arretées* (arrested development), according to which new forms arose when the embryo failed to complete the full course of its development, a theory that, like Cuvier's requirement for every part to be represented in every animal, he would later abandon as his own ideas took shape.[47]

Though unfailingly courteous to his students, Knox could be scornful of the competition: he dubbed John and Alexander Lizars's Argyle Square School, where anatomy was taught by means of large, brightly coloured pictures, the "Infant School of Anatomy", not because he disapproved of illustrations as adjuncts to learning – he was involved in the publication of several series of anatomical drawings, known as "Knox's plates" – but because he saw oversimplification as "an illegitimate mode of instruction": direct observation of nature was the proper scientific method. He liked to puncture academic pretentiousness, and in his translation of Cloquet's *System of Human Anatomy* (1828), for which he was paid £150, he poked fun at Philippe-Frédéric Blandin (1798–1849) for referring to the head as the "Encephalic extremity of the trunk".[48] Another target for satire was Liston, who, he wrote, "plumes himself on the wonderful strength of his hands and arms, without pretension to head", and who he alleged had killed a patient in a botched operation while assisted by a former butcher's boy.[49] The notoriously rude and combative Liston gave as good as he got, and told his own students that there was no-one more ignorant than a "Doctor" (*i.e.* an MD).[50]

Large classes, translating and museum work kept Knox almost constantly occupied, but when his "academic seminary" closed in late April or early May he would shake off the effects of "[m]ental fatigue and bodily toil, carpeted rooms, dining in and dining out" by walking and fishing in the highlands, usually with his brother or another male companion.[51] These holidays afforded an opportunity to collect specimens of birds, snakes and fish for his private museum, and to continue his racial studies.[52] He sought out Town Yetholm in the Cheviot hills near the English border, where a "great gipsy family" had their "winter encampment", in the hope of seeing "a good specimen of the race", a mission that required some patience as they were "[t]imid and sensitive, like wild animals", and shunned contact with outsiders. During a second visit, hoping for a closer look, he knocked at the door of one of their "hovels" on the pretext of asking for directions, and was rewarded with the sight of an "extremely beautiful" young woman, "the finest of the race I ever saw", but as she raised her arm to point the way he observed "a circular leprous spot, not to be mistaken": she might have been the embodiment of the nineteenth-century fear of contagion from the "dreadful lepra" concealed by dark-eyed, beautiful youth.[53]

Although "little or nothing" was taught about the subject in British medical schools, "race" was "as familiar as household words" to Knox's students who, one of their number recalled, spread his "novel" theories "far and wide".[54] Charles Darwin, an Edinburgh medical student in 1826–7, *may* have attended some of Knox's Saturday lectures on ethnology, but it is unlikely that the two men made much impression on one another: in later life Knox kept up with the progress of former students and boasted about the successful ones, but though he praised Darwin's *Journal of Researches into the Geology and Natural History of the various countries visited by H.M.S. Beagle* (1838) as the work of a "talented and acute observer", he never mentioned having taught him.[55] For his part, Darwin read Knox's works, but made scant reference to them.[56] Another latterly famous visitor to Edinburgh in 1826 was John James Audubon, seeking subscribers for his *Birds of America*, who called at 10 Surgeons' Square where Knox, "dressed in an overgown and with bloody fingers", showed him the dissecting theatre: "The sights were extremely disagreeable, many of them shocking beyond all I ever thought could be. I was glad to leave this charnel house and breathe again the salubrious atmosphere of the streets." Knox paid a return call on Audubon, pronounced his drawings "the finest in the world", promised to introduce him to the Wernerian Society, and talked "very scientifically indeed – quite too much so for the poor man of the woods".[57]

Knox's school thrived, and in 1828 he took on three assistants: William Fergusson (1808–77), Alexander Miller and Thomas Wharton Jones (1808–91).[58] Fergusson, a talented student who had abandoned law for medicine, was chief demonstrator or first assistant, in which capacity he gave demonstrations of surgical anatomy three times a week, and shared in Knox's limited surgical practice.[59] All three assistants left soon after the West Port scandal: Fergusson was destined for a distinguished career, Miller practised as a surgeon and took up mesmerism, and Jones eventually became professor of ophthalmic medicine and surgery at University College London, where his taciturnity earned him the nickname "Mummy Jones".[60]

Lonsdale made a valid, though rather invidious, point when he wrote that a teacher's influence is apt to be exaggerated and that in most instances it is the student's industry that leads to success.[61] Nevertheless, the roll call of Knox's pupils demonstrates that his classes were favoured by those who went on to enjoy successful careers, even if his teaching was incidental to their progress. Edward Forbes (who pronounced his name "four-bees"), a medical student impressed by the "subtlety, suggestiveness, and ingenuity" of Knox's teaching, developed an interest in transcendentalism and went on to become, just prior to his early death in 1854, Regius Professor of Natural History at Edinburgh.[62] Other Knoxites who achieved academic preferment were the Edinburgh professor of surgery, James Spence, and professor of obstetrics and pioneer anaesthetist (Sir) James Y. Simpson, while a future Director General of army medicine, Thomas Alexander, owed his start to Knox's influence with Sir James McGrigor, to whom Knox sent specimens for the army museum at Chatham. Two pupils whose renown was unconnected with Knox's teaching were Stephen Stanley, who won first prize for dissection in 1836, and Harry Goodsir, brother of Knox's would-be biographer John Goodsir, who were both lost in the ill-fated Franklin expedition to the Northwest Passage. Among the other scholars, lawyers, clergymen, artists, men of letters and "scions of the nobility" who attended his lectures were the phrenologist and anti-sabbatarian Robert Cox (1810–72), the writer and historian John Walker Ord (1811–53), and the parliamentarian, courtier, bibliophile and antiquarian Lord Glenorchy (later Marquis of Breadalbane), who joined Knox's class in 1827 and sent him "[t]wo very fine specimens of the wild cat, shot in the forests of Glenorchy" for his museum.[63] Knox's loyal students knew him affectionately as "Old Cyclops": to his enemies, he was Robert the Devil.[64]

CHAPTER SEVEN

The West Port Murders, 1828–1829

It is often noted that Knox became involved in the West Port murders by chance, when on 29 November 1827 William Burke and William Hare, seeking Monro's dissecting-rooms, were directed instead to 10 Surgeons' Square by one of Knox's students, though even without this chance meeting they would probably have ended up dealing with Knox, who had the largest class and paid the best rates for the subjects he guaranteed his pupils. At Knox's school, Burke and Hare met his assistants, Jones, Miller and Fergusson, who told them to return after dark. Much was later made of the young men's admission that they did not ask the pair how they had come into possession of a corpse, though even the most callow medical student would have seen the futility of directing such a question to a pair of presumed resurrection men. Burke and Hare returned that night with a body in a sack and were told to lay it on the dissecting table. The dead man was still wearing a shirt, and it was obvious that he had never been buried. Knox arrived, looked at the body – a candlelight inspection to assess its "freshness" – named £7 10s as the price, and asked Jones to pay, which he did, remarking to Burke and Hare that he would be "glad to see them again".[1] Knox had purchased the body of a pensioner named Donald, who had died a natural death at William Hare's house in Tanner's Close (a Close in Edinburgh being a narrow alleyway). Donald owed Hare £4, and selling his body for anatomy was a way of recouping the debt.

The Athens of the North was a city of contrasts: it presented an impressive prospect from a distance, but a visitor to the Old Town, South of the castle, and especially to the West Port area, where Tanner's Close lay, was likely to be "miserably disappointed". These "filthy and squalid" districts had no proper drains, and the air was "contaminated" by a "sublimation of mephitic effluvia" from the open channels in the streets and closes, which served as latrines,[2] for there were none inside the houses: "[i]n a word, the excrementitious matter of some forty or fifty thousand individuals is thrown daily into the gutters". The task of cleaning these narrow streets was almost impossible: the houses, some of which were over ten stories high, were so jammed together that a person might step through his window into the house of his neighbour, and the common stairwells became as filthy as the streets outside. The slums were seen both as a health hazard and a place of "moral evil", where "people, old and young, become familiarized with the spectacle of filth, and thus habits of uncleanliness and debased ideas of propriety and decency are ingrafted."[3]

It was in these degrading conditions that Hare, an Irish labourer often said to have been something of a simpleton, lived with his wife Margaret Laird in a single ground-floor room which, at least after his crimes became known, had broken windows and no furniture except a bed of straw. Nearby was the tiny, filthy room that his friend and fellow countryman William Burke (1792–1829) shared with his mistress Helen McDougal, and from which he carried on his trade as a cobbler. It contained no furniture except a "crazy" chair, two broken stools, and a bed that was merely a wooden frame filled with straw and old rags.[4] When Lonsdale had cause to visit West Port during the relapsing fever epidemic of 1843 he found it "indescribably brutal and debased": the people passed their time drinking and carousing, and, apart from surgeons, few outsiders ventured there.[5]

That the substantial sum of £7 10s could be earned from a corpse came as a revelation to Burke and Hare, who devised a brutally simple *modus operandi*: tempt in vagrants or prostitutes, ply them with drink (and possibly opiates), and murder them by asphyxiation. Over the next eleven months they sold at least sixteen victims to Knox, the last of whom proved their undoing, as the body was seen in Burke's room before it could be taken to Surgeons' Square. So ample is the literature on these crimes that they will be considered here only in respect of Knox's personal involvement. He met the pair for a second time on or about 12 February 1828, when they brought the body of their second murder victim, pensioner Abigail Simpson, to his school. It was cold and stiff, and Knox, it was later reported, "approved of its being so fresh, *but did not ask any questions*", though it is difficult to imagine what questions he could have asked that would have exposed the crime.[6]

Their most notorious victim was Mary Paterson, a prostitute about eighteen years old and "well known" to Burke, who was "cut short in her sinful career" on 9 April 1828.[7] The hundreds of prostitutes in West Port were noticeably better dressed than the factory girls, who were paid a pittance and whose few scraps of clothing were "wretched in the extreme", and Mary Paterson's youth and beauty made her a particularly conspicuous figure.[8] Knox's doorkeeper David Paterson (no relation) admired the "beautiful symmetry and freshness of the body" and the students were similarly struck by her "handsome" corpse, some even making sketches of it. After the murders became known, a story circulated that one of Knox's students had been on "terms of more than ordinary intimacy" with Mary, as Leighton delicately put it, only hours before she died.[9] According to David Paterson, it was Fergusson who had been "acquainted" with her, though he knew her as Mary Mitchell.

The emotive image of the "voluptuous" young woman in the

dissecting-room became widely associated with the crimes of Burke and Hare – an early example of the association of prostitution, dissection, and (venereal) contagion that was to become a cliché of nineteenth-century sensationalist writing – and several of those caught up in the scandal tried to present themselves in retrospect as Mary's defenders.[10] David Paterson claimed he had asked Burke how he obtained the body, and Lonsdale reported that Fergusson too had questioned Burke. Both, apparently, received the same answer: Burke had purchased the body from someone else, and Mary had died of drink.[11] Robert Liston was said to have remonstrated with Knox about Mary Paterson in front of his class before knocking him down and removing the body for burial, but this chivalrous incident probably never happened: Burke claimed in his confession that Mary's body was dissected and Lonsdale confirmed this.[12] More recently, Knox has been accused of indulging himself by preserving Mary's body in alcohol for his lectures on muscles,[13] a course he would hardly have taken had he suspected the true cause of her death.

At the beginning of October another well-known corpse was brought in, that of James Wilson, a local character known as Daft Jamie. Paterson later claimed that he and several students had recognized Jamie, and that Knox insisted they were mistaken and arranged for Jamie's body to be dissected out of turn, after the head and malformed feet had been removed.[14] In all, Knox purchased some sixteen bodies from Burke and Hare over a period of eleven months, which Lonsdale estimated was one-sixth of the total for that session, a claim supported by official figures.[15]

The final victim, "Madgy or Margery, or Mary M'Gonegal or Duffie, or Campbell, or Docherty", an old Irish beggarwoman, was murdered at around eleven o'clock on the evening of 30 October. Shortly after midnight, Burke brought Paterson to his house, where he had hidden the body under his bed. Paterson apparently approved, and after Burke and Hare delivered the body to Surgeons' Square the following morning he accompanied them to Knox's home at 4 Newington Place, a large three-storey town house about ten minutes' walk away, where Knox handed over £5. They were to receive a further payment once he had seen the corpse for himself.[16] Knox went early to the school, but the police were there shortly after him: James and Ann Gray, temporary lodgers at Burke's house, had reported seeing the body stuffed under the bed, and at 7 a.m. a police Lieutenant and Sergeant Major had called on Paterson, who took them to 10 Surgeons' Square. Knox was initially reported to have received the police with the "utmost civility", though a subsequent claim that he swore at them from a window and then threatened "to blow their brains out" suggests a more characteristically Knoxian reaction to the agents of authority.[17]

For weeks the talk in Edinburgh was of nothing other than the impending trial, and "fearful disclosures" concerning the "Daemon Burke" were eagerly anticipated.[18] By the time the case came to trial, on

24 December 1828, Hare and his wife had decided to turn "approvers" and give evidence for the Crown, without which there would have been little chance of a conviction. Despite his best efforts, which included beating corpses in the dissecting-room to determine whether they could be bruised post-mortem (an experiment that Conan Doyle had Sherlock Holmes repeat at Barts), Robert Christison, professor of medical jurisprudence at Edinburgh university, was unable to be certain that various marks on the victims' bodies had not been produced when their corpses were forced into boxes for transportation. He visited Knox, who told him he acquired subjects "by his providers watching the low lodging houses" and purchasing bodies immediately after death.[19]

Christison mistrusted Knox's explanation on the grounds that the relatives of Irish Catholics would not have countenanced such a transaction, but he may have had too sanguine a view of human nature: doctors, ministers and sextons sometimes tipped off resurrectionists before a body was buried, and there were many Irish folk prepared to sell their "friends and relatives" for dissection. James Somerville, a future Inspector of Anatomy, told the 1828 select committee on anatomy that "the lower order of Irish" commonly sold bodies to anatomists once the wake was over, and there was a regular traffic of dead bodies from Ireland to Edinburgh.[20] We cannot know if Knox truly believed that Burke had obtained bodies by purchase, wanted to believe it, or merely wanted Christison to believe it, but it was not an unwarranted assumption to have made. For his part, Christison supposed that "Knox, a man of undoubted talent, but notoriously deficient in principle and in heart, was exactly the person to blind himself against suspicion, and fall into blameable carelessness. But is was absurd to charge him with anything worse."[21]

In the absence of conclusive evidence of murder, the court relied heavily on the testimony of the obliging Paterson, who described himself as the keeper of Knox's museum. He gave evidence that Burke and Hare had "frequently" brought in subjects that appeared not to have been interred, though he implied he had not always seen them; "other people", he claimed, had also brought uninterred bodies, and medical men had sometimes given Knox the addresses of poor patients who had died.[22] The Lord Advocate asked Paterson a series of leading questions culminating in: "You are a medical person. Did that appearance of the countenance [of Mary Docherty] indicate strangulation?" Paterson's confident answer, which the court probably expected, was that she had in his opinion been either strangled or suffocated. After this much needed corroboration of Hare's testimony, Burke had no hope of deliverance.

On Christmas morning, the court sentenced Burke to be hanged and dissected. The case against his partner Helen McDougal was found "not proven" and she walked free, to loud applause. A transcript of the trial was promptly made available to an eager public by the shorthand writer John Macnee, with a matter of fact preface exculpating the medical profession on the grounds that "subjects must be had to lecture upon" and urging readers to bequeath their own "miserable carcase" for dissection, with the exception of "refined" women, who were expected to preserve their modesty to the last, the deficiency being made up from the "poor-house".[23]

Aside from Hare, who enjoyed a degree of official protection for having turned King's evidence, it was Paterson whom the press considered most likely to have been complicit in the murders. The *Caledonian Mercury* reported that he had tried to sell the body of Mary Docherty to "a highly respectable" anatomy lecturer for £15, £3 more than Knox had offered, though Paterson denied it.[24] There was also a question mark over his relations with Burke and Hare: he had met them many times, and had visited Hare's house, which was less than seventy yards from his home. A dissecting-room porter usually looked at bodies before buying them to avoid handing over money for a rotten corpse, or no corpse at all (in Mrs Kelly's novel *The Fatalists*, a resurrection man sells his friend's body to a surgeon; once the surgeon has paid the "body" gets up, boxes the surgeon's ears, and runs off[25]), and his duties included "washing and cleaning subjects preparatory to their being brought into the class room", yet when Paterson went to Hare's house after the murder of Mary Docherty,[26] whose body he subsequently testified showed marks of violence, he allegedly did not look at the corpse: why then had he gone there?

It was in Paterson's interest to present himself as submissive to Knox's orders, and on 15 January 1829 he wrote to the *Mercury* accusing his former employer, under whose "guidance and direction" he claimed to have acted, of neglecting his promise to "espouse my cause"; he denied that he had been dismissed by Knox, though the *Mercury* claimed to have heard this "from Dr Knox's own lips", and claimed he was "the scapegoat for a personage in higher life". Paterson sent the *Mercury* a letter written to him by Knox on 11 January, in which he offered "to do every thing in my power to prevent you taking wrong steps", though this was hardly, as Paterson claimed, an invitation to return to his service; indeed, it sounds suspiciously like the reply to a blackmailer.[27]

Knox's assistants, who had left the school after the scandal broke, weighed in with the observation that Paterson had not been "keeper of the museum", but "a menial servant hired by the week", though this point may have been counterproductive as servants, like women, were presumed to be subject to the will of their masters. They also alleged that Paterson had been "so far associated" with Burke and Hare as to have been on the point of accompanying Burke to Ireland "to procure a greater supply of subjects".[28] In reply there appeared a sixpenny pamphlet, written under the pseudonym "The Echo of Surgeons' Square", in which Paterson claimed he had raised doubts about the provenance of the corpses, only to be silenced by Knox. He took no further part in the anatomy trade but remained in Edinburgh, and offered to sell his "invaluable collection of anecdotes" to Sir Walter Scott, who commendably ("curse him... and damn him") turned him down.[29]

Burke's execution in the Lawnmarket on 28 January 1829 was marked by "universal shouts and yells of execration" from the 25,000-strong crowd, which continued even as he knelt to pray and, according to one account, as he struggled for "many minutes" at the end of the rope, "each violent motion calling forth renewed shouts of triumph."[30] "Hang Knox", screamed the crowd, "He's a *noxious* morsel!".[31] Burke's body was dissected in Monro's classroom the day after his execution, when for the first and only time a vast crowd, clamouring for admission, besieged Monro's rooms. Among the thousands of people who streamed past the dissected remains were "seven females", who were "roughly handled" by the mob.[32] As Richardson observed, the irony of Burke's fate was that it reinforced the notion of dissection as a posthumous punishment: "a strong feeling against dissection, in the event of death in hospitals, has often been expressed by patients and their friends, because it was treating them like murderers."[33]

The lone figure of Burke on the gallows also strengthened public feeling that full justice had not been done, and Knox was the only other person who could conceivably have been brought to trial, though any prosecution would certainly have failed. Burke had been convicted because Hare confessed and Paterson perjured himself, but the medical witnesses had produced no proof of murder, and there was no evidence that Knox had known the deaths were unnatural. In particular, the often repeated allegation that Burke killed one young boy by breaking his back, in which case Knox could not have failed to notice marks of violence, was, as Edwards concluded, mere fiction.[34] A broken back would not have been immediately fatal and it would have been uncharacteristic for Burke to kill a defenceless child in a detectable way when he had not left any marks of violence on his adult victims.

In early February, the court lifted its interdict on the publication of Burke's official condemned cell confession, which he had made on 3 January, but this did little to settle any remaining suspicions: the point had been well made at his trial that lies and perjury were presumably of little consequence to a man who had murdered in cold blood. Burke clearly wished to incriminate Hare, who he said he would be happy to see hanged, while as far as possible he exculpated Helen McDougal, Hare's wife, Paterson and Knox. This was certainly a magnanimous gesture as far as the two women were concerned, for they must have known of their partners' crimes. Burke claimed that he and Hare had "very little communication" with Knox, whom he mentioned having met only twice: once when they delivered the body of Donald, who had died of natural causes, and again when they brought the body of "a woman from Gilmerton", and Knox had approved of its freshness.[35]

Burke made a second, more detailed confession, known as the *Courant* confession as it was published in the *Edinburgh Courant*, on 21 January, in which he described sixteen murders in a different order from the fifteen in his earlier confession. He claimed that Hare had committed one murder while he was away and denied it on his return, whereon he had gone to "Dr Knox, who told him that Hare had brought a subject".[36] Burke also described their having "entered into a contract" with Knox and his assistants, who promised to pay £10 in winter and £8 in summer for "as many subjects as they could bring". At the end of this final confession, perhaps mindful that these disclosures could incriminate Knox, Burke added in his own hand:

> Burk declares that docter Knox Never incoureged him Nither taught or incoreged him to murder any person nether any of his asistents that worthy gentleman Mr Fergeson was the only man that even mentioned any thing about the bodies He inquired where we got that young woman paterson
> SINED WILLIAM BURK PRISONER[37]

Following Burke's execution and Hare's escape to England, and obscurity, Knox became the preferred target of popular loathing: a mob of "[t]he lowest rabble of the Old Town" hanged, burned and tore apart his effigy on 12 February 1829 and broke most of the windows of his and his neighbours' houses.[38] To Knox's family, trapped inside while a mob trampled the tiny garden and threatened to lynch him, these events must have been terrifying, and it is to his credit that in the following months he neither moved from Edinburgh nor missed a lecture, but continued to walk the streets, armed with a sword and pistols. Lonsdale recalled that for some weeks there were cat-calls from a mob gathered outside the dissecting-room, which were answered by cheers from the students within, and that some "persons" kept watch for Knox in the High School Yards, the only exit from Surgeons' Square, after his evening lecture, though his students easily frightened them off.[39]

Knox's home and professional addresses, and his movements between the two, were well known, and a determined crowd could easily have murdered him given the will and spirit for it, but the mob seems to have been composed largely of boys and idlers, probably the same lads involved at other times in "town and gown" fights with the students, who were looking for trouble only if it came at no risk to themselves, and Knox must have realized that, for all the shouting, there was no real danger if he kept his countenance. There was a second effigy burning at Portobello on 3 March, but the public soon tired of these antics and the crowds melted away. Marquis Spineto, lecturing on ancient Egypt at London's Royal Institution, probably had Knox in mind when he told his audience that the rôle of the "Dissector" during mummification was "considered so vile and degrading, as to oblige him immediately to betake himself to flight, as if he had committed a crime, to escape the pursuit, and, if caught, a severe punishment from the bystanders".[40] Knox was characteristically indifferent to the general outcry, though Lonsdale told a well-known story of his being moved to tears when a child, unaware of who he was, expressed a fear that he would sell her to Dr Knox.[41]

Literary attacks on Knox's reputation were potentially more consequential, since they would be read by the middle classes, from which most medical students came. The *Caledonian Mercury*, still hoping to see Hare punished, asked who had taught Burke the "science" of murder, and provided its own emphatic answer, "IT WAS HARE!" But its readers were not expected to believe that an Irish labourer had devised an undetectable method of killing unaided: "who taught Hare", the *Mercury* asked rhetorically, "a person of the very same country and class with Burke?" Without naming Knox, the *Mercury* was accusing him of being an accomplice to murder.[42]

On 17 March, Knox wrote to the *Mercury*:

I have a class of above 400 pupils. No person can be at the head of such an establishment without necessarily running the risk of being imposed upon by those who furnish the material of their science to anatomy teachers; and, accordingly, there is hardly any such person who has not occasionally incurred odium or suspicion from his supposed accession to these violations of the law, without which anatomy can scarcely now be practised. That I should have become an object of popular prejudice, therefore, since mine happened to be the establishment with which Burke and Hare chiefly dealt, was nothing more than what I had to expect. But if means had not been purposely taken, and most keenly persevered in, to misrepresent facts, and to inflame the public mind, that prejudice would at least have stood on right ground, and would ultimately have passed away, by its being seen that I had been exposed to a mere misfortune which would almost certainly have occurred to any body else who had been in my situation.

But every effort has been employed to convert my misfortune into positive and intended personal guilt of the most dreadful character. Scarcely any individual has ever been the object of more systematic or atrocious attacks than I have been. Nobody acquainted with this place requires to be told from what quarter these attacks have proceeded.[43]

He concluded by saying that this was the first and last time he would make a public statement in his own vindication, and for once he was as good as his word.

The March edition of *Blackwood's Magazine* carried a dangerously intelligent attack on Knox in the *Noctes Ambrosianae*, a popular series of imaginary conversations between Edinburgh wits penned by Professor John Wilson (1785–1854) under the alias Christopher North.[44] Wilson, a stalwart contributor to this Tory periodical, had been appointed to the university chair in moral philosophy, by a Tory town council, in 1820, and although, as an advocate and journalist, he was scarcely qualified for the post (his was precisely the type of political appointment to which Knox vehemently objected), he had made a success of it due to his oratorical and literary powers. Wilson used his *Blackwood's* column to accuse Edinburgh's anatomists of gross insensitivity: the cheers of Knox's students were, he wrote, "calculated – whatever may be their effect on more thinking minds – to confirm in those of the populace the conviction that they are all a gang of murderers together, and determined to insult, in horrid exultation, all the deepest feelings of humanity . . . ". He demanded that Knox should "open his mouth and speak" and so "prove" that "it was impossible he could suspect any evil", but Knox prudently declined the challenge and excused himself in a letter to the *Mercury* by saying he had avoided giving evidence in court because "the disclosures of the most innocent proceedings even of the best-conducted dissecting-room must always shock the public".[45]

Many medical men probably agreed with Thomas Wright, whom Knox had befriended as a student, when he wrote after the West Port scandal that "[t]he unprofessional part of the community are by the very nature of the system most inadequate judges of occurrences in a dissecting-room".[46] Knox's class greeted the "the hero of the day" with three rousing cheers, and presented him with a golden cup.[47] Human nature is such that the scandal probably boosted Knox's appeal as a teacher, and in 1829–30 he had 504 pupils, the largest anatomy class ever assembled.[48] He presented himself as a "martyr" for the cause of anatomy, and "electrified" the class with tales of earlier anatomical martyrs, such as the apocryphal story, first put out by Ambroise Paré and frequently repeated, that Vesalius inadvertently dissected a nobleman who was not yet dead and so was hounded out of Spain by the Inquisition.[49] Knox doubtless had little difficulty in convincing his students that his own sufferings were equally undeserved, and it was certainly no exaggeration to claim that nineteenth-century anatomists risked their lives for their work, though it was typhus, erysipelas, or blood poisoning, contracted from dissecting fresh cadavers with unprotected hands, rather than the angry mob, that threatened to make them "a sacrifice to their love of science."[50]

According to Lonsdale, immediately after the discovery of the murders Knox's "rivals in the Anatomy School" tried to "damage his reputation to the utmost".[51] Dirty tricks among the private teachers were not unheard of – Knox had previously accused one Edinburgh teacher of arranging for a warrant to be served so the authorities could seize bodies destined for a competitor[52] – but the struggle to overcome the restricted supply of cadavers tended to unite them in opposition to what they saw as unreasonable impediments to dissection. Surgeons, and their patients, also stood to lose if they had to learn anatomy while they operated ("the poor will . . . have their living bodies mangled, in order to save their dead bodies from examination"[53]), and so anatomy scandals usually prompted the medical profession to close ranks. When, in 1828, a London student was convicted of a misdemeanour for having purchased a body for dissection, London's medical men, including such luminaries as Sir Astley Cooper, organized a subscription to defray his expenses.[54]

When Knox proposed, early in 1829, that a committee should investigate the allegations against him, he could hardly have expected anything other than exoneration, as no-one could reasonably censure him for having failed to detect signs of murder when even the professor of forensic medicine had found nothing conclusive. He turned to Edinburgh's Royal Society, but it proved difficult to gather support: the President, Sir Walter Scott, refused, calling the enquiry a "whitewash" and saying that Knox would "ride off on no back of mine" (he also blocked an attempt by Knox "to read an essay on some dissections" which he thought "very bad taste"), and the committee's first chairman, the 6th Marquess of Queensberry, resigned after a month for undisclosed reasons.[55] Sir John Robinson (1778–1843), the Society's General Secretary, replaced him as the chairman of an eight-man group of Edinburgh worthies who, when they reported on 13 March, censured Knox only for carelessness: the "notoriously bad character" of persons engaged in supplying subjects for dissection had demanded, they said, "greater vigilance".[56]

Edinburgh's people were divided between those who agreed that Knox had been merely careless, perhaps culpably so, and those who thought the inquiry a whitewash. In January 1829, David Macbeth Moir had written to Robert Macnish as one literary doctor to another:

> Seriously, however, nothing ever gave me a viler opinion of medical morality, than the conduct of the Profession on this atrociously memorable occasion; and nothing, I am sure, since the days that old Herophilus dissected living men, has ever occurred, which should – and will more effectually humble it in public estimation ... how much greater reason have the British public to dread and detest a science, which in its abominations, has trampled morality, religion, and every feeling of common humanity under foot, which has countenanced a tragedy to which the fiction of Bluebeard in his bloody chamber, is but a foil, – and which now unblushingly comes forward to defend on the plea of the advancement of knowledge, the perpetration of cold-blooded murders.[57]

Many people in Edinburgh thought that anatomists had been complicit in the crimes committed on their behalf, but when Thomas Wright recorded in his diary that "the name of Dr Knox has sounded from one end of the empire to the other with all the opprobrium which public hatred could attach to it ... ", he exaggerated.[58] The West Port murders were reported in the world's newspapers but personal attacks on Knox were largely restricted to the Edinburgh press. London newspapers were more concerned with denigrating the Scots nation than their anatomists: the crowd's jeers as Burke knelt to pray showed, according to *The Times*, that the Scots were "unsophisticated", and the *Sun* made much of Burke and Hare's Irishness because their murderous schemes had been "far *too original* for the *inferior conceptions* of Scotchmen."[59]

A possibility that few were keen to consider was that murder for dissection was not an isolated crime. Early in 1815 a body had been found "shockingly mutilated" in a hamper that had been sent by two "despicable-looking" men from Smithfield, London to "Mr Wilson", the "janitor" at Edinburgh University who acted as Dr Monro's "resurrection-man". The body showed no signs of having been buried, and a London jury returned a verdict of wilful murder.[60] There were occasions, according to Somerville, when a body in a London dissecting-room was suspected of being "a victim";[61] indeed, "[t]he belief that such horrors were practiced led some anatomists to express concerns to the government in November 1828, previous to the detection of Burke, but their statements were thought so far to exceed the extent of human depravity, that they were deemed incredible."

Knox was probably not the first anatomist to buy the corpse of a murder victim, and he would not be the last. In 1831, two seasoned London resurrection men, John Bishop and Thomas Williams, were found guilty of murdering the so-called "Italian boy" (actually a Lincolnshire cattle drover), whose body they had attempted to sell to anatomist Richard Partridge, and while awaiting execution they confessed to other killings. "Surely", wrote Somerville to the Lord Chancellor, "no-one will now presume to assert that the monopoly of murder was in the hands of Bishop and his associate . . . others, better skilled in the diabolical act . . . are now thriving in their trade, for the exercise of which London furnishes such infinite and unsuspected resources."[62]

In 1861 Leighton published an allegation, which he had apparently heard from a former medical student, that six months before the West Port scandal the assistant of another Edinburgh anatomist had been offered the corpse of a prostitute killed by a blow from a blunt instrument. He had angrily refused it, but the sellers "soon found a less scrupulous customer"; it was possible, suggested Leighton, that "equally suspicious cases were by no means rare".[63] Nor was it supposed that these "horrid feats of cannibals" had ended with Burke's conviction: "Let it not be presumed," observed the *Lancet*, "that with the extermination of Burk [*sic*], the crime to which he has given an undying name has ceased to exist; or because the vigilance of the civil authorities is not bringing to light such damning deeds, that they are not now committed."[64] John Macnee, who published the transcripts of Burke's trial, thought it "very likely" there would be more murders, but he was sanguine concerning the repercussions for the medical profession:

> as for the medical men, nothing in this case can possibly affect them; though

after such an affair, vulgar prejudice may class them for a time with cannibals and banditti, who use choke pears, opiates, poisons, the wet cloth, and a *certain acid*, to procure what is indispensable to their profession, they may despise the unfounded clamour – yet let them not remit in their caution as to their dangerous purchases, nor trust at all to their unprincipled purveyors – "lest a worse thing befall them".[65]

The allusion was to John 5:14 – "Behold, thou art made whole: sin no more, lest a worse thing come unto thee".

CHAPTER EIGHT

A Nation of Cannibals

Thomas Hodgkin, an enemy of strong drink, told a tale of a drunken wretch, by implication a medical man, who "made his way into an anatomical museum; where he drank the spirit in which the preparations were preserved, until he became completely intoxicated; in which state he fell upon the fire, and was burnt to death." Intemperance, warned Hodgkin, could lead to the gravest moral degeneration imaginable: "It is not merely a tincture of human flesh which the drunkard has been known to swallow: his vitiated appetite has not revolted at the flesh itself: and in this way, cannibalism, the mention of which, as committed by ignorant and barbarous heathens, excites our horror, has been perpetrated in England and France, the most polished nations of the civilized world." For Hodgkin, the West Port murders had their origins in intemperance: "The most atrocious and revolting murders committed within a few years, for the purpose of selling the bodies of the unfortunate victims for dissection" were the work of "persons who had not only stifled their consciences, but destroyed the common feelings of humanity by the continued influence of ardent spirit."[1]

To be likened to a cannibal, as Knox was in the reference to "the court of Cacus" on the title page of Macnee's *Trial of William Burke* (1829) and as other anatomists were in the satirical press (at "Mr Rapp's farewell feast" the lecture-room skeleton was placed "in a classical attitude" in the banqueting room, while the students performed "dissections" on the meat, carving it up into "anatomical preparations"[2]), could be regarded as the worst vilification imaginable; yet the conceit of anatomy as cannibalism was not confined to scurrilous invective but was deployed by Hodgkin and other medical men forcibly to express their concerns over the prevailing means of obtaining bodies for dissection: "practices which would disgrace a nation of cannibals."[3]

For the citizens of Edinburgh, the most serious repercussion of the West Port scandal was a breakdown in public order: "a reign of social terror" that left whole families afraid to go at night, not because they feared being murdered and sold for dissection, but because gangs of thugs had taken to sticking pitch-plasters over the faces of pedestrians, particularly girls, who dared venture out after dark.[4] With susceptible members of the public worked up into a fever of "Burkomania", this diabolical prank could have terrible results: "Idiocy, insanity for life, nay, almost

78

instantaneous death have often been its dreadful consequences".[5] The journalist Albany Fonblanque linked Edinburgh's exaggerated concerns over murder for dissection and cannibalism ("pork sausages were made of the flesh of little children . . . sold by their own parents") with the fear of revolution:

Where'ere you are lurking,
Behold but the *Burking*
That's now going onward in every quarter!
See poor Constitution
'Neath fell Revolution,
Pitch-plaster'd and pinion'd, prepared for the slaughter.[6]

Reports from revolutionary France had already given the reading public cause to associate social disorder with a release of unnaturally savage appetites; the sansculottes, metaphorical *mangeurs de rois*, were accused in the British press of literally turning to cannibalism: cutting up their victims, roasting and devouring their limbs, drinking their blood and turning them into soup.[7] They were compared to "Hottentots", creatures so primitive they dined on "guts and garbage", a bestialising diet even if eaten from necessity.[8] In turn, the Revolutionaries dubbed the aristocracy *mangeurs de peoples*: "This cannibal is now prevented from drinking French blood" proclaimed the August diet on the suspension of Louis XVI in 1792.[9] Even so ardent a radical as Knox thought that European revolutions were caused by periodic upsurges of Man's "savage nature", which erupted in "brutality, ferocity, frivolity, and a base and dreadful fanaticism".[10] In this respect, the European lower orders were potentially every bit as savage as natives of Africa or the South Pacific: was it not ironic, wrote the tuppenny blood novelist and social reformer George Reynolds, that the British were busy converting "savages" in far off lands while there were the "swarms" of "infidels" in the slums of their own cities.[11]

Cannibalism, more than any other behaviour, was characteristic of savages, who as Samuel Johnson had remarked "are always cruel", and in nineteenth-century Britain tales of cannibal excess from around the globe served to bestialize peoples that the British sought to subdue.[12] Fresh back from the Cape in 1849, Lt. Col. Elers Napier mounted a devastating literary attack on the natives – ignorant, atheistic, dirty, cruel to animals, immoderate in appetite – especially his erstwhile enemies the "Kaffirs", who he described as ferocious, bloodthirsty cannibals.[13] Drawing on his own experiences, Knox replied to this kind of propaganda by insisting that "[in] Africa no such practise [as cannibalism] exists"; furthermore he "doubted the fact of cannibalism having ever existed": it was "a romance, but it has served its purpose with those that think the end vindicates the means."[14] The cannibal libel was, however, pervasive and by the 1870s even the initially sceptical David Livingstone imagined such "depravities" as human sacrifice, premature burial and a "depraved taste" for human flesh occurring in the Dark Continent.[15]

Regardless of whether Western accounts of savage cannibals were literally true, cannibalism became a trope for the cruel and uncivilized behaviour of others. Burke and Hare, though poor, had by no means lived at the lowest level: Burke was literate and charmed his gaolers, Hare was capable of a subtle cunning, and both had once been hard working; nevertheless, their Irish Celtic origins made it easier to dismiss their crimes as acts of inherent barbarity, and reports of the West Port murders in Scotland tended to emphasize the murderers' Irishness, as though to exculpate the Scots from complicity in their crimes. Some blamed a popish plot, while others, including Knox, saw the Celtic race as innately savage. Irish Celts, like Alexander Pearce who was hanged in Hobart in 1823 for murdering and eating a companion, whose flesh he had found "by far preferable" to pork, were assumed to be inclined towards cannibalism: Carlyle had accused the survivors of the Great Irish Famine of the 1840s of subsisting by "*eating* the slain", and the nineteenth century's most durable fictional cannibal, Sweeney Todd, was given a distinctively Irish name.[16]

The English press, which tended to regard all Scots as Celts (a claim many lowlanders vehemently repudiated), likened the "complicated atrocity" of the West Port murders to the crimes of Sawney Beane.[17] "Sawney" was a common satirical epithet for a stereotypical Scotsman – when Richard Owen confused the skulls of a Scotsman and an African, *Punch* made mock of the similarity between "Sawney and Sambo" – and English readers would have been familiar with colourful tales of Sawney's clan of Celtic cannibals, and others like them.[18] Within living memory, it was said, benighted travellers who stopped at a certain inn on the way to Edinburgh were offered human flesh baked in a pie before being hunted down and killed by the "dark and uncouth" proprietors of the house.[19] Malchow, who saw the legend of Sawney Beane as a link between cannibal savages in other lands and a savage Scots underclass, noted a similarity between the claustrophobic interior of Sawney's cave – a "foetid" den of darkness fit only for a savage – and middle-class descriptions of slums.[20] It might also have been a description of the dissecting-room, the "fetid laboratory", or the "dingy, disreputable" school of anatomy – places morally contiguous with the slums from which Burke and Hare gleaned their victims.[21] Anatomy, which destroyed the integrity of the body, appropriated the dead for the use of the living, and treated flesh as food for the intellect, was often likened to cannibalism, and, as with Sawney Beane, the figure of the cannibal anatomist could be seen as both satirical humour and a veiled accusation. Most tales of supposed anatomical cannibalism were clumsy affairs in which, for example, medical students ate human steaks, but they may well have reflected real anxieties at the license anatomists were permitted in the dissecting-room.

By the nineteenth century, Egyptian mummy (*mummia*) had been dropped from the pharmacopoeias, and medicinal consumption of even tiny quantities of processed human flesh, a valued cure-all in previous centuries, had become unacceptable.[22] Anatomists, however, still had access to a sophisticated tasting menu of refined and liquefied corporeal essences: Edinburgh lecturer in anatomy and physiology John Gordon noted that the "nervous matter" of the brain assumed the appearance of "fresh cheese" when partially "digested in alcohol" and could then be evaporated to leave an "oily substance" that tasted of "boiled meat"; Monro *tertius* reported that the fluid within the ventricles of the brain was tasteless, while according to Grainger, blood was "nauseous", lymph "saltish" ("with a strong spermatic odour"), human fat had "a mild and insipid taste", synovial fluid was "saltish" and extract of macerated muscle tasted "acrid".[23]

The quantities of human remains ingested in the cause of science were infinitesimal, but the process of dissection, like the cannibal savage, consumed the body entirely leaving no identifiable remains. It was never clear exactly how many murders there had been in West Port, or what became of the *disjecta membra*, but the dissectors were "as thorough workmen as putrefaction and the worms",[24] and in several cases the identity of the victim was never known; thus the murders exemplified the worst horror of the dissecting-room: loss of identity.

> Here was a shaking down of man's presumption. O misery, here you stood, naked, barefaced, flaterless! Look at these lumps – bits of different bodies mixed in one foul heap; how like butchers' offal! Here is a bit that would once have summoned you before a magistrate for giving it a kick. – Look, here is an eye – mysterious heaven! This might have been my own. What lover wants this mirror of his soul to make him sensible of the beautiful form and loveliness of woman? ...
>
> Here comes a hardened, blood-bespattered menial, to carry away the refuse of a novice's knife. O wretched necessity of the sciences – O melancholy humiliation of the soul's sepulchre – here's a pretty mess of life's worn-out habiliments, all hacked and tossed, as if they had never felt, or wept, or loved, or worshipped God![25]

To this commentary on his poem *Othello in Hell*, Michael Constable added a (probably superfluous) note warning the reader to "never go into a dissecting-room" lest they see their friends and relatives "sliced and mauled about, till their sexes and ages are lost in shapeless atoms", by "callous-minded" anatomists wielding the "unpoetic knife" among the "clammy" corpses and "jeering" over the "reeking fat".[26]

Just as cannibalism was both a sign of a savage temperament and a cause of "ferocity",[27] anatomy, it was feared, not only attracted the callous minded but also brutalized the honest student's character. The savage was cruel by nature, but the anatomist acquired inhumanity with the practice of his profession. At a time when patients had to be gagged and held down with their hands tied for the duration of an operation, there was some benefit to surgeons in achieving what William Hunter notoriously referred to as "a necessary inhumanity", but the insensitivity needed to treat diseases that were often painful, disfiguring and incurable had to be balanced against patients' and colleagues' expectations that medical men should demonstrate a gentlemanly sensibility. Anatomists, however, were noted for the kind of cold-bloodedness usually associated with murderers – one lurid crime report included the horrific detail that the murderer had cut the victim's throat and drunk his blood "with the coolness of an anatomist at a dissecting table" – and in popular fiction they readily became murderers: in one story a murderous Irish surgeon was apprehended after rashly boasting of the skill with which his victim had been dissected.[28] It entered into folklore that surgeons, like butchers, were forbidden from serving on Coroners' juries, since "a frequent contemplation of sanguinary scenes, hardens the heart, deadens sensibility, and destroys every tender sensation", though no such law ever existed.[29] In the wake of West Port, a *Lancet* editorial condemned "the possessors of the practical insensibility, acquired in the dissecting-room", and in his later writings Knox tended to dwell excessively on the demoralizing effects of exposure to "forms which Nature never intended should be seen".[30]

As a young man, Knox's anti-vivisection stance had been a very public demonstration of the moral sensibility that patients expected from a physician: animal experimentation, he wrote, was "a practice I could never witness, and have always held in extreme abhorrence".[31] Though he advanced arguments, similar to those used by his friend Charles Bell, that "cruel vivisections" added little to anatomical knowledge, he seems to have had a "natural horror" of cruelty and, according to Lonsdale, "shuddered" when he spoke of vivisectionists' experiments.[32] Nowadays, it would be assumed such sentiments were prompted by sympathy with animal suffering, but Knox was more likely to have been troubled by the potentially brutalizing effect of vivisection on the experimenter: The *London Medical Gazette's* condemnation of those who objected to vivisection, though done for "the profit of others", but indulged in the "manly sports of fishing and shooting" and destroyed life for "pleasure", might have been written with Knox in mind.[33] In addition to his fondness for blood sports, Knox occasionally performed vivisection in the field, though never in the classroom, where some practitioners advocated it to habituate medical students to suffering and pain.[34]

In its use as a posthumous punishment for murderers, dissection came uncomfortably close to human vivisection: in Hogarth's popular engravings *Four Stages of Cruelty* (1751) the sadistic Tom Nero begins by torturing a dog and ends up in a dissecting-room where a dog devours his worthless, discarded heart while anatomists dismember his corpse, its face contorted in anguish.[35] The belief that the dead remained, in some way, sentient to injury or pain was (and is) a common reason to shun dissection; relatives still refuse permission for hospital autopsies on the grounds that the deceased has "suffered enough". As well as linking anatomists with callous cruelty, vivisection had awkward overtones of butchery. William Hamilton Drummond, in his anti-vivisection monograph *The Rights of Animals*, contrasted the avoidance of vivisection by the "practiced anatomist" with its acceptance by the "bungling blockhead, whom nature designed to be a butcher".[36]

Malicious comparisons of anatomists to butchers, which date back to the time of Tertullian, not only slighted their professional standing, always a sore point for surgeons (in the 1850s a Norfolk butcher turned the tables by advertising himself as a "zootomist"), but also made the damaging point that anatomists treated human and animal bodies the same, a practice that still arouses powerful opposition: at a recent exhibition of human anatomical specimens in Munich a dissected horseman riding a dissected horse was banned because it was thought to offend human dignity by degrading man to the level of a beast.[37] Ballads and cheap prints concerning the West Port murders played on such fears by depicting the anatomist's subjects as animals: Knox was "the boy that buys the beef" and was shown dissecting a pig, an image reused in the 1945 film *The Body Snatcher*.[38]

As a revelation of contemporary savagery, the West Port murders resonated far beyond the narrow world of Edinburgh's anatomists and their suppliers: the enormity of murder for dissection, the disclosure that the poor were worth more dead than alive, and the realization that no-one apparently cared where the subjects in the dissecting-room came from, implied a breakdown in social order as great as that during the French Revolution, when according to Thomas Carlyle society had become cannibalistic.[39] West Port was not merely a setback to humanity's optimistic hopes for the intellectual enlightenment, or a shocking exposure of the dark foundations of medical science, for it had long been understood that enlightened science required knowledge of the structure and mechanisms of the body: it was a blow to society's faith in its own moral progress.[40]

The radical publisher Richard Carlile perceptively blamed the murders not on individuals but on the double standards of the system of Edinburgh medical training, which gave no incentive for an anatomist to be "virtuous", but required him, if he wished to succeed in his profession, to submit to "a continual war of suppressed convictions, resisted evidences, stifled sentiments, compromises, connivances, collusions, and violences" against nature and morals.[41] In retrospect, Carlile's indictment of the hypocritical disregard with which Edinburgh's most acclaimed area of teaching was carried on, Hodgkin's condemnation of intemperance, and the *Lancet*'s concerns over the demoralising effect of dissection all offer some insight into the tragedy that so shockingly exposed the undercurrent of brutality beneath the city's civilized surface. Burking was a "worse than cannibal crime",[42] "whose comparison doth blanche the feats of cannibals and anthropophagies into innocence", yet it had happened in the "Christian Athens, the centre of civilization, the core of orthodoxy, the pith of piety, the marrow of morals, the God-fearing, Kirk-going, Sabbath-keeping, Bible-circulating, Missionary-sending, *Edinburgh*".[43]

CHAPTER NINE

The Most Popular Teacher in Our Metropolis, 1830–1836

After his vindication by the committee of enquiry, Knox carried on his professional life outwardly unperturbed. He took less interest in the study of human anatomy – the notes on human dissection in his private museum catalogue stopped in 1828[1] – but whether he became averse to it, or whether there were simply more opportunities in the field of comparative anatomy, we can only guess. In December 1829, he addressed the Royal Society of Edinburgh on the Dugong, a marine mammal the head, heart, stomach and genital organs of which, presented to the Society by one Mr Swinton, had been passed to him for dissection. Though he thought the resulting anatomical preparations far superior to those in the university museum, whose dugong skeleton had apparently been put together by someone "unfit for real anatomical research",[2] his work remained largely unnoticed outside Edinburgh, and failed to win him recognition where he most coveted it, in France. His evidence that the dugong did not belong to the order of *Cetacea* (whales and dolphins), to which Baron Cuvier had assigned it, was ignored by Cuvier's brother Frédéric, a slight on which Knox, who had spent hundreds of pounds on whales for dissection, found it "painful to dwell".[3] Though cetology did not earn him the international recognition he hoped for, he monopolized the subject at the Royal Society of Edinburgh, where he exhibited what he claimed were "the only authentic drawings" of the rorqual. When Professor Traill indignantly asked what he thought of *his* drawings of that species, Knox told him: "very like a whale".[4]

Relations between Knox and the Council of the College of Surgeons had worsened in 1829 when his "rival" James Syme, who had opposed his appointment as Conservator in 1826, became one of the museum's Curators.[5] One of Knox's duties as Conservator was to act as Registrar for the students, who paid five shillings to use the College facilities and Museums. It appears that some of this money went to Knox, and the College's resolution in February 1829 to waive the fees (which he did not hear about until November) looks like a spiteful move to take away one of his few perks. Thereafter, the Curators seem to have made his life increasingly difficult, insisting on one occasion that newly acquired specimens were laid out for their inspection "in the kitchen of Dr McCansh's

85

house".[6] In 1831, after a "misunderstanding" over the display of a specimen, Syme publicly "admonished" Knox for not showing "the respect which was due to the Curators": the museum committee reprimanded him for being difficult, but Knox told them he saw "no prospect of a cordial co-operation".[7]

That summer, just as New Surgeons' Hall in Nicolson Street was almost completed, Knox abruptly abandoned his efforts to move the College's collection there, "in consequence of the entire want of water and the danger of even moving about in the New Hall". When the College wrote to his school to enquire what he was doing, Frederick replied that Robert had decided to resign and had gone to stay in the country. Under the terms of Barclay's bequest, Knox had a job for life if he wished, but he called his resignation "a measure I have for a long time contemplated".[8] It has been suggested that, after the West Port scandal, Knox's "affronted" colleagues in the College had "ostracized" him:[9] there are favourable references to his Conservatorship in the College minutes, which contain no criticism of his work as a private teacher and no mention of West Port, but the possibility that he was forced to resign by pressure applied behind the scenes is difficult to rule out. Other causes of dissatisfaction with his work are suggested by the College's decision prospectively to clip his successor's wings by banning private practice and forbidding the Conservator to leave Edinburgh without permission.[10] Despite his characteristically volatile relationship with his employer, Knox had given good service: he left the College museum greatly expanded and scientifically catalogued, and continued to take an interest in the collection, on which he worked from time to time without remuneration until his departure from Edinburgh in 1842.[11]

On 17 November 1831, Lord Fitzroy Somerset wrote to Sir James McGrigor regarding Knox's Army commission, which he was obliged to resign in order to avoid further service in the Cape. He left the Army on 2 August 1832 and received a commutation of a hundred pounds.[12] His resignation removed his last guaranteed income, though as he had been on half-pay for more than ten years (latterly at four shillings a day) he had no cause for complaint and, with record class sizes, the private school alone provided an adequate income. For a professional man he was living quite frugally, spending some three hundred pounds a year on himself and his family and reinvesting his remaining profits in the school.[13] In October 1831, he and Frederick spent "the trifling sum of £10" on the skeleton of "a whalebone whale of vast magnitude" that had been washed up west of North Berwick, where thousands turned out to see the "monstrous fish".[14] At Robert's request, the obliging Hodgkin sent a description and measurements of a similar specimen in London, thus enabling them accurately to reconstruct the twenty-eight-ton skeleton.[15] Robert presented an account of the whale's anatomy at the Royal Society of Edinburgh, and Frederick exhibited the articulated skeleton to the public at the Royal Institution in Princes Street and the Pavilion, North College Street, before Robert finally sold it to the University Museum.[16]

These zoological investigations were not merely the disinterested pursuit of science: an academic reputation would have helped attract non-medical pupils to Knox's summer courses on comparative anatomy,[17] and even medical students demanded research-based, up-to-date teaching, which for the many radicals amongst them, fired up by the July Revolution, meant the latest Parisian ideas. In London, Professor Granville Sharp Pattison's (1791–1851) students rioted in protest at his "*total ignorance of* and *disgusting indifference* to new anatomical views and researches", and in 1831 a combination of student pressure and bad press in the *Lancet* forced him from his post.[18] In a competitive marketplace, it paid to teach radical anatomy.

Knox first mentioned philosophical anatomy in print in 1831, in a paper on (of all things) the stomach of the Peruvian llama, interest in the subject having been raised by the celebrated Cuvier–Geoffroy debate in Paris the previous year. Appel and others have shown that it is an oversimplification to regard the debate as a straightforward contest between Cuvier's functionalism and Geoffroy's formalism, with Cuvier victorious, for though it was a professional triumph for Cuvier, it was Geoffroy who won the popular *success d'opinion,*[19] an outcome that may have inspired Knox to present his own theories directly to the public once his academic career had stalled.

Knox had long been critical of the extreme functionalism of the Cuvierian school; according to his own account he had been denouncing their "pretensions" in conversation as early as 1821 and in the lecture room since 1825.[20] Functionalism was based on the "natural" assumption that "every part of the animal economy must have its use", but Knox argued against attempting to find a use for parts that "obviously serve no immediate purpose", and he found Cuvier's celebrated claim to be able to reconstruct a whole animal from a single bone overambitious, since it assumed that animal form was governed by laws as absolute as those of mechanical physics. For Knox, the search for rigid physical laws was "impracticable", because animals were "regulated by the mysterious principle of life", and he rejected the well-worn comparison, popular with creationists, between an animal and a machine (usually a watch) as a non sequitur, since a machine is created for a specific purpose, whereas "The animal machine abounds with structures, the reason for which he [the anatomist] cannot guess at, neither can he calculate what might be the result of their absence or destruction." Geoffroyan formalism could account for functionless structures as expressions of an underlying common plan, but Knox's position in 1831 cannot simply be equated with that of Geoffroy, and he was sceptical of over reliance on unity of plan. "Mr HUNTER said that 'Nature was fond of analogy,'" he wrote scathingly, "and so, I presume, in sport, placed organs in animals which seemingly performed no functions . . . ".[21]

For the time being, however, his work left little time for philosophical speculation. At numbers 10 and 3 Surgeons' Square, which he rented for £270 a year, he gave classes in "Practical Anatomy and Operative Surgery", which included a daily demonstration of the soft tissues and a session on the anatomy of the bones.[22] There were lectures on the human brain and nervous system every Friday, a course on surgical anatomy and operative surgery, and daily "examinations" and "conversations" on anatomy in the practical rooms, where Knox and Fergusson undertook to be in constant attendance.[23] It was a full schedule, but Knox felt vindicated now that he had the largest class in the city: "I know it will give you pleasure to hear that my attending class is 504", he wrote to Hodgkin in January 1832: "so much for Edinb[urgh]".[24] He also took on occasional surgical cases, and on 3 March 1831 advised Fergusson on what was apparently the first successful operation for imperforate anus.[25]

Between 1829 and 1832 the anatomy school's accounts, kept by Fergusson, record payments to shadowy figures such as the "Black Bull man" and the "Man at Canal" for bodies from as far afield as Manchester, Glasgow and Dublin.[26] The West Port murders had probably deterred the local resurrection men from dealing with Knox – in 1829 one alleged grave robber testified that he wanted nothing to do with him[27] – though in the struggle to obtain subjects for his record class, the Asiatic cholera epidemic of 1832 proved an unexpected boon. Fergusson confessed with remarkable candour – albeit in a medical journal – that victims of the epidemic often ended up in dissecting-rooms because the medical profession frightened people into believing the bodies were too contagious to await proper burial, and so they were hurried into unhallowed, and no doubt shallow and poorly guarded, graves, from which they were easily removed. Sometimes, according to Fergusson, they were buried "before the vital heat was extinguished" and even, "before the breath was out of the body", though we can only guess how he came by this information.[28]

The winter of 1831–2 was the warmest Knox could remember, and outbreaks of cholera all around Edinburgh – divine wrath over the Reform Bill, some said – caused "great alarm". A board of health was set up, the poor were supplied with warm clothing, and in January the University considered closing for the term, but the danger passed and classes were not interrupted.[29] Fortunately, despite the origin of some of their subjects, no-one working in the city's dissecting-rooms became infected, and Edinburgh was spared the cholera riots that broke out elsewhere in Scotland and in Liverpool when word got out that doctors were carting away the dead or dying for dissection.[30]

The surrounding towns and villages were not so fortunate: one Sunday, the only day on which they were free to leave town, Robert and Frederick walked to the village of Fisherrow, where, on enquiring about a family he knew, Frederick was told "They are all dead, save one who is now dying." Later, during a walking and fishing holiday on the Solway, where Robert "continue[d] a series of observations on the salmon", they saw "in the extreme distance, seemingly over the town of Dumfries, a vast cloud in motion; it extended from earth to Heaven. In one sense it was stationary – that is, it remained on the same place, but every particle of it seemed to be in motion." The cloud was made up of millions of flies, and the next day they heard that the cholera "had rested on the unhappy town of Dumfries, the population of which it had decimated."

The "eastern plague" spread to the Marquis of Lothian's estate, where the district surgeon was one of Knox's former pupils. When the local authorities tried to set up a *cordon sanitaire* he complained to Knox, whose advice to the locals was to walk straight up to the constables set to guard them, who would be so afraid of being infected that they would turn and run. "This is the way I always treat the impertinent interference of impertinent government officials", he wrote, some twenty years later. To further demonstrate his contempt for the interference of the "supine, grasping, grovelling, money-getting magistracy" in matters medical, he visited the affected villages himself and touched the sick to prove there was "no danger of contagion".[31]

Anatomists were just the sort of "active, pushing, intelligent" people whom proponents of the Reform Bill anticipated would shake up local government.[32] In June 1832, the Scottish Reform Act enfranchised the professional classes and increased the electorate from around 4,500 to over 60,000, but radical anatomists had little time to celebrate as the passage of the Anatomy Act the following month posed a new threat that alarmed them into closing ranks. Ruth Richardson's *Death, Dissection and the Destitute*, which recognized the Anatomy Act as a pivotal event in the regulation of medicine, provides a comprehensive analysis of the Act's origins, which will be only briefly summarized here.

In March 1829, in the wake of the West Port murders, the radical MP Henry Warburton drafted an Anatomy Bill, "to legalize and regulate the supply of dead bodies for the purpose of dissection", but it failed to reach the statute books, owing to opposition from the Church of England and others to its "cannibal-like" proposal that subjects for dissection be obtained from hospitals and workhouses.[33] In vain did the astute Scottish MP Sir James Mackintosh argue that, since a "decline" in anatomy would impair surgical training and lead to patients' lives being lost, it was not the means by which corpses were obtained but "legal impediments to anatomy" that merited the charge of "barbarity". Was it worse, he asked, for the body to be given up to the "noble science" of anatomy, or for the grave "vindictively" to devour it?[34] The *London Medical Gazette* carried an editorial in a similar vein, contrasting the "honourable and useful purpose" of anatomical dissection with the horrors of inhumation:

> Here we have the putrefactive and disgusting process of the common grave, with specimens of *rats' dissection*; the liquifactive process in the leaden coffin; broiling and burning; the effects of a watery grave, adipocere; drying in vaults; suffering the moist parts to exhale and be dissipated in the atmosphere; mummy, in all its unnatural hideousness, &c.[35]

Parliament admitted the necessity of dissection, but baulked at the provisions of Warburton's bill; the real question, as the *Christian Examiner* perceptively put it, was not "whether any bodies should be dissected, but what bodies".[36]

Legislators were inspired to fresh urgency by the murder for dissection of the "Italian boy" and others in London, after which metropolitan outrage all objections to a new Anatomy Bill were swept aside. The essence of the 1832 Anatomy Act was that, instead of dissecting corpses privately obtained, anatomists were to be allocated the bodies of those who died destitute.[37] To many people, this was simply "inhuman", and it would be difficult to exaggerate popular revulsion at the new law. So great was the horror of being anatomized that when gibbeting was (briefly) reintroduced as a judicial punishment to replace public dissection, the *London Medical Gazette* speculated that many people considered the gibbet a less fearful prospect than "the daring scrutiny of the unfeeling dissector."[38]

The humanitarian B.M. Forster (1764–1829), who added opposition to anatomy school "abuses" to his abolitionist, anti blood sport and philanthropic portfolio, asked whether it was *necessary* to procure sufficient bodies to instruct a thousand pupils a year in anatomy in London alone.[39] To some, the Anatomy Act seemed a wanton outrage to the feelings of "the poorer classes of His Majesty's subjects":

> The body of the friendless and unclaimed pauper (mark the total dereliction of humanity, the contemptuous defiance of all the better feelings of our nature, displayed by the abettors of this measure in the selection of the friendless and the destitute for their horrid purposes!) is to be hacked and hewn into small bits for the purpose of gratifying the cannibal propensities of a cruel, unfeeling, and bloodthirsty profession!

Thus *Blackwood's Magazine*, which anticipated that subjects for dissection would soon ("alas!") be "too plentiful",[40] though as we shall see, this was not the case.

Much has been made of the control the Anatomy Act gave medical men over the bodies of the poor. It also gave the state an unprecedented degree of control over anatomy schools, and it is notable that few anatomists came out in support of the Act. From the perspective of Britain's private teachers, a worrying aspect of the Parisian system, despite the ready availability of subjects, was that the *Ecole de Médecine* was an "engine of the state", subject to "the surveillance of police officers".[41] Now, in 1832, British anatomists found themselves entirely dependent on the whims of government in allowing them corpses with which to teach. The law, "that odious chain, contrived by men of detestable characters to fetter and enslave humanity",[42] had empowered the authorities to take away their livelihood, and Edinburgh's anatomists, geographically and politically a long way from London, were having none of it.

In September 1832, the physician and editor of the *Edinburgh Medical and Surgical Journal* Dr David Craigie (1793–1866) was appointed to the unenviable position of His Majesty's Inspector of Anatomy for Scotland. His first task was to inspect the schools of anatomists who had applied to the Home Secretary for a license, as required under the Anatomy Act, but only three – Monro, William Mackenzie and Robert Liston – had done so. The remaining out-lecturers called the government's bluff and won: Craigie backed down and, citing "difficulties" in inspecting the other schools, granted them all temporary licenses.[43] On 27 November, Knox was licensed to teach at 3, 4 and 10 Surgeons' Square, three attractive Georgian houses on either side of Old Surgeons' Hall.[44]

For the time being, the independent lecturers could afford to be blasé about the Anatomy Act, since bodies could still be obtained via the traditional route. Legally, however, there were now only three sources of supply: the Royal Infirmary, the gaols, and the five Edinburgh parishes, *i.e.* the City, St Cuthbert's, Cannongate, North Leith, and South Leith. Summing up the situation ten years on, Craigie's successor, James Somerville, recalled that the Infirmary was the most "acceptable" source, and that its managers "gave instructions that the unclaimed bodies should be given up for Anatomical Examination". The distribution of these bodies was devolved to the College of Surgeons, and "[t]he consequence was a loud complaint on the part of the Extra Anatomical Teachers against the monopoly of the College, but as the managers did not yield, recourse was had to other sources."[45]

It is not clear how Craigie, who had no experience as an anatomy teacher and could be "distant and cold" towards his colleagues, obtained his appointment as Inspector of Anatomy, though there were rumours it was "a Whig job" arranged through his connections with the Home Secretary, Viscount Melbourne.[46] Craigie took his work, and himself, extremely seriously, but it soon became clear that his political masters would provide little practical support, and when he voiced concerns that "offences against the Anatomy Act" were being committed in Edinburgh, Melbourne blandly instructed him to cooperate with the Lord Advocate in "bringing the guilty Parties to Punishment."[47] In December 1832 a body was found in a crate in Perth, awaiting shipment, but Craigie was unable to discover for whom it had been intended.[48]

When the Inspector of Anatomy for England, James Somerville, heard that resurrection men were still at work, he was concerned that

Edinburgh's anatomists were not giving the Act "fair play".[49] By the beginning of 1833 he had become exasperated with Craigie's handling of the matter ("we are kept painfully in the dark as to your proceedings in Scotland . . . ") and wrote to remind him of the Home Secretary's "strong determination to abolish all sources of illegal supply",[50] to which end he suggested that Craigie "place a Police man at the door of each Dissecting Room, in order to suppress and prevent at one the introduction of subjects in any other mode than according to the Provisions of the Anatomical Act."[51]

Lord Melbourne, "aware of the feeling which exists in Edinburgh with respect to Schools of Anatomy", thought Somerville's suggestion "most improper",[52] and merely advised Craigie to "make every possible enquiry" into reports that Edinburgh schools were obtaining bodies from London and to "strongly impress upon the Professors of Anatomy the illegality of obtaining bodies in the manner above alluded to – and the severe penalties imposed by the Act for regulating Schools of Anatomy for obtaining Bodies otherwise than in the way pointed out by that statute."[53] Apparently mindful that threats alone would be unlikely to succeed, he exhorted Craigie to rely on "the engagement of honour which the Anatomy and Surgery Teachers at Edinburgh have entered into" for "satisfying the public feeling", and to set about "removing the obstacles" to their obtaining bodies.[54]

To ensure an adequate and equitable supply of subjects, Edinburgh's extramural anatomy teachers organized themselves into an Association of Teachers of Anatomy and Surgery, whose members were Knox, Fergusson, Robertson, Sharpey, Handyside, Mackenzie, Turner, and John and Alexander Lizars. Sharpey was Knox's "particular friend", a transcendentalist who had dedicated his MD thesis to Knox and who, in 1831, had moved in next door at 9 Surgeons' Square, where he taught anatomy until offered a London chair in 1836.[55] Mackenzie seems to have joined reluctantly and Monro refused any part in the Association, and so in Melbourne's opinion was not entitled to "any share in the distribution of the bodies."[56] Craigie, however, seemed more concerned with reining in the private lecturers, and in January 1834 he wrote to Melbourne accusing Knox and Fergusson of "having obtained a Body irregularly for dissection".[57] It is not clear how exactly they were supposed to have broken the rules, but Craigie was a stickler for compliance and had added some extra regulations of his own to the Act, such as a requirement that bodies should be dissected within three days. When his edicts were flouted, he complained ineffectually to Melbourne that "some individual ought to possess the power of repressing the contumacy in any Teacher, or of inflicting some penalty . . . for every similar act of insolence or audacious defiance of authority, or otherwise small irregularities will pass by insensible degrees to gross violations", but his "dictatorial and petulant" manner when visiting the schools only antagonized the teachers further.[58]

Beneath the bluster, Craigie had no real authority: at a meeting on 6 February 1834 (the earliest for which minutes are preserved), with Knox in the chair, the Association of Teachers unanimously resolved to inform Craigie that "Anatomists and Surgeons should have a prior claim to one male subject each to illustrate their lectures", which Knox duly did by letter. On 10 March, again under Knox's chairmanship, the Teachers set up a committee to decide "the best means of procuring and distributing bodies". Craigie was invited to attend a meeting on 24 March, but he cannot have made a very good impression, as two days later the teachers "unanimously agreed that Dr Craigie be relieved of the duty of distributing bodies, which hereafter is to be conducted by the Office under the superintendence of a Committee of Members of the Association".[59]

His Majesty's Inspector of Anatomy for Scotland replied that the Association "is not competent . . . to propose or carry into effect any alteration in the present arrangement . . . ". Relations between the private schools and their inspector had irretrievably broken down, but for once Knox, who had been absent when the meeting voted to relieve Craigie of his responsibilities, was conciliatory, and abstained from an inflammatory motion passed on 7 April that called upon Craigie to declare "upon what grounds [he] claims the power of distributing bodies". A week later, Knox was tasked with communicating the Association's grievances directly to the Home Secretary, and he drafted a letter calling for Craigie's removal, which was signed by everyone except Sharpey and sent to Lord Melbourne on 4 June. Craigie counter-attacked by accusing the teachers – "calumniously and falsely" in their opinion – of having supplied him with class lists "exaggerated in regard to numbers".[60] This was a dispute in which it would have been difficult for either side to prove their case, as the only independent register of medical students, kept by the College of Surgeons, was not signed by all.

Knox's school, which in 1833 moved to the grander premises of Old Surgeons' Hall (currently the home of the University of Edinburgh Faculty of Social Sciences Graduate School), was sufficiently thriving to take on a third lecturer, John Reid (1809–49), who paid £250 for a third share in the profits.[61] Reid, another of Knox's former pupils, had recently returned from two years in Paris, during which time he had kept in touch with Knox, sending him an account of an unsuccessful operation for strangulated hernia performed by Dupuytren at the *Hôtel Dieu*.[62] Knox's manner towards his new assistant could be condescending – it was said that when Reid consulted Knox after failing to find the brains of two sharks he was dissecting, Knox remarked that if he desired to see sharks with no brains he need only pay a visit to parliament – but Reid was well liked by his students, who collected over £30 for a presentation when he left the school, his duties being taken over by Frederick Knox.[63]

In 1834, shortage of subjects for dissection forced up prices to £5 for an "entire adult", £3 for an adult that had been "opened" and £1 for a child under eight years old. Although this was considerably less than before the Anatomy Act, when prices had reflected the risks involved in obtaining cadavers illegally, in those days expense had been no obstacle to Knox, who as the most successful teacher could afford to pay well. Now he had to wait his turn, since on 20 October 1834 the Association of Teachers had agreed that the surgical teachers should have first claim on two bodies each in a fixed order of precedence – Ballingall, Lizars, Fergusson and Robertson – followed by the anatomists in the order Knox, Lizars, Sharpey, Handyside and Sherriffs. Though Knox's precedence among anatomists and leading rôle in the Association indicates his respected position among his colleagues, the limited supply of subjects was beginning to hamper his work as a teacher.

The principal beneficiaries of the Anatomy Act were Craigie, whose salary was increased in 1834 from £100 to £400,[64] and Monro. Lampooning lecturers has always been the stock-in-trade of student magazines, but the students had a particular grievance against Monro, who they felt abused his position by charging fees for lectures at which attendance was compulsory without giving adequate return:

> The *first*, the glorious of the three,
> The founder of the M_____os, He!
> Who not content to be himself resplendent,
> Made and left fame *enough* for each descendent;
> The second got it – used it too,
> But still *he* added something new;
> He gave his lectures to the third,
> This one *can read* them every word;
> And though he reads them mighty ill,
> Yet manages the place to fill
> Which M_____os long have fill'd – and longer will.
> The Gown an heir-loom in their race,
> Which once they honour'd, *** ********
> ...
> Force, force thy students to attend,
> And there unwilling listeners send;
> But were the lecturer worth a plack [a small coin],
> The students would not be so slack.
> Compell'd by roll-calls to attend –
> Merit alone once gained that end;
> Doubled the fees,– though more than halv'd the merit,
> Say, did he, too, his love of cash inherit?[65]

"Stupid Stingy M[onr]o"[66] could afford to be indifferent to such contumely as the University took roll calls in his lectures, and he had the lion's share of the subjects for dissection while the extramural teachers went without. In the 1833–4 session, Knox had received only nine cadavers by Christmas, and more than two hundred dissatisfied students petitioned the town council to increase the supply. Mackenzie criticized the grammar of their petition, the students criticized the grammar of Mackenzie's lectures, and deadlock ensued.[67]

One anonymous out lecturer was so dissatisfied with the status quo that he published a pamphlet, *An Examination into the Causes of the Declining Reputation of the Medical Faculty of the University of Edinburgh* (Edinburgh: Burgess, 1834), criticising the university's teaching and providing figures from the College of Surgeons showing that the extra collegiate anatomy schools had more than twice as many students as the University.[68] It is the sort of thing Knox might have written, and the pamphlet has come to be associated with his name, though there is no direct evidence he was the author.[69] Stylistically, the pamphlet could be by Knox, and it inveighs against two of his particular bugbears: the appointment of professors by the Town Council and compulsory attendance in classes. One pupil told his father that Knox laughed at the Edinburgh MD, an opinion shared by the author of *An Examination*: "The writer has known many who have received their degrees in Edinburgh, who were not to be trusted with the life of a cat, and who could not write a decent letter in the mother tongue . . . although they wrote, or rather got the credit of writing, a dissertation in Latin!" Many students, he alleged, were "inattentive", "dissipated" and "stupid", yet graduated MD with the help of a paid "grinder" to coach them and ghost write their thesis.[70]

There were some students whose "admiration" for Knox and desire to avoid Monro's tedious classes led them to study for a surgical diploma rather than an MD. One such was John Goodsir (1814–67), a bright young man with wide-ranging interests in metaphysics, aesthetics, and transcendentalism, who was unsurprisingly bored with his work as a dental apprentice, and who became one of Knox's favourite pupils: he prepared skeletons for his private museum (on which Knox spent at least eighteen hundred pounds) and was invited to become vice-president of the Anatomical and Physiological Society, which Knox founded in 1833 with himself as president.[71] The Society, not to be confused with the larger Anatomical Society of Edinburgh (of which Reid was president), appears to have been an attempt to establish a coterie of pupils (Lonsdale also joined), but it never flourished and soon lapsed into desuetude.[72] Goodsir was astute enough to follow his own path, negotiating for himself the Conservatorship of the University museum and later succeeding Monro as professor of anatomy, one of an ever-growing band of "Knoxites" whose worldly success outstripped that of their teacher.

Knox's students were active in Edinburgh undergraduate life through the Royal Medical and Hunterian Medical societies, and in the Maga Club, founded in the winter of 1834–5 by Edward Forbes and others, which produced a magazine that pricked the pomposity of the "asses and boobies" of the town council ("Let fame her 'posterior trumpet' sound loud, then / And show to the world this astonishing crowd, then") with barbs of Knoxian wit. Forbes went on to found the Edinburgh Oineromathic Society, also known as the Brotherhood of the Friends of the Truth or the Brotherhood of the Magi, whose symbol was a silver triangle on which was engraved ΟΙΝΟΣ, ΕΡΩΣ, ΜΑΘΗΣΙΣ (wine, love and learning), and who wore across their breasts at all times the "Roseate Band", a silken ribbon woven with the "mystic letters" OEM in black.[73] They met in John Goodsir's top-floor rooms at 21 Lothian Street, known as "the barracks", where he lived with his younger medical-student brothers Harry and Robert, and it was from here that the Arch Magus and his Triangles – the Society's officers – issued their edicts. Knox was an evening visitor to the fraternity, where he spoke about his African experiences and discussed nature and philosophy after his day's work was done.[74]

Henry Lonsdale, an Englishman from the Scottish borders and Knox's future biographer, joined Knox's class in 1834 and, mindful of the "shadows" in his mentor's past, found himself studying his character.[75] Knox made his students welcome, addressed them as equals, and enjoyed their company. In 1834, for example, Andrew Whelpdale, a medical student newly arrived in Edinburgh, told his father in Cumberland that Knox was the only one of the city's "savans" with whom he had become acquainted, though Knox was perhaps too eager to please: there were dangers, wrote Whelpdale, for a lecturer who "exults in entertaining an admiring audience".[76] Knox's "flowery and poetic language" in the lecture room was reminiscent of the Theatre Royal Drury Lane, and the applause was just as loud. Another easy way of courting popularity was to ridicule the other teachers, particularly Handyside and Alexander Lizars, or Peter and Sandy, as Knox called them: "By G[od] it saves a world of talk / To resort to board and chalk" he quipped of their "washing-tub diagrams". Knox talked non-stop, often going on beyond his allotted time, and some found him complacent and over-fond of the sound of his own voice.[77]

Despite his rather bombastic style of lecturing, Knox's provision of dissecting-room microscopy shows that he did not neglect technical advances, at least if they facilitated precise observation in the Parisian style. Edinburgh's extramural teachers had been the first to introduce the microscope to British medical training: the anatomist and embryologist Allen Thomson taught microscopy in the 1830s, and after taking up the chair in physiology he offered Britain's first university course on "microscopic anatomy", in 1842.[78] Though Knox did not teach microscopy as a separate subject, it was familiar to all who studied in his dissecting-rooms: Frederick was "much versed in the examination of minute objects under the microscope", and his discoveries included a parasitic worm, which he identified after examining the muscles of over 130 cadavers "publicly, and with the greatest care, in presence of numerous classes".[79] Knox may have "satirized" the microscope,[80] as he did many things, but his appears to have been the first British anatomy school to invest in this expensive instrument and use it routinely.

After the 1835–6 session, Knox no longer offered "practical" as well as descriptive anatomy, presumably for want of subjects for dissection.[81] According to returns made under the Anatomy Act, the university received thirty-five bodies during this session and the extra-mural schools only eighteen between them, though of course these figures took no account of the unofficial sources of supply that, at least in Monro's case, still existed.[82] At the conclusion of the previous session, a committee of Edinburgh medical students had again expressed their dissatisfaction in a petition to the Home Secretary, only to be advised that "public discussion" would be "extremely prejudicial to their objects" and that they should "rely on the unostentatious exertions of Individuals...".[83] Finally, on 15 October 1836, the new Home Secretary, Lord John Russell, mindful of the "considerable irregularity in the distribution of bodies" and of Craigie's conduct in the dissecting-rooms, which was "calculated to give offence to the Teachers" in the presence of their pupils, dismissed him from his post for "misconduct" and "gross neglect of duty".[84]

By this time, Knox and his brother were working alone: Reid had resigned his partnership in May 1836 to take up a post as lecturer in physiology, and Fergusson had given up anatomy due to increasing hospital commitments (he had been surgeon to the Edinburgh Royal Dispensary since 1831).[85] It was rumoured that Knox was considered for a chair at University College London when Dr Jones Quain resigned in 1835, and that one of the London professors visited Edinburgh incognito to hear the various anatomy lecturers and liked Knox the best, but nothing came of this. It was perhaps small consolation that the *Lancet*'s Edinburgh correspondent called Knox "certainly the most popular teacher in our metropolis".[86]

CHAPTER TEN

A Scandalous Monopoly, 1836–1840

After Craigie's dismissal, Somerville, the Inspector of Anatomy for England, took on the remit for Scotland, and struck an encouragingly conciliatory note in his initial circular to the Association of Teachers, whose "zealous cooperation" he optimistically anticipated.[1] He sympathized with them over the limited supply of bodies and "the inequality of the distribution", and promised reform, but was leery of their proposal for "a course of popular anatomy", which sounds like a Knoxian scheme, because of the "deep seated prejudice against anatomy in this City".[2] Somerville was aware that pauper cadaver acquisition was especially problematic in Edinburgh: "my conclusion from the observations I have been able to make is that enough has not been done at Edinburgh to conciliate that class of persons who by their influence with the lower orders caused much of that extreme repugnance to anatomy which at present exists".[3] The Association of Teachers apparently threatened to take matters into their own hands, and in a letter to Knox, dated 25 March 1837, Somerville acknowledged "the great injury inflicted on the private schools" but counselled against adopting "extreme means".[4] At least he did not favour the university, as Craigie had, and in September Monro heard from the Home Secretary that Somerville had complained of "the manner in which the practice of Anatomy is carried on in the Dissecting Room under your charges [*sic*]".[5]

The more-or-less equal allocation of bodies among the members of the Association made it difficult for an exceptional teacher to enlarge his class. The records of pauper funerals at St Cuthbert's paid for by anatomy teachers suggest that, if anything, Knox's classes were declining: he dissected more bodies from the parish than Lizars in 1836, but fewer in 1838 and 1841.[6] In 1837, Knox had seventy-one enrolled students, compared with Lizars's ninety-eight and Handyside's fifty-one, each of whom paid three guineas for the complete anatomy course. Fifteen bodies cost £3 each, leaving Knox £178 13s out of which his other expenses had to be met.[7] He supplemented his income by performing minor surgery and bone setting, and "never resigned altogether the practice of a surgeon", though he "disliked the knife".[8] In addition, he sometimes performed autopsies in cases where women had died in childbirth and their accouchers feared the viscera might be contagious,[9] not work an anatomist would willingly undertake unless short of funds.

He continued his attempts to find an academic post, and in July 1837 wrote to the Lord Provost and Town Council to apply for the university chair in general pathology, which had been vacated by the resignation of John Thomson (1765–1846) due to ill-health:

> Of my qualifications as a Teacher of the most important branch of Medical Education, viz. Anatomy, the public has long ago given a favourable and far too flattering verdict, in the numerous Classes of Medical Students I have had the honour to teach, — Classes probably exceeding in numbers those taught by any individual in Britain in proportion to the time, and comprising, in addition to the strictly professional student, a large proportion of gentlemen in other ranks of life, and following other professions, such as distinguished Clergymen, Professors in the University, Advocates, &c., together with the sons and relatives of a great proportion of the Clergy of Scotland.[10]

Knox did not supply any testimonials, but added defiantly that "the determined opposition and hostility of numerous individuals . . . and corporate bodies" was the surest proof of his attainments. Despite his now habitual tone of haughty disdain, the letter put his case well and, as he pointed out, his "scientific status" was such that his candidature could hardly be "overlooked".[11]

The next day, as soon as they heard of Knox's application, a "junto"[12] of Edinburgh professors – Sir Charles Bell, W.P. Alison, Robert Christison and James Syme – wrote to the Council to propose the abolition of the chair, claiming that its continued existence would be "injurious to the interests of the Medical School". Six other professors – James Howe, George Ballingall, T.S. Traill, Thomas Charles Hope, R. Graham and James Hamilton – added their names to the letter, expressing "approbation", while Monro *tertius* merely concurred.[13] So keen were they to suppress the unwanted chair, they offered to pay Thomson's £150 annual retirement allowance, which would normally have been found by his successor, out of their own pockets.[14]

His prospective colleagues' antipathy to the post, which had been established by Royal Commission in 1831 against the wishes of the University Council, posed a problem for Knox, and in his application he imprudently advertised his disapproval of compulsory classes in pathology, which, he suggested, offered a crutch for "a Professor [who] cannot, by his own exertions, maintain the numbers and respectability of his class . . . ". The other professors may have agreed in principle that: "the medical student, like every other class of society, is entitled to obtain his education *where and how he likes*, and that to render any Chair whatever imperative is to create a scandalous monopoly, and is to a certain class of the community the height of injustice",[15] but it was the "imperative" subjects, for which students were obliged to purchase lecture tickets, that provided many of them with a guaranteed income.

Knox admitted having been "personally opposed" to Dr Thomson, and he may well also have opposed the creation of the very post for which he was now applying: the pseudonymous "Philo Scotus" who complained in the *Lancet* about the chair "unnecessarily" created for Thomson, "who never succeeded in teaching one of the many branches of medical science which he professed, nor in obtaining any place but by intrigue", certainly sounds like Knox.[16] Most men would have recognized that they could not expect to join the establishment and remain critical of it, but Knox, characteristically, stuck to his guns. His impolitic first letter was a model of restraint compared with the second, in which he described the creation of imperative chairs as "Diffusion of Useless Knowledge", the Chair of Clinical Surgery – held by his old rival Syme – as "odious", and "compulsory attendance on the lectures of *particular individuals*" and payment of fees "to *particular colleges*" as "oppressive in the highest degree, iniquitously unjust, and simply devised to suit the views of corrupt corporate bodies."[17]

In his own letter the Lord Provost, Syme proposed that the chair be abolished and the lectures divided up between the other professors. He was dismissive of independent teachers, and argued that a "public" appointment, rather than popularity, betokened academic authority: the extra-academical lecturers, he wrote, clearly with Knox in mind, "led away" students "through the inducement of smaller fees, the influence of private solicitation, or the deception of popular arts, making arrogant assumption take the appearance of qualification to instruct."[18] Although the Town Council was keen to suppress the chair for financial reasons, the Home Secretary insisted that it remain. Thomson therefore withdrew his resignation, and it was agreed that his son William would give the lectures.[19]

Lonsdale noticed a "marked change of feeling" on the part of the Fellows of the Royal Society of Edinburgh towards Knox in or around 1833, though he was sure the rumour that this was due to the West Port murders "need not be entertained for a moment". That the University of London considered Knox for a chair in 1836 indicates that he was not *persona non grata* in the wider academic world, and suggests that any ill feeling in Edinburgh was personal. Lonsdale attributed the falling out between Knox and his colleagues to his sharp tongue and pen.[20] He was certainly a vocal critic of the Royal Society, though despite asking why anyone should "throw away" money on an organization that was "rapidly hastening to the guidance of banker's clerks, fifth-rate medical practitioners and the like", where they would gain "nothing of science, and as little honour", he continued to pay his dues.[21]

Caustic wit in academic settings adds spice to otherwise dry proceedings, and is often relished by those who are not its targets, but Knox, who enjoyed playing to the gallery, overindulged. On 4 December 1837, the hall of the Royal Society was crowded with members eagerly anticipating not the advertised paper on herring and salmon, but an outburst from Knox, which was widely applauded when it came. Charges of plagiarism and inaccuracy made against him by John Stark, a printer and amateur naturalist, brought down a scathing rebuke on this "dabbler in science", who "appeared *Stark* raving mad", and who, to the indignation of Professors Christison, Syme and Traill, Knox accused of being the cat's paw of a "professorial clique".[22] While Lonsdale may well have been correct in his claim that Knox's performance was funnier than a music hall turn, the use of the kind of rhetoric enjoyed by students in the setting of a learned society was an error of judgement. It seems Knox's delight in winning arguments by sheer force of oratory got the better of him, for he had mastered his temper since his days in the Cape, and had earned a reputation for being impossible to provoke: when one of Monro's students called him, to his pocky face, "the ugliest fellow I ever saw in my life", Knox patted him on the shoulder and replied "then you cannot have seen my brother Fred".[23]

Meanwhile, Somerville continued with his apparently well-meaning efforts to help the private teachers. He proposed allocating bodies according to the number of pupils registered at each school, which might have gone some way towards alleviating the inequalities of distribution: "if the supply received by the Schools at Edinburgh is not yet fully adequate to the demand", he wrote optimistically in 1838, "it is at least satisfactory for me to be able to report a gradual increase . . . ".[24] When the Anatomy Act had been passed, Somerville had been among those who anticipated "abundant opportunities" for anatomists to dissect unclaimed bodies from the "various charitable institutions".[25] According to Jones Quain, the professor of anatomy at University College, the "unclaimed bodies" from two London parishes alone would have been sufficient to supply all the metropolitan anatomy schools.[26] It turned out, however, that although many Edinburgh folk ended their days in institutions – mortality at the Royal Infirmary was one in eight, and the House of Refuge for the destitute, opened in 1832 during the cholera epidemic, admitted sixteen hundred persons annually – the number of unclaimed bodies was "very small": about a hundred a year.[27]

In the winter session of 1837–8, a total of eighty bodies were dissected in the Edinburgh schools: fifteen at Knox's school in Old Surgeons' Hall, thirty-two at the University, twenty-one at Lizars's Argyle Square establishment and twelve at Handyside and Robertson's school at 4 Surgeons' Square. The number of bodies dissected in the private schools continued to decline over the next three years, and although the number of dissections at the university increased, Edinburgh was beginning to lose students.[28] Apart from the lack of bodies – he presided at a students' meeting on the subject – Lonsdale blamed the longer and more expensive curriculum, "senile" professors, and competition from London, Dublin and the English provincial schools for the city's failing fortunes.[29] Anatomy was "the Alpha and the Omega" of medical training, the only "proper" way to study it was "by actual dissection of the dead body", and London, where 322 bodies were dissected in a year, was the new anatomical capital of Britain.[30]

Knox was leading "a most laborious life" in 1838, though he found a few weeks of leisure in the summer to visit Wales and Holland, where he saw Fremery's "very beautiful" museum in Utrecht, and pursued his racial studies in Amsterdam's bustling Jewish quarter, where he entered a crowded synagogue and was rewarded by standing "almost within reach" of a youth who was a "perfect likeness" of the Ancient Egyptian Memnon.[31] In 1839, he left Old Surgeons' Hall and took over the School at 11 Argyle Square (he was licensed there on 16 October[32]) from Alexander Lizars, who had moved to Aberdeen as professor of anatomy. Though Knox's classes were no longer the largest (he had 103 pupils to John Lizars's 125,[33]) he was still "exceedingly occupied" with lecturing, which left him little time for academic work, and he completed a translation of de Blainville's lectures with the merest nod to transcendentalism: "with respect to this subject, almost as many different views are held, as there are distinguished comparative anatomists in Europe".[34]

The Knox brothers continued to add to their private museum: the unambitious Frederick, a skilled preparator who rarely lectured, dissected exotic animals and mounted their skeletons for display while Robert published the descriptions.[35] "Brother Fred's" reluctance to allow students to use his carefully prepared specimens could be exasperating, but his tranquil nature was a welcome relief from his impulsive brother.[36] It appears, however, that the school's income was inadequate to support them both, for in March 1838 Robert approached his ex-pupil the Marquis of Breadalbane (like many radicals, he dearly loved a Lord, and frequently dropped Breadalbane's name in lectures[37]) in an attempt to secure for Frederick a place as "Naturalist and Surgeon" on an expedition to Northern Australia: a passage on a convict ship, he suggested, would enable Frederick to make the trip "free of expense".

Robert's letter to Breadalbane is a typical specimen of his peculiar combination of hectoring and pleading: having apologized for troubling him with such a request, he then bemoaned at length the iniquities of the patronage system through which "Chairs in Our University" are "bestowed in the most reckless and shamefull [sic] manner", which sounds like sour grapes after his own repeated failure to obtain one.[38] Knox's ambitions for a university career in Edinburgh had been effectively ruined by his letters to the Lord Provost, but he continued to air his grievances against "scientific coteries" who, he wrote in the *Lancet*, were aware of his "contempt for them, and the thorough acquaintance I have of the mean arts by which they have foisted themselves into notice . . . ".[39]

In April 1839, anticipating the loss of Frederick's services, he solicited John Goodsir to join him, but he declined.[40]

Knox continued to take a leading rôle in the Association of Teachers, and was in the chair on 20 September 1839 when they passed a motion to raise a subscription of £2 from each teacher of surgery and £4 from each anatomist for "funeratories": mortuaries in which unclaimed bodies could be kept prior to dissection. The cost of a funeratory was estimated at £400, which the teachers expected to recoup from their pupils.[41] Ten days later, Knox chaired a second meeting at which it was agreed that, as the funeratories would also be of benefit to the university, its teachers should be asked to contribute. James Hope Jr, the Clerk to the Royal Infirmary, replied on Monro's behalf that a contribution would be forthcoming only if the Association promised to avoid any "interference" with bodies at the Infirmary – where mortality had now risen to one in six – "until the wants of the University are satisfied".[42] Alexander Lizars agreed to these terms on behalf of the Association, on the understanding that the University would be supplied "upon the same terms as the Teachers of Anatomy and Surgery".[43]

It was an uneasy compromise, and at the start of the 1839–40 session, Somerville visited Edinburgh to hear the teachers' grievances. The result was "the Regulations for the Equitable Distribution of Bodies", which stated that all unclaimed bodies, including those from the Infirmary, were to be moved to the funeratories and distributed among the teachers in order of "seniority", taking into account the number of pupils in each school.[44] The teachers agreed to this, and to fines of £5 and £10 for those who infringed the new regulations.[45]

The funeratory system was unique to Edinburgh, where "[a] very unconscionable number of the Poor . . . find refuge in the Workhouses". If they died there "there was no system of removal by Parish Undertakers as in London"; instead, the Kirk Session (the equivalent of the parish council in England) provided a coffin and a grave, and the "rites" were "usually conducted in a very dense meshbrushead [sic] followed by a Concourse of friends and neighbours who considered it a mark of respect to follow the funeral." In the presence of so many witnesses, it was "impossible to remove bodies directly" to the anatomy schools, hence the need for "a Public Dead House for the Parish to be called a *Funeratory*", to which "all Bodies whatever in the Parish requiring gratis funerals" were taken "prior to interment". The funeratory was to be "sufficiently capacious to contain a supply of Coffins, provide for the residence of a Keeper, and afford room for the assembly of friends to follow the funerals."[46] Relatives or friends could claim a body from the funeratory if they were prepared to pay for the funeral, while all unclaimed bodies were taken to the dissecting-rooms, and thence to Greyfriars Kirkyard, to be buried at the anatomists' expense.[47]

What is not clear from Somerville's account is why it was thought easier to remove *unclaimed* bodies from the funeratory than from hospitals or workhouses. The Edinburgh poor, who dreaded dissection – there were rumours that the remains were made into "'natomy pie" and returned as an unwelcome supplement to the meagre workhouse diet[48] – probably kicked up a fuss whenever they saw a body being unceremoniously carted away to Surgeons' Square, but if they could prevent bodies being taken to the anatomy schools directly from the workhouse, they could presumably also have prevented their being taken there via the funeratory. One possibility is that, as funeratories were in churchyards, which were deserted at nights, bodies might have been removed without the relatives' knowledge and the coffins filled with sand and nailed shut. There is no evidence to confirm such a theory, but it is difficult to imagine how else the relocation of pauper dead houses would have served to increase the anatomists' haul.

The Edinburgh out-lecturers enthusiastically commended the funeratory system to the Home Secretary; the Government, Kirk Session and parishes supported it, thus relieving themselves of the expense of pauper funerals, and Somerville thanked the "Lords Provost, Magistrates and Clergy of all denominations" for their "enlightened zeal" in "promoting the objects of the [Anatomy] Act." The City funeratory proved "very successful", though "the supply of bodies was still insufficient for the purpose" and, in view of this "emergency", Somerville and the teachers opened a second funeratory in St Cuthbert's parish. The anatomy teachers argued that having to pay for so many pauper funerals would "write a prohibition against the practice of Anatomy instead of encouraging it" and they applied for, and were granted, four hundred pounds a year from the exchequer "to promote the operation of the Anatomy Act in Edinburgh."[49]

CHAPTER ELEVEN

Nature's High Priest, 1840–1844

The Argyle Square School of Medicine, where Knox taught anatomy, Dr Sillan materia medica, and Dr Alexander Ward, medicine,[1] was run down by contrast to the grander and more spacious Old Surgeons' Hall: the dissecting-room was "dirty" and the subjects "stale", but Knox's rooms "attracted numerous visitors", who came to see his comparative anatomy specimens, and the *Medical Times* wrote very favourably of his classes, especially his short course on general anatomy. They also praised his textbook *The Edinburgh Dissector*, despite the errors that had found their way into that hastily printed volume. Knox disliked book learning of anatomy (in his introductory lecture in 1837 he had thrown a copy of the newly-published *Pocket Anatomist* contemptuously to the floor) and he somewhat shamefacedly published the *Dissector* anonymously ("by a Fellow of the College of Surgeons"), which may have accounted for its poor sales.[2]

The transcendentalist slant of Knox's lecturing was seen by some as a fault, as he tended to "diverge" onto philosophical questions and "shirk dry anatomical details", though he knew how to keep an audience attentive, and it was rare for a lecture not to include some "humour and ridicule". He told how, in the Cape, he had fired a musket at an elephant to test Monro's claim that the animal's skull was "bomb proof": unfortunately, he said, the ricocheting musket ball had struck the posterior of a nearby woman, thereby demonstrating "the interesting physiological fact that Hottentot ladies are not *bum proof*."[3] Those who have taught medical students will appreciate that a higher level of wit would have been wasted.

Students in general were less enthusiastic in the 1840s than when Knox had first returned from Paris: forced to collect certificates from a prescribed number of anatomy courses in order to enter for their examinations, they attended perfunctorily, or not at all, and lacked interest. The London schools were prospering at the expense of Edinburgh, and everywhere the Anatomy Act was squeezing out the independent teachers, whose dissecting-rooms were "so very badly supplied, that their work is almost at a stand-still: they cannot compete with the schools to which, being attached to hospitals, a certain, though still a very insufficient number of bodies, *must* come."[4] The private schools' predicament led to rumours that body snatchers were again at work, and when the mutilated bodies, or parts of bodies, of murder victims turned up, they were examined by the police for signs of dissection.[5]

That the police suspected anatomists of dumping corpses in the street indicates the low esteem in which the profession was now held. Anatomy shocked Victorian sensibilities, which found the erstwhile beautiful science as unpleasant as it was irreligious. In 1843, William Greenhill recalled listening to his first anatomy lecture as a medical student with a "swimming head" and being disgusted by "a wax model of some of the internal organs": for the evangelical Greenhill, these were "fearful studies".[6] Even those who got through their obligatory anatomy classes without fits of fainting or religious doubt found them disagreeable and dangerous:

> Man doth shun the slimy frog,
> Croaking in the damp dark bog;
> But in the dissecting-room,
> There is more of filth and gloom;
> More of filth, with danger thick,
> If you do your finger prick.[7]

Declining student numbers at least left Knox more time for writing: he dashed off a monograph on the human ovary during a "few days of leisure" over the Christmas holidays,[8] and in the same year he wrote papers on gibbons, the heart, the placenta, and puerperal fever. His practical knowledge of human and comparative anatomy and of individual museum specimens was probably unrivalled in Britain, and his commentary on de Blainville's account of the orangutan and chimpanzee, published in the *Lancet* in May 1840, reads like a master correcting his pupils, though in his haste to disagree with Owen, Knox blunderingly stated that the orangutan possesses a *ligamentum teres*.[9] According to the *Medical Times*, he demanded "excessive" fees for his commissioned writing, though as that journal subsequently published a series of his articles he presumably became less demanding after his move to London in 1844.[10]

On 9 July 1840, Frederick Knox set sail for New Zealand aboard the six-hundred-ton barque *Martha Ridgway*, on her maiden voyage from London, with his wife and five children. As Surgeon Superintendent his passage was free but his medical skills were called upon almost immediately after leaving England, when smallpox broke out. There were no deaths from the disease, but they had to spend three weeks in quarantine on arrival at Wellington after more than four months and eleven thousand miles of sailing.[11] Frederick was one of Wellington's first doctors, and Hodgkin, who had contacts in the antipodes through the Aborigines Protection Society, provided him with some letters of introduction, and sent him books and instruments "for the benefit of the natives".[12] For a while he did not see any "bright prospect" there, but in time he settled into the routine of expatriate life, taking up, in addition to his medical practice, the post of librarian, and pursuing his interest in comparative anatomy.[13] He regularly exhibited his anatomical preparations to the Wellington Philosophical Society, until his death at the age of 82.[14]

His place as "demonstrator and partner" was taken by Lonsdale, who had worked as Knox's assistant during his student days but had returned to Cumberland after qualifying in 1838, suffering from "overwork".[15] Partnership with Knox was not the plum it had once been: the Argyle school was allocated only four bodies during the 1839–40 session, and in October 1840 Knox failed to pay his subscription to the funeratory fund. It is not clear whether he could afford to pay, but he made it a matter of principal not to, alleging that Monro had also failed to contribute.[16] He complained to Somerville that the fund was being mismanaged, and implored him to enforce the "Regulations for the Equitable Distribution of the Bodies in Edinburgh" sooner rather than later, but Somerville supinely awaited instructions from the Secretary of State.[17]

Somerville's insistence that Knox pay into the fund must have been infuriating as Monro, who the funeratory's manager William Campbell claimed had "contributed next to nothing", received "a much larger proportionate number of bodies" than the other teachers. Monro treated the funeratory system with contempt and "stood aloof from its concerns and arrangements": he could obtain bodies directly from the infirmary, which supplied about half of the total number, and there were rumours he was importing more from Paris.[18] Somerville told the Home Office that there was an "adequate" supply of bodies, and merely noted "some dissatisfaction" among the private teachers "at the University Professor being permitted to receive all the Bodies from the Royal Infirmary . . . at a time when bodies are scarce."[19]

Between 1839 and 1841, a group of extramural lecturers briefly combined their forces in a new venture, "Queen's College, Edinburgh", which despite its grand title was no more than a loose coalition of struggling teachers. "Dr Knox, Q.C." offered "anatomical demonstrations" and classes in "practical anatomy" and "operative surgery", the two last in conjunction with Lonsdale. Despite high overheads (bodies were £3 each), Knox's courses cost a guinea, among the cheapest on offer: most other medical subjects cost three guineas and mathematics, four.[20] As he struggled to keep the school going, Knox continued to provoke the scientific establishment: in correcting, for the *Lancet*, some passages in Meckel's *Comparative Anatomy* that he felt did not give sufficient credit to his own work, he took the opportunity to express his contempt for "members of the numerous scientific coteries of Britain".[21] Even the *Medical Times*, which was generally favourable towards him, saw that he was "hated by many of his contemporaries" and that he relied on "withering sarcasm" to browbeat his critics: "Many a cur would snarl – many an ass would kick – if they dared . . . ".[22]

Knox's critics got their opportunity to kick when he unwisely became embroiled in a row over plagiarism with his former assistant John Reid, who since 1838 had been pathologist to the Edinburgh Royal Infirmary. In a paper in the *London Medical Gazette* in October 1840, Knox described the anatomy of some vascular tufts in the placenta, which he claimed to have first observed in a specimen shown to him by Reid. His stated intention in publishing was to allow "the scientific public . . . to decide previous to the publication of Dr. Reid's memoir, in how far these observations of mine agreed, or were at variance, with the discoveries of [Ernest Henry] Weber", and he apparently intended to steal Reid's thunder:

> At the time I originally made these observations, I withheld their publication on the grounds . . . that they seemed to me to have been anticipated in all essential points by Weber. In what respect they may be found to coincide with Dr. Reid's more elaborate researches into the same subject, I cannot pretend at present to say, having seen but a very brief abstract of the memoir (in the Athenaeum) read by him to the meeting of the British Association held during the present autumn in Glasgow.[23]

It is not clear what reaction Knox expected from Reid after having announced that the latter's soon to be published observations were probably not new, and that even if they were, they were actually Knox's own. Nor is it clear why he was keen to dispute priority for a discovery that, but for the controversy it attracted, would hardly have been noticed. He did not betray any personal antipathy towards Reid, whom he called "my most esteemed friend and former pupil", but Reid delivered a stinging rebuttal, in which he began by putting Knox's accusation plainly: "the obvious and unavoidable inference must be, that I had pointed out at the British Association certain anatomical facts as having been ascertained by myself, while in truth I was indebted to Dr. Knox for them; and that he, from a feeling of delicacy, refrained from charging me openly with plagiarism."[24] Reid denied that the vessels were the same as those previously reported by Weber, and condemned the "deceitful conduct" of Knox in claiming that *he* had performed the dissections: Knox, said Reid, had been "merely a spectator, I can with all the solemnity of an oath declare, *that the various dissections stated by Dr. Knox to have been made on that occasion were not then made.*" He backed up this damaging claim with statements, signed by eleven medical colleagues, to the effect that it was he who had demonstrated the placental vascular tufts to Knox, who had reacted as though they were new to him.

Reid's crushing *ad hominem* attack on his "deceitful" former employer suggests that there was already no love lost between them: "if Dr. Knox's statements", he continued, "contained in the MEDICAL GAZETTE, had been restricted to Edinburgh, where he is well known, they would only on this, as on former occasions, have afforded subject of amusement to my friends and myself."[25] Reid may have over-reacted, but Knox's attempt to push his name forward lost him credit with the Edinburgh medical fraternity: it had not taken Reid long to find eleven colleagues prepared to put their names to a statement that effectively called Knox a liar. Chagrined that so many medical men had taken Reid's side, Knox avoided their company, preferring "to have no friends than doubtful ones"; he even cut John Goodsir in the street, until Lonsdale effected a rapprochement.[26] Reid went on to become professor of anatomy at St Andrews, where his promising career was cut short by cancer of the tongue at the age of forty. His biographers passed over the dispute with Knox, and posterity has not judged that either of the protagonists discovered anything of significance in the placenta.

In 1841, Knox made a final attempt to join the faculty of Edinburgh University by applying for the chair in physiology. Edinburgh's professors were chosen by the "provost, bailies, counsellors, and deacons" of the town: the university faculty could exert influence – as they had to prevent Barclay's appointment – but the decision rested with the Town Council. To some critics, and especially to Knox, it seemed "a great absurdity" for "ignorant men" to appoint "professors of learning". Knox's "biting, sarcastic" letter of application, in which he criticized the testimonial system and called attention to the failings of the other three candidates, two of whom, W.B. Carpenter and John Reid, were his former students, was characteristic of his inability to be diplomatic even when his career depended on it: not surprisingly, "[n]o one attempted to reply".[27] The appointee was Allen Thomson (1809–84), whose career until that point had mirrored Knox's: an Edinburgh MD, Fellowship of the Royal College of Surgeons of Edinburgh, training on the continent and an extra-mural anatomy lectureship in partnership with Knox's "particular friend" Sharpey at 9 Surgeons' Square. It must have been galling to lose out to a man whose anatomy class had ranged from twenty-two to twenty-eight students, while hundreds, according to Thomson's obituarist, had "flocked to the brilliant but egotistical lectures of the famous Robert Knox".[28]

Undeterred, Knox put himself forward for a lectureship in anatomy at the Scottish Academy, but failed to gain a single vote. Lonsdale, whose own candidacy had prompted Knox to apply, magnanimously called his mentor "unquestionably the fittest man" but both lost out to James Miller, who was shortly to become professor of surgery.[29] Other extra-mural anatomy teachers who found opportunities in academe were Alexander Lizars (1809–66), (Sir) William Fergusson (1808–77) and John Lizars, who became professors at Aberdeen, King's College and the College of Surgeons, respectively. In 1842 the ailing John Thomson finally resigned the Edinburgh chair of pathology, and though Knox did not reapply, he would hardly have been pleased to know that his old friend

Hodgkin had written to the Provost and Town Council to recommend the self-important ex-Inspector of Anatomy, David Craigie.[30]

Lonsdale maintained afterwards that Knox's pursuit of an Edinburgh chair had been thwarted by the Town Council's "religious scruples". The Council also appointed ministers of the Kirk, and Knox's avoidance of conventional religious observances may indeed have counted against him: he did not have a Kirk wedding or have his children baptized, and as far as we know he never attended church. Perhaps the established status of the Kirk deterred him, for he held firm Protestant views, which included a dislike of religious images and Scottish Catholicism.[31] Lonsdale also claimed Knox's marriage held back his career, and that he was so ashamed of his wife that he kept two establishments, a private family home and a professional address, where he lived with his sister.[32]

The 1841 census locates him ("Professor of Anatomy") at his official residence, 4 Newington Place, along with his sisters Mary aged "45" and Jessie, "41" (Mary was in fact 60 and Janet, 52), both of whom were described as being of independent means. Also resident were Jessie's orphaned son Thomas Birnie, aged 14, a 20-year-old Englishman named William Hunter (presumably a student), and a female servant.[33] Knox's wife and children were living out of the public gaze in the coastal parish of North Leith, on the Southern shore of the Firth of Forth, in Lilliput Cottage. It is to be hoped the name was meant ironically, since it was home to fifteen people, including the customs officer and his wife, five female servants, the 34-year-old Susan Knox and her six children: Mary (aged 14), Susan (12), Isabella (10), Robert (9), John (3), and one-year-old baby William. The Knoxes later had a seventh child, but only two survived into adulthood.[34]

Many friends and associates were probably unaware that Knox had a family: when he wished to entertain, he did so at Newington Place, which was the scene of many convivial evenings. Here he was free to present himself as "a man of refined taste and accomplishments": a classical scholar, conversationalist, lover of music, and dancer of anything from a graceful measure to an Irish jig. As a host, he was suave and diplomatic, smoothing over disputes with a ready wit and always *en rapport* with his audience, gently turning the conversation his way, monopolizing it, beguiling and winning over his listeners: a polyglot, polymath, and urbane sophisticate with polished Parisian manners, he was an incorrigible dandy, whose few remaining locks of brown hair were carefully coiffed with Mary's curling tongs before his visitors arrived. His reputation caused newcomers some qualms that his physiognomy – he looked like a "coarse and ugly revolutionist" – did little to dispel; but his strong personality, fund of stories and way with women usually charmed them in the end. "Have you heard the latest news?" he would enquire, before producing some piece of scandalous medical gossip. And then there were tales of his exploits in the Cape, "galloping among the vanguard across the plain" while the rest succumbed to sunstroke or enemy attacks. Young men new to Edinburgh were taken in by his traveller's tales and thought him unquestionably at home in "elegant society", but to those who knew better, he could seem selfish, indiscreet, evasive, even untrustworthy, and prone to hide the truth, except perhaps in matters of science.[35]

Though Susan Knox's secretive existence was never allowed to spoil her husband's polished performances, her death in 1841 from puerperal fever devastated him. "She is gone, she is gone!" he repeated to Lonsdale over and over again,[36] and this from a man famous for never losing his composure. In his bereavement, he considered emigrating to Australia, where he might have escaped not only Edinburgh's painful memories but also the worsening financial situation. The combination of an excess of medical graduates and a weak economy was making it difficult even for those with "connections" to get a living: one of Monro's medically qualified sons left Edinburgh in 1842 for New Zealand, where he eventually became speaker of the House of Representatives.[37] The London *Medical Times* used rumours of Knox's imminent departure as an opportunity to praise his work:

> He is a pre-eminently able and indefatigable anatomist; he has done more for his pupils than any other man. . . . He encouraged the industry of the tyro, not as Professor Monro and many others did, but by setting the example of industry *himself*. . . . he made use, during the scarcity and dearness of subjects, of every auxiliary means of plates, his museum, and constant attendance in the dissecting room, at that time [sic] could supply to make up for the inevitable deficiencies. . . . He was coldly regarded by some of the professors, and by others as an innovator, and probably from those feelings of envy and jealousy, which are so notoriously characteristic of the MEDICI FAMILY.[38]

Yet despite "many" deprivations, the "great teacher of anatomy" chose to remain in Edinburgh, and in 1842 he suffered a further blow when his four-year-old son John died of scarlet fever. Lonsdale and Knox were the only mourners.[39]

In the same year, the decline in Knox's professional fortunes was hastened by Somerville's dismissal as Inspector of Anatomy for complicity in transgressions of the Anatomy Act in London.[40] Though he had failed to uphold the letter of the Act, Somerville had at least been mindful that the situation in Edinburgh called for particular "judgement and caution". His successor Rutherford Alcock reintroduced a separate anatomy inspectorate for Scotland, which he placed under the charge of Dr Alexander Wood, an inflexible bureaucrat who set himself the task of "assisting the Lecturers to extricate themselves from the load of debt which had occurred from mismanagement of the Funds".[41] Wood's campaign effectively ended Knox's teaching career, in the course of which, he later estimated, he had taught some five thousand students.[42]

Though the supply of bodies for the 1841–2 season, the last full session Knox taught in Edinburgh, had been inadequate, he had nonetheless been in a favourable position compared with the other lecturers: in the first quarter he had received eleven bodies, more than anyone else except Monro, who received fifteen, and in the final quarter, from February to April, he received ten bodies to Monro's sixteen, the other extramural lecturers sharing fourteen between them.[43] The crisis came at the start of the 1842–3 session, when Knox abruptly moved to 31 Nicolson Street. David Skae succeeded him at Argyle Square, and Lonsdale, who had recently been licensed as a teacher at Argyle Square in his own right, joined Handyside at 1 Surgeons' Square. Lonsdale later told how Knox had offered an anatomy course in Edinburgh in the winter of 1842, "[r]egardless of both legal and moral obligations . . . but got no class".[44]

The most probable explanation for Knox's legal difficulties is his failure to make payments to the funeratory system. Wood was most particular about this, and though no relevant correspondence with Knox has survived, we know that when his successor at 31 Nicolson Street, Dr Macdonald, failed to make timely payments, Wood refused to send any bodies until he signed "a written agreement to conform to the rules of the funeratory".[45] Macdonald, who on his arrival in 1843 had "unfortunately mislaid" his license to teach anatomy, and who left the school after only one year, referred Wood's enquiries to Knox, who seems still to have been involved behind the scenes.[46] Even after Knox abandoned his attempts to lecture, his popularity with the Nicolson Street students was undiminished, and a toast to his name at a student dinner was "warmly responded to".[47]

Fifty years later, the acerbic Sir John Struthers, who attended Monro's lectures during the 1843–4 session ("a dreadful drone he was"), recalled hearing that Knox "had announced 'Anat[omy] & Phys[iology]' and was interdicted from proceeding after the intro[ductory] lecture".[48] This may have been the lecture that, fifty years afterwards, William Richardson remembered attending in or after November 1843.[49] Lonsdale, who was secretary and treasurer of the Associated Professors and Teachers of Anatomy and Surgery, who financed the funeratory system, must have known the facts underlying the failure of Knox's school, but chose to omit them from his biography.[50]

In 1843, with no class to teach, Knox accepted a commission from the *London Medical Gazette* to write a series of articles on transcendental anatomy, a subject "well known to most of my hearers", but hitherto hardly mentioned in print: the only British book on the subject was *Rudiments of Physiology* (1835) by John Fletcher, an Edinburgh MD who had taught anatomy at Argyle Square from 1828 until his death in 1836.[51] An early article in the series discussed the "tiger arm" – actually a human arm in which an aberrant foramen in the humerus mimicked a structure normally present in big cats – an obscure anatomical detail of no practical importance, which Knox had first noted in 1841, and which was to become his best-known anatomical discovery.[52]

For Knox, the significance of such functionless analogies between species lay in their suggestion of reversion to a more primitive type. In his *Medical Gazette* articles, he argued that "deformations" such as the tiger arm and variant forms of the human pelvis, which reproduced structures found in "animals placed lower than man in the scale", were the result of an "arrest of development", or persistence of the foetal type.[53] This was a well-established Geoffroyan theory that Knox invested with a degree of spurious novelty by disingenuously describing it as a "considerable modification" of the views of Goethe. As he churned out more articles, he refined and reconsidered his opinions: he expressed reservations about "arrest of development", and claimed there was "no truth" in the idea that the human embryo was "necessarily forced" to pass through a series of "metamorphoses". As an alternative, he adopted the *Naturphilosophische* idea that the interaction of pairs of opposing laws controlled development: deformations were produced when the "transcendental law" of "unity", which yielded a generic body plan, prevailed over the law of individuality, which gave rise to the particular form of a species.[54]

Knox found support for his rejection of arrest of development in his studies of hermaphrodites. Male and female genital organs were not formed by "metamorphoses" during embryonic life: both were present in the early embryo, but during the normal course of development one set disappeared. If this regression failed to occur, an hermaphrodite resulted.[55] This situation, he claimed, blithely disregarding any difference between sexual differentiation and species formation, was similar to that of the organs of respiration: initially, embryos had both gills and lungs, but as development proceeded one set of organs disappeared. In general terms, the embryo harboured multiple developmental possibilities of which only some were realized: a "bold hypothesis" that Knox alleged had first occurred to him as long ago as 1827.[56]

"[T]he philosophy of the animal organization, founded on an ideal analogy of organs, cannot be trusted", he wrote in 1843. Instead of a hypothetical ideal archetype, Knox attributed homologies between animals to their common origin from the embryo, which "embraces within its range all possible structures . . . ", including apparently functionless ones such as the human appendix, which he interpreted as "organs required by that portion of the animal kingdom which has ceased to exist."[57] It was crucial for transcendentalists to account for the existence of such vestigial structures, as their presence was a major embarrassment for the Creationist argument that perfect correspondence between form and function was evidence of intelligent design.

The arguments for purposeful design had recently been aired in a series of treatises published under the legacy of the Rev. Francis Henry Egerton,

Earl of Bridgewater, which were intended to show "the Power, Wisdom and Goodness of God as manifested in the Creation". Though Knox sneered at the "Bilgewater treatises" as "ingenious" but "downright nonsense" he did treat the natural world as evidence of a "creative idea" that was "essentially complex, yet simple, sublime, all foreseeing". However different in philosophical terms a "creative idea" was from a Creator, his thinking was apparently teleological, and his conception of Nature "foreseeing" that some animals would need lungs and "aiming" at beauty of form hovered uneasily between pleasing metaphor and pantheism.[58] He was, however, writing to order, under pressure of time – misspellings of names and failure to cite even his own papers correctly suggest that he had limited access to libraries – and the imperfect theories advanced in his *Medical Gazette* articles were themselves as yet embryonic.

Over the years, Knox kept in touch with Hodgkin in London; often treating him like a pupil – sending him requests to copy out information from a book "not worth purchasing" or to measure the skeleton of a whale – but uncharacteristically recognizing his "superior knowledge & judgement".[59] In 1843, Knox joined Hodgkin's newly founded Ethnological Society and, though not able to attend meetings in London, made useful "exertions" on its behalf, presumably by working to "procure an accession of members."[60] In January 1844, reduced to such financial straights that he skipped meals to save money and desperate for employment, Knox approached Hodgkin with a proposal for an expedition to the Cape.[61] Nineteen years earlier, when he had refused to help publicize the "very horrible" treatment of its indigenous peoples, Knox had told Hodgkin he would "never more mention even the name" of the Cape Colony. Now he suggested that if he were to "receive an appointment & be sent into the country amongst chiefs & people with whom he was formerly acquainted" he could assist the colonists in reaching an "understanding" with the "several tribes". It is unlikely that Knox, who had little contact with races other than the Khoi, except as an adversary, would have been accorded any special reception twenty-two years later, but he managed to convince the idealistic Hodgkin that he was "greatly attached" to the Cape, and had been "for years desirous of revisiting it."[62]

While Hodgkin tried to enlist the support of the Colonial Secretary, Lord Stanley, Knox approached the brother of Whig politician Lord Murray, "with whom I have the honour to be well acquainted". When things did not move swiftly enough, Knox goaded Hodgkin into action with tales of colonial atrocities of the kind he had once refused to make public: "You cannot credit the enormities now committing on the coloured races of Southern Africa and yet I can grant *these are the facts*", which are "perhaps better known to me than to any other now in Britain." He added a canny warning that Southern Africa "abounds with Jesuits", and suggested that the Society of Friends might prove more "efficient" than the Society of Jesus if they sent out "a small mission, which I should much prefer accompanying to any other body of men: Men of Peace – Something for the good of Mankind."[63] Knox seems to have been genuinely interested in a Quaker mission to the Cape, which he had first proposed as long ago as 1825, but he was clearly desperate for employment in any capacity: in September he tried to persuade a Glasgow merchant to fund a cattle and sheep rearing project in "extra-tropical South Africa".[64]

In the event, no support was forthcoming for the unlikely missionary, and Knox ventured less far afield, taking out a license to teach anatomy at the Portland Street School of Medicine in Glasgow, where, though classes were small, he "delighted" his audience, despite poor facilities and a lack of subjects.[65] The latter of these difficulties was due to the influence of the officious Wood, who refused to supply bodies because the school's surgical lecturer, Dr Lyon, had omitted to re-license himself for the Portland Street address.[66] Consequently, Knox received only three subjects for the 1844 session; in November the course had to be abandoned and he returned the students' money.

"[A]nything so low, so disgraceful, so entirely unprofessional as the state of the educational establishment and of the Medical and Surgical Faculty generally of Glasgow never did before exist in the world", Knox wrote to one of his erstwhile colleagues in Portland Street from London, where, disillusioned with "the state of things in Glasgow, Edin. and the North", he had decided to try his luck.[67] He disposed of his private museum, which "absolutely did not realize the price of the glass in which the preparations were placed", and he and his sisters gave up 4 Newington Place.[68] In 1844, his membership of the Ethnological Society was terminated because his annual subscription of two pounds remained unpaid.[69] "Poor Knox", wrote Struthers, "had become 'low' & a wanderer on the face of the earth".[70]

CHAPTER TWELVE

Popular Anatomy, 1845–1848

Though he remained licensed to teach in Glasgow, after 1845 Knox abandoned medical schools in favour of public lecturing, choosing as his subject "the races of men". Assisted by his son-in-law, W. Syme Wilsone, he gave "various courses of lectures", beginning with a series of six at the Philosophical Society of Newcastle and moving on to Birmingham, Manchester, Liverpool, Colchester, Sheffield, Chelmsford and Warrington, where his audiences were predominantly self-improving artisans.[1] He was never one to despise working-class audiences, for, as he wryly observed, the Apostles had mostly been "mechanics".[2] In London he addressed more genteel assemblies at the Royal Institution and the Athenaeum, but there were scant opportunities for medical teaching, as the profession was overcrowded and the number of students was in decline.[3] The University of London, the "godless college in Gower Street", which might have been a congenial employer, had already rejected him, and its Professor of Surgery was his old adversary Robert Liston. Professionally frustrated, Knox characteristically blamed his lack of connections: "mediocrity is your only chance, it secures your entrance into good society . . . in universities it is the only sure passport to a chair."[4]

A series of articles for the *Medical Times* provided much-needed income as well as a belated opportunity for sour grapes over the "snug but excessively paltry jobs" enjoyed by "Professors of pictorial anatomy".[5] After his rejection by the Scottish Academy, Knox was not inclined to be lenient towards artists who ventured into anatomical territory, and he published a scathing review of the first volume of Benjamin Haydon's *Lectures on Painting and Design* (1844):

> Mr. Haydon's Latin is like his English: *pisiform* is translated "neat little bone!" The number of bones in each finger is not even hinted at, nor the remarkable differences their joints exhibit; the forms of these even in a general way are not even hinted at. His theory as to the cause of the afflicting deaths of Lord Castlereagh and Sir Samuel Romilly (a brain overcharged with blood) is not new. We remember hearing a surgeon of some influence now, (Mr. Syme), bring it forward, and explain thereby the effort of the suicide as an attempt merely to relieve the overcharged brain. It is a poor theory; the Parisian leaps into the Seine in quest of death; women drown and poison themselves in a variety of

ways; men fire pistols at their own heads, all according to this theory to let the blood out and the cold air in. It will scarcely do.[6]

He could not have known that, within a year, Haydon would test the theory for himself: on 22 June 1846, he cut his throat and then shot himself in the head.

Knox's personal tragedies continued: his daughter Isabella, whom he had left behind in Edinburgh with her aunt Mary, died on 15 December 1845 at the age of fifteen.[7] That winter, he revisited Paris to inspect Felix Thibert's collection of anatomical models, and on returning to the *Jardin des Plantes* was disconcerted to find Cuvier's museum "gloomy, deserted, mouldering, decayed".[8] As a business venture, however, the trip was a success, and Knox was engaged to manage Thibert's museum in London, which was to display models of "the more instructive parts of the human anatomy to popular audiences."[9]

The museum, which opened in the spring at the Cosmorama Rooms in Regent Street, home in happier times to such attractions as "the singing mouse", comprised two rooms: a "popular" display of coloured models of fruit, fish and birds, and a "museum of anatomy", which ladies were not permitted to enter, wherein were found models of venereal and skin diseases, monstrosities, and microscopical preparations.[10] Knox took his responsibility for promoting the museum seriously: in a lecture to the Pathological Society of Birmingham he stated that attempts to preserve the original colour and appearance of real anatomical specimens were doomed to failure, and that anatomical waxworks were expensive, fragile, and able to shed light only if "converted into tapers". The only models he recommended were, of course, those to be seen in Thibert's museums in London and Paris.[11] At the first annual meeting of the British Association for the Advancement of Science, in September 1846, he demonstrated coloured models of "all kinds of fishes", but when questioned about Thibert's method of manufacture replied obtusely "that he was not at liberty to state more than that it was a plaster cast painted."[12]

Possession of a museum was still regarded as a *sine qua non* for an anatomy teacher, and since it required much labour and "considerable expense" to prepare and preserve real specimens the manufacture of wax or plaster substitutes was potentially lucrative.[13] Many continental medical schools used anatomical models, but British schools tended to regard them as an inferior option and they were mostly to be found in public museums rather than professional settings.[14] In Britain, the popular audience for anatomy was much larger than the professional one: in two months during 1847, 974 members of the public visited the museum of the Edinburgh College of Surgeons compared to only forty-nine medical students.[15] Like other forms of working-class education, popular anatomy was linked to a radical agenda, and while it was "nonsense", according to the American founder of the Working Man's Party, Thomas Skidmore, to suppose that men acquired rights by being lectured on anatomy, medicine, painting, or anything else, self-knowledge *was* a step towards self-determination.[16] The chartist William Lovett published *Elementary Anatomy and Physiology* to promote social "improvement" as well as physical well being: knowing one's own body and mind were prerequisites for assuming social responsibility.[17]

The ethos of popular anatomy exhibitions was one with which Knox may well have sympathized, since an acquaintance with the basics of anatomy and physiology empowered visitors to exercise control over their own health. Unfortunately, such public exhibitions were usually short lived, as visitor numbers dwindled after the initial enthusiasm had passed. Thibert's models were fêted in France, where the *Institut* awarded him a Monthyon prize, but the London museum survived for only a few months: it quickly moved to more modest premises at 29 Bridge House Place, Newington Causeway, where it was open from 11a.m. to 4 p.m. three days a week, and in August 1846 all 1,200 models were advertised for sale.[18] Shortly afterwards, Knox's association with the collection seems to have come to an end. It briefly reopened at 7 Westminster Road, but failed to prosper and in 1848 it was again put up for sale.[19] Sarti's Museum of Pathological Anatomy, back in London after eight years on tour, replaced Thibert's in the Cosmorama Rooms, where it promised to teach the visitor "the absolute necessity of putting implicit faith in those men who have made Anatomy and Physiology the study of their lives."[20]

The status of popular anatomy museums has been much debated: were they, as medical authorities at the time alleged, "indecent and demoralizing", a pretext for sensation and titillation, or was "the universal study of anatomy" really the best way to avoid diseases of "a sexual nature"?[21] Perhaps Knox's earnest efforts to popularize anatomy were not sensational enough: Joseph Kahn, whose Anatomical Museum opened in Oxford Street in 1851, when London was thronged with visitors to the Great Exhibition, lectured on "Abuses of the Generative Organs", spermatorrhoea, venereal disease and "Men with Tails", and his museum survived, largely on profits from the sale of quack remedies, until 1872, when the medical profession declared it obscene and forced it to close. To present anatomy to the public, as Knox did, was to court professional disapproval: one of the earliest erasures from the register of the General Medical Council for conduct unbecoming a medical practitioner was for publishing an "Illustrated and Descriptive Catalogue of the Subjects Contained in the London Anatomical Museum".[22] With most professional avenues closed to him, however, Knox had little option but to capitalize as best he could on his reputation as the best-known anatomist in Britain.

In the autumn of 1846, he wrote to the prime minister Lord John Russell and the colonial secretary Earl Grey to propose a survey of Africa, but despite the support of the Marquis of Breadalbane and Sir George

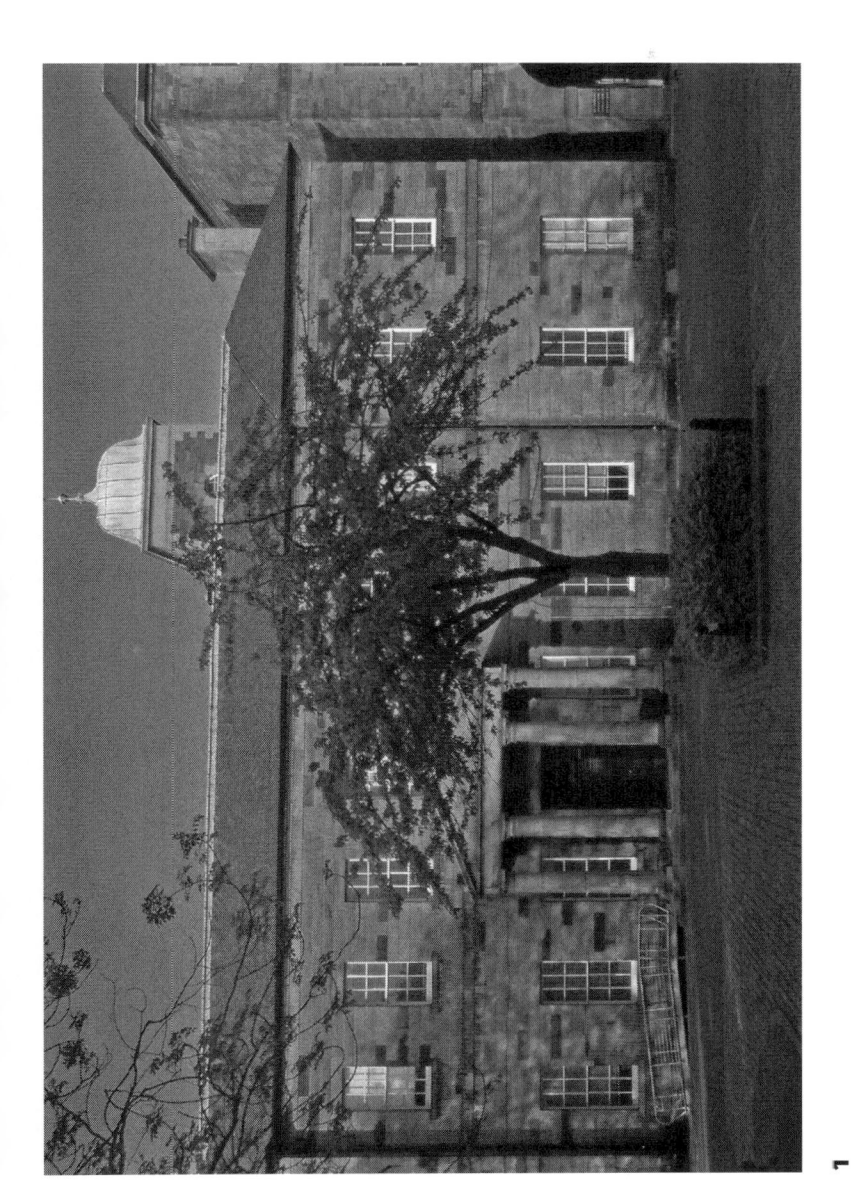

1
Edinburgh's High School, which Knox attended from 1806 to 1810. The building is now part of Edinburgh University
(photograph by the author)

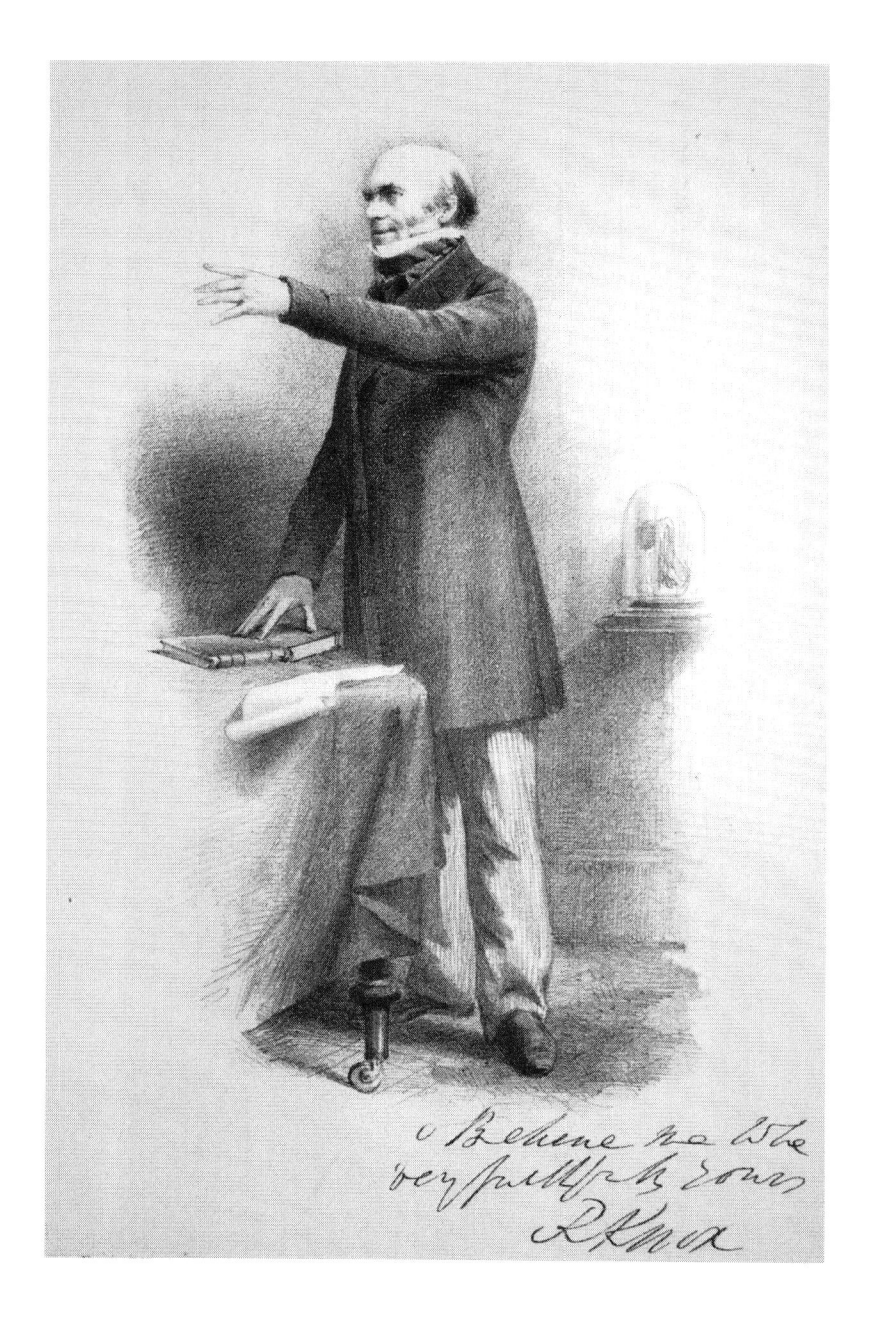

2
Dr Knox lecturing
(from the author's collection)

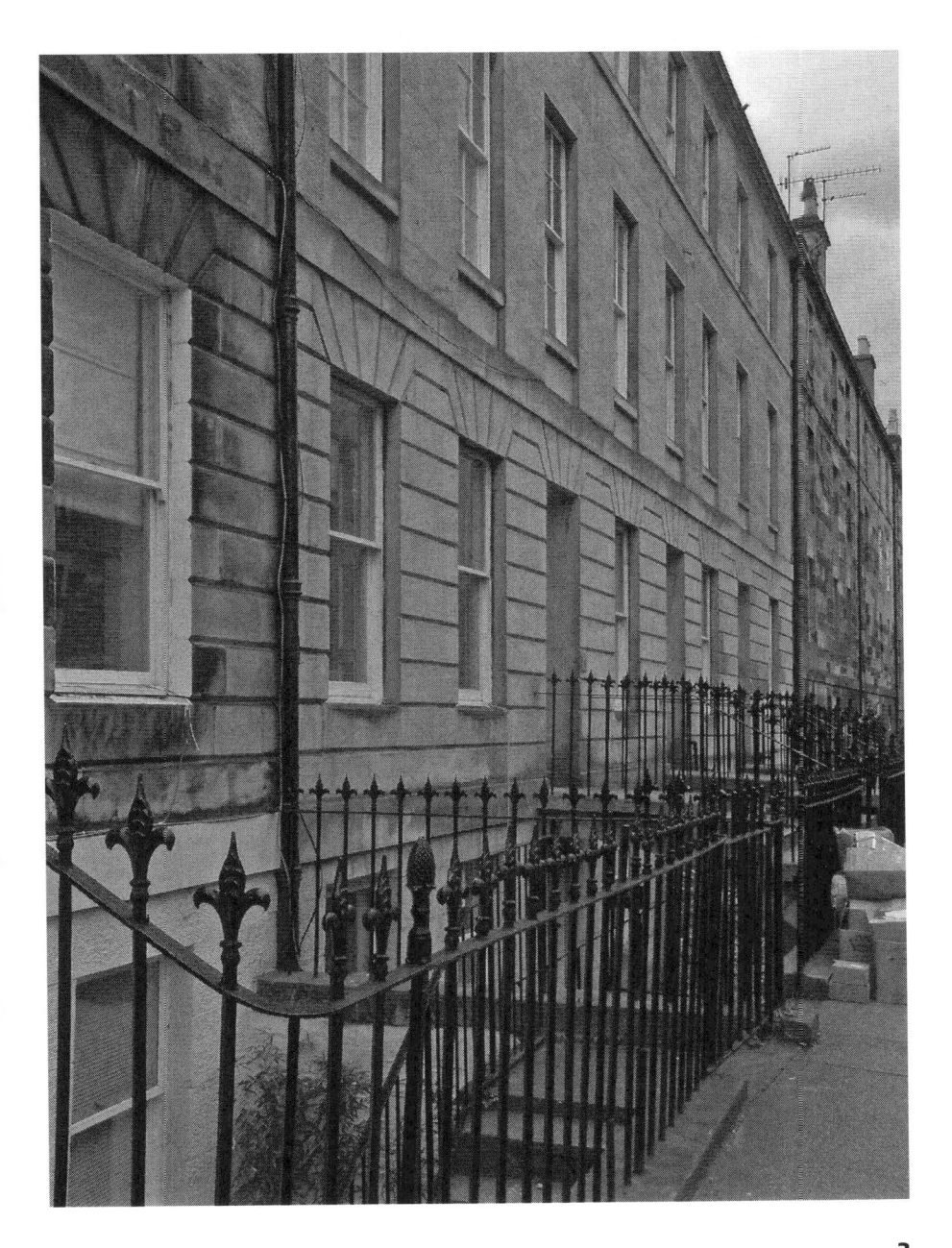

3
Knox's official Edinburgh home at
4 Newington Place
(photograph by the author)

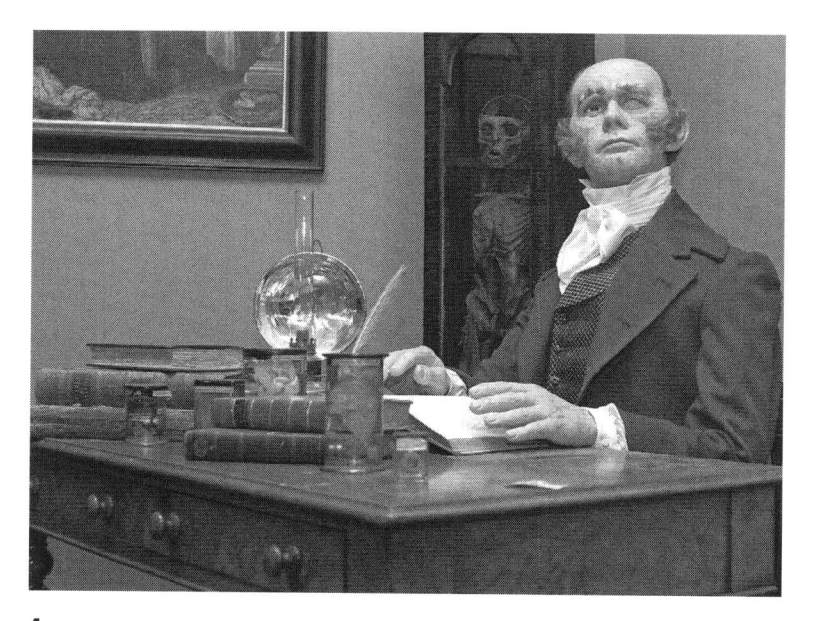

4
A display from the Jules Thorn Museum of the Royal College of Surgeons of Edinburgh, showing Knox with his textbook of anatomy.

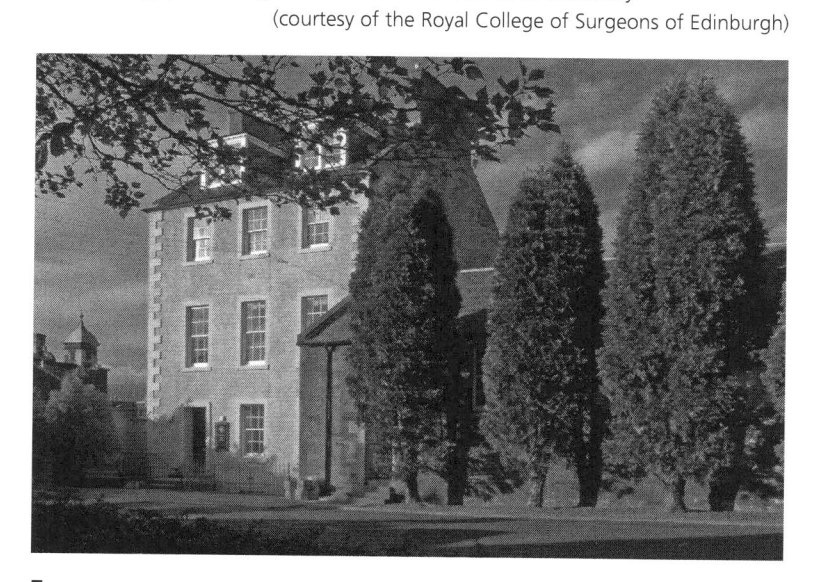

(courtesy of the Royal College of Surgeons of Edinburgh)

5
One of the few remaining houses in Edinburgh's Surgeons' Square; No. 1, formerly Handyside's school of anatomy, which Lonsdale joined after leaving Knox

(photograph by the author)

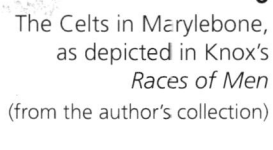

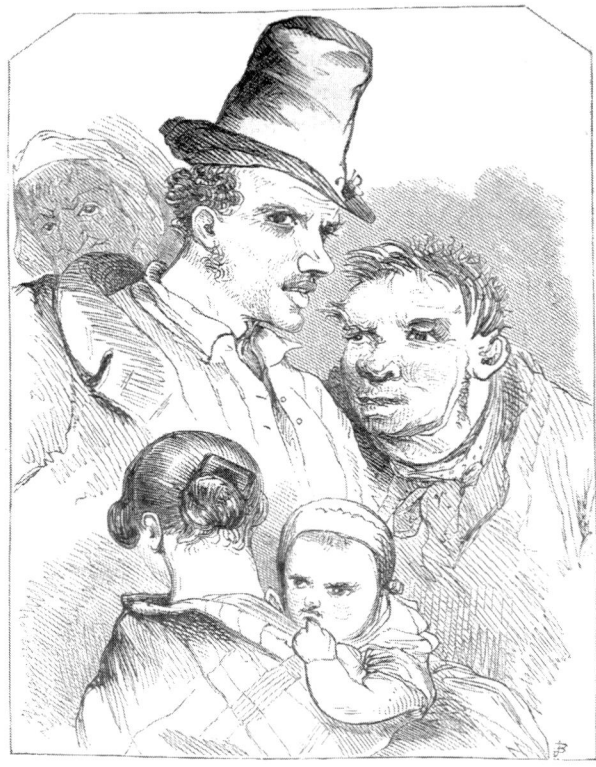

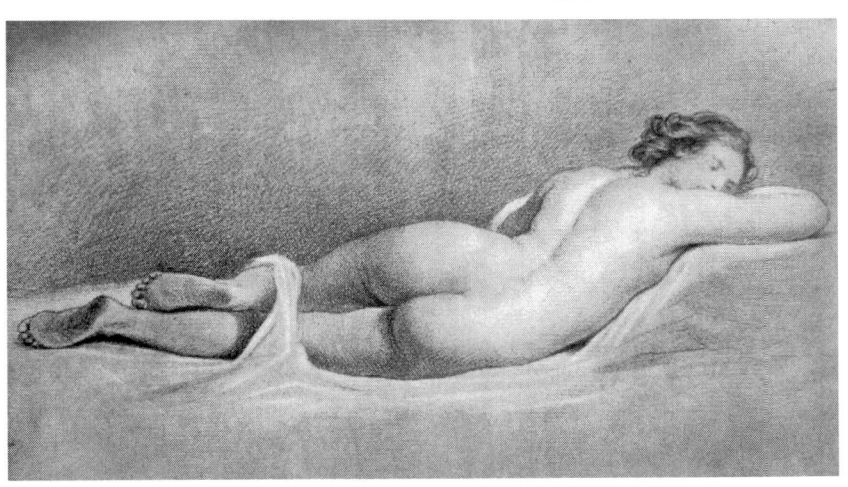

6
The Celts in Marylebone,
as depicted in Knox's
Races of Men
(from the author's collection)

7
Mary Paterson as Venus in the dissecting room;
from a drawing, now lost, by John Oliphant
(from the author's collection)

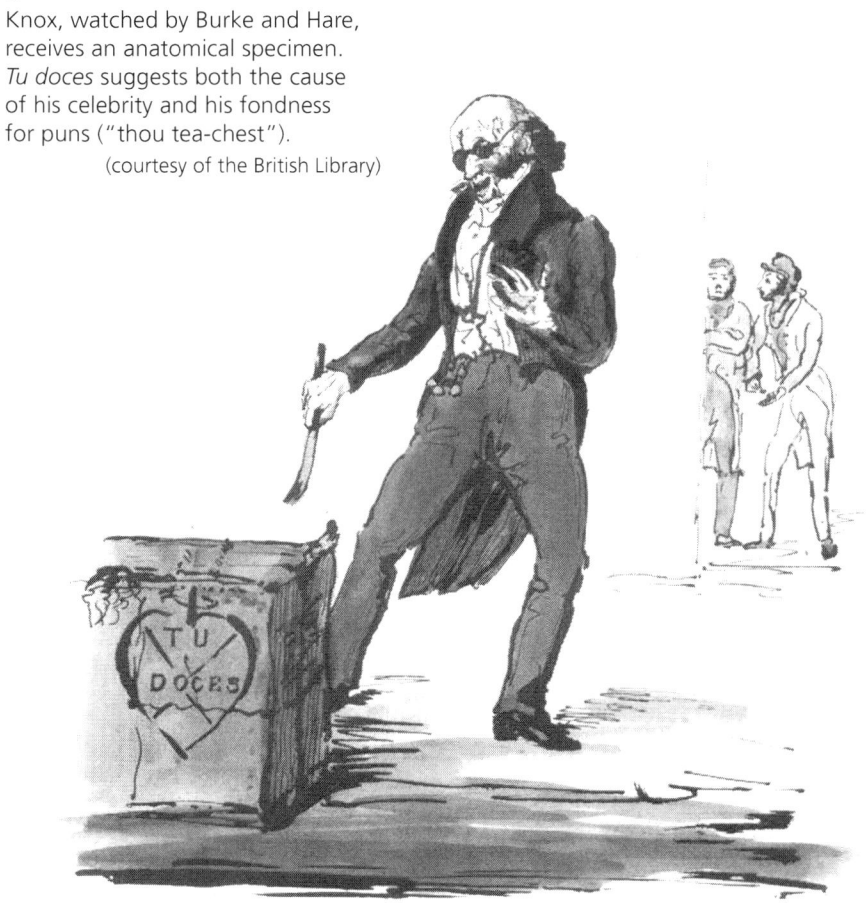

8
Knox, watched by Burke and Hare, receives an anatomical specimen. *Tu doces* suggests both the cause of his celebrity and his fondness for puns ("thou tea-chest").
(courtesy of the British Library)

Sinclair he failed to win government backing. Undaunted, in August 1847 he sent Lord Lincoln, the commissioner for woods and forests, his plans for the colonization of South Africa, and at Christmas, while staying with Mary and the family at 15 Clarke Street, Edinburgh, he approached the wealthy scientific amateur David Milne (later David Milne Home) with a proposal for "an Agricultural School or College" in the city.[23] Though all these projects concerned matters within the ambit of Knox's extensive professional experience, his willingness to move from one abortive scheme to the next suggests intellectual and possibly financial desperation. He seems to have accepted any public engagement he could: in Liverpool he addressed the Mechanics' Institution on "the structure of the human frame" and in Bristol the "celebrated anatomist" witnessed a performance of mesmerism in the presence of the "World's Sweetest Singer", the soprano Jenny Lind.[24]

The customary outlet for Knox's energies was controversy, and in 1846 he found himself, uncharacteristically, on the side of the authorities. James L. Warren, late surgeon of the 7th Hussars, had accused coroner Thomas Wakley of misconduct during an inquest into the death of Private Frederick John White. The case was a *cause célèbre*, with both press and public outraged that White had received a hundred and fifty lashes for striking a sergeant: he had walked away whistling after the punishment, but within a month he was dead. At autopsy, the cause of death was found to be inflammation of the pleura and heart, "in no wise connected with the corporal punishment", but the coroner's jury thought otherwise, and Wakley certified death as due to flogging.[25] Warren accused Wakley of publicly admonishing him and his fellow officers for complicity in White's death and of instructing counsel to draw up charges against them before the jury had reached its verdict. Warren's allegations were supported by affidavits from a varied group including Knox, Sir James McGrigor, Lt. Col. Shirley, the surgeons Francis Reid and Horatio Grosvenor Day, Sergeant Potter, and Privates Kelley and Weir, but Wakley denied any wrongdoing and the court found no evidence against him other than hearsay.[26]

The following year, Knox once more found himself the subject of scandal, this time concerning his certification of the attendance of one John Henry Osborne at his anatomy classes. Osborne had qualified "College and Hall", with diplomas from the Royal College of Surgeons of England and the Society of Apothecaries, but some of his colleagues were suspicious that the certificates he had produced in order to sit the examinations must have been false, since he had attended only six months of lectures. John Edward Fosbrooke, a Nottingham apothecary, wrote to the Apothecaries' Court of Examiners to draw their attention to Osborne's supposedly bogus certificates, including one signed by Knox on 1 May 1840, which stated "that Mr. John Henry Osborne attended my anatomical demonstrations at the School of Queen's College, Argyle-

Square, Edinburgh, from the fourth day of November, one thousand eight hundred and thirty-nine, to the first day of May, one thousand eight hundred and forty; that this course included 100 demonstrations; and that he carefully dissected during the same period."

This could not possibly have been true: for part of that period Osborne had still been at school, and at no time during the 1839–40 session had he been in Edinburgh. The Apothecaries found no proof of fraud, and upheld Osborne's qualification to practise, but Fosbrooke was not prepared to let the matter drop and sent a mass of documents to the *Lancet* to substantiate his charge. It is a wonder he found time for his medical practice in between gathering evidence – Knox was abroad, but Fosbrooke corresponded with several other Edinburgh medical men, one of whom suggested that Osborne had "probably" obtained Knox's certificate from Mr Maddence, one of his demonstrators, though Fosbrooke apparently heard from Knox that the certificate was "substantially correct".[27] The *Lancet* took up the cause: Osborne had certificates that attested to his having been in two or even three places at once, and as Knox maintained that his signature was genuine, the *Lancet* concluded that "All the suspicion which attaches to this part of the case consequently lies at the door of Dr. Knox". This seems an unjustified assumption, since Osborne's other certificates could also have been false, and it is possible that the mercurial Wakley had been prejudiced by Knox's support for Warren during the White case.

There is no proof that Knox's certificate was a calculated fraud; he may simply have made a mistake and signed without checking the records. The certificate system, however, was inherently open to abuse, as neither teacher nor student benefited from being too scrupulous. Lecturers were well liked by students if, like Dr Philanthus, an "exceedingly good-tempered" lecturer in a *Medical Times* skit, they "filled up all their schedules [*i.e.* certificates] whether they attended or no, and put 'very diligently' to all".[28] At the shadier end of the scale there were those who, for a few guineas, were prepared to sign up students they had never seen for lectures that may never have been given, though even this deception was purely an offence against bureaucracy, as a student could qualify only if, like Osborne, he passed his examinations.[29] Unfortunately for Knox, the newly regulated medical profession was particularly sensitive about "false certificates" – qualifications were, after all, what separated them from quacks – and his carelessness in signing them earned him a reputation for being "wholly unscrupulous".[30]

As a consequence, the Edinburgh College of Surgeons refused to accept Knox's certificates in future, and notified the other British examining boards of their decision, which effectively barred him from teaching medical students anywhere in Britain.[31] In 1847, his subscription unpaid, he was "ejected" from the Royal Society of Edinburgh and his election was retrospectively cancelled,[32] though despite, or perhaps because of, this mean-spirited decision, Knox continued to claim the fellowship of the society that he had often pretended to despise. He made London his home, and though, amid the "miles of hideous brick walls", he dreamed of Scotland and the Cape, he never left England again: the nearest he came to his homeland was Macready's *Macbeth* at the Princess's Theatre, but the "horrible burlesque" failed to move him, and to his experienced eye the blasted heath looked "very awkward".[33]

CHAPTER THIRTEEN

The Races of Men, 1848–1851

One of the enduring Knoxian myths is that he ended his days as "showman" to a "travelling party of Ojibbeway Indians".[1] His involvement with popular ethnological shows certainly seems, at times, to have been other than scientific: a group of "Bushmen" – two men, two women, and an infant – who arrived in London in 1846 were shown in the *Pictorial Times* performing a "native dance" under his direction, and he lectured on them at Piccadilly's Egyptian Hall, which had recently hosted such attractions as a "mammoth horse", a "polar dog", and "Professor Kist's Poses Plastiques".[2] Whatever the intent of this exhibition, there is little doubt it confirmed many people's prejudices: Charles Dickens remembered their "horrid little leader . . . in his festering bundle of hides", and wished that such people might be "civilized off the face of the earth".[3]

For an anatomist of Knox's standing to be associated with these "human zoo" exhibitions was something of a fall from grace, but as he had no English medical qualification his status in London was on a par with other foreign MDs, many of whom resorted to public lecturing or quackery as the only forms of practice open to them. Popular "a-shilling-admission-lectures" brought out the worst in lecturers, who eked out their "slender acquirements" with magniloquent talk;[4] though Knox would scarcely have accepted such work had he held a university post, it did have the merit of allowing him to speak on the subject of race, a topic he had had been obliged to pass over when training students for their examinations, and the lectures he gave were adapted and published, as a series of twenty-four, in the *Medical Times*.

Knox's studies were in the tradition that would later be called physical anthropology, which had its origins in the eighteenth-century, when philosophical speculations backed by observations of savages and feral children had called into question the assumption that humans were by definition rational creatures. If savages lacked both language and understanding, what was it that made them human? The challenge was to locate human characteristics of the body rather than of the intellect or spirit: to be human, and to belong to a particular race, became matters of morphology, and distinctions between apes and men, and between one race and another, were sought in the body's interior.

The quantification of anatomical differences between races was first attempted through studies of cranial morphology such as the Dutch anatomist Pieter Camper's (1722–89) "facial angle" – a measurement of the slope of the face that was supposedly greatest in Negroes and least in classical statuary – which promised to put racial distinctions on a measurable, scientific footing, as phrenology was attempting to do for character and intellect. John Hunter, who was probably influenced by Camper, presented a graded series of skulls, from ape to man, when he lectured at the Royal Academy – the series can be seen in the open book in Reynolds's famous portrait – and the German physiologist and collector of human crania Johann Friedrich Blumenbach (1752–1840) noted that "seen from above and from behind, placed in a row on the same plane . . . the racial character of skulls . . . strikes the eye so distinctly at one glance, that is not out of the way to call that view the vertical scale".[5]

By the nineteenth century, the racial scale based on a skull series had become something of an anatomical cliché. Guy's Hospital museum, under Hodgkin's curatorship, contained twenty-five Caucasian skulls arranged in series according to their resemblance to other "varieties" (*i.e.* races), including "Indians", South Sea Islanders and Knox's "Caffre".[6] Camper, Hunter, Blumenbach and Hodgkin made no claims for the superiority of particular races or for transmutation of one to another over time, but human skulls arranged in sequence with those of apes were easy to (mis)read as a hierarchy: if human races were part of the great chain of being, might not some "inferior" races constitute separate species between apes and civilized men? This was how it appeared to Charles White, a Manchester physician who heard Hunter lecture and was inspired to write *An Account of the Regular Gradation of Man* (1799), in which he proposed "a gradation from the European man to the brute", with the "African", who was not descended from Adam, interposed between "civilized" races and the rest of creation.[7]

White had no apparent political motive for advocating either polygenism – the theory that human races did not all share a common ancestor – or racial inferiority, and he prefaced his book with a strong anti-slavery disclaimer. Like Camper, his notion of a racial series was primarily an aesthetic one – Camper had placed apes at one end of the scale and Apollo at the other – and White naturally considered his own, European, race the most beautiful, particularly the "women of Europe", whose "nice expression" and "general elegance of features and complexion", not to mention their "plump and snowy white hemispheres", were without equal elsewhere on Earth.[8] White remained a little known figure in the scientific world, but many nineteenth-century anatomists from Cuvier down came to accept his premise of a graded racial series. In his *Règne animal* (1812), Cuvier called the Caucasian head the most "beautiful",[9] and his statement in *Discours sur les révolutions du globe* (1817) that some races were "condemned to an eternal inferiority" by the shape of their skulls was, as Stocking concludes, tantamount to polygenism.[10]

Knox had maintained a longstanding interest in race throughout his years in Edinburgh and Glasgow, and in 1841 had translated Quetelet's *Treatise on Man*, which argued that each race was immutable, and adapted to a specific climate. Whilst *Treatise on Man* cannot be taken as an expression of Knox's own views, Quetelet's use of moral statistics, patterns of behaviour, and anthropological measurements may well have inspired Knox's own venture into cranial morphology.[11] With the assistance of the phrenologist Phineas Deseret, Knox examined some 260 skulls and plaster casts belonging to the Phrenological Society of Edinburgh in an attempt to estimate brain bulk in different races.[12] He was never an enthusiast for phrenology, with its emphasis on correlating skull shape with sentiments and character, but he was attracted to craniometry as a means of demonstrating measurable differences between skulls of known racial provenance. This limited quantitative evidence of supposed racial differences was, however, tangential to his aesthetically understood, ideologically motivated and much misconstrued theory of the biological basis of race, as set forth in *The Races of Men*, his most original and influential book.

The ambitious aim of *The Races of Men* was to offer a "Zoological history" of mankind, and its central thesis was that the immutable biological factor of race determined human history, which would otherwise be nothing more than "a chapter of accidents". "With me", declared Knox, "race, or hereditary descent, is everything." Its influence was not confined to skin colour, skull shape, or other anatomical characteristics – human behaviour, history and politics were all racially determined. Knox claimed to have predicted the 1848 European revolutions – which, he maintained, were essentially a struggle between races – on the basis that "human character, individual and national, is traceable solely to the nature of that race to which the individual or nation belongs ... ". Politicians, historians and journalists, he alleged, deliberately avoided the "great subject of race" because it constituted an insurmountable barrier to colonialism and nation building, and was "unpalatable" to "dynasties lording it over nations composed of different races".[13] "The idea that any race can be governed by laws, customs, and manners opposed to its physical nature", wrote the *Medical Times* in support of Knox, was "a delusion which seems almost confined to the English press."[14]

Written at a time of aggressively jingoistic European politics, *The Races of Men* can be seen as an attempt to supplant bellicose nationalism ("Nationalities are always odious") with "the profounder matter of race".[15] It also placed anticolonialism on a biological footing: all races were suited to their own environment, and each was "perfect in its own way" and best adapted to its land of origin.[16] The Saxon, with his "savage energy", had succeeded in "exterminating and enslaving" the "simple aborigines" of the Cape because they were "inferior" to him in "physical structure and mental qualifications"; he had plundered their lands and massacred them almost to extinction, but he had not been "placed there" by nature, and could not live, as the "Hottentot" and "Caffre" did, "in harmony with all around him".[17] This image of a peaceful, paradisiacal wilderness despoiled by Europeans was in stark contrast to the descriptions of uncolonized lands as "primitive, unruly and unstable" that were customarily used to justify Western intervention.[18]

The Races of Men did not confuse what was with what ought to have been: Knox's personal position was that slavery and colonialism violated the rights of man, and he dismissed the British government's argument that empire-building protected aboriginal peoples as the hypocrisy of wolves offering to guard sheep. But his experiences in the Cape had convinced him that the domination of one race by another was both inevitable and racially driven:

> The doctrine which teaches us to love our neighbours as ourselves is admirable, no doubt; but a difficulty lies somehow or other in the way. What is that difficulty, which all seem to know and feel, yet do not like to avow? It is the difference of race. Ask the Dutch Boor whence comes his contempt and inward dislike to the Hottentot, the Negro, the Caffre; ask him for his warrant to reduce these unhappy races to bondage and slavery; to rob them of their lands, and to enslave their children; to deny them the inalienable right of man to a portion of the earth on which he was born?[19]

Knox had noticed that, when he lectured on race, whether to scientific or popular audiences, it was easier to secure their attention when speaking of Europeans than of the "dark races", presumably because they thought the latter "not of our kind". "Practically," he claimed, "all men believe in the element of race", though they might hypocritically deny it.[20] In its claim that a preference for one's own race, and antipathy towards other races, are natural sentiments, *Races* constituted a forewarning of the dangers of what later became known as "racialism". As one obituarist put it "we see in [Knox's] outspoken utterances the real motives which have actuated so many of our most profound anthropologists".[21]

The more than usually breathless confusion with which Knox presented his work left it particularly vulnerable to selective, out of context quotation, and contemporary ideologues drew on *The Races of Men* in support of theories and attitudes very different from Knox's own. Later commentators have deprecated the uses to which Knox's writings were put and condemned his "faulty logic":[22] Philip D. Curtin called Knox "the real founder of British racism and one of the key figures in the general western movement towards a dogmatic pseudo-scientific racism", and Sven Lindqvist wrote that *The Races of Men* "reveals racism at the actual moment of birth, just as it takes the leap from popular prejudice via Knox's conceded ignorance to 'scientific' conviction".[23] The scientific import of Knox's pronouncements on race was largely obscured by a cloud of moral disapproval until Laura Callanan, apprised of Knox's anti-imperialism, untangled the transcendental theories underlying his racial studies, which can be adequately understood only in the context of his wider views on the formation of animal varieties and species.[24]

In the 1850s, Knox's subsequently notorious statement that "race is everything"[25] was not an extreme attitude but a fashionable view that had been expressed, for example, in Disraeli's *Tancred* (1847):

"All is race; there is no other truth."
"Because it includes all others?" said Lord Henry
"You have said it."[26]

To the modern reader, Knox's classification of race, a nebulous concept at the best of times, seems little more than a hotchpotch in which the supposed distinguishing characteristics of Saxons, Celts, Gypsies, Jews and many others are determined according to the author's personal whims. This unsystematic impression is exacerbated by *Races* Knoxian humour, often on the edge of persiflage: for example the Saxon (in which race, with its instinct for "soul-consuming, body-wasting labour" Knox counted himself) "invents nothing", "has no musical ear", lacks "genius", and is so "low and boorish" that "he does not know what you mean by fine art."[27]

Knox particularly relished twisting the tails of the Celts, whose "unalterable character" made it impossible for them to progress, and whose peasantry lived in "hovels they chose to call farmhouses".[28] Like many nineteenth-century lowland Scots, he denied his Celtic roots, preferring the idea that the lowlanders were a Teutonic or Germanic people: in calumniating the "lazy, worthless" Celt in his "dark and filthy hovel",[29] he was following in the footsteps of the likes of Edinburgh antiquarian John Pinkerton (1758–1826), who claimed that the lowland Scots were Goths, and the Celts a race of "inferior" interlopers. The former Lord Chancellor, Lord Lyndhurst, who had been much criticized for calling the Irish "aliens in blood, in language, and religion", took comfort from Knox's Celtic caricature and, not surprisingly, "wished... to see the [*The Races of Men*] freely circulated in the best English society."[30]

The book generated more interest during Knox's lifetime than any of his other works, and he anticipated criticism: "Each race treated of in this little work will complain of my *not* having done *them* justice", he wrote disingenuously, "of all others they will admit that I have spoken the truth."[31] An anonymous reviewer in the *Gentleman's Magazine* considered that a subject "of the highest interest and importance" had been ill-served by Knox's "abuse of all men and things which come his way, and by the dogmatism of his unsupported assertions", and complained that, though Knox wrote with style and eloquence, "he does not inquire thoroughly into anything, he only concludes", a criticism applicable to much of his work.[32] *Bentley's Miscellany* called it an "offensive" book. So it was, and no-one was spared:

> To be brief: the book teaches nothing, and denies every thing; it abuses men and institutions, families and governments, with wonderful prodigality; calls the King of Prussia an infamous coward, the King of Greece an idiot and a vulgar Goth, and the modern Greeks serfs by nature and slaves of the horrible and brutal superstitions of the Greek Church. As for the Saxon nations in Europe, enslaved as they are, they basely hold their lives and properties at the mercy of five or six . . . families or dynasties, paltry families, unknown to fortune or renown.
> The English are the grand tyrants by sea, and as to the civil and religious liberty we assert we possess, it is a fallacy altogether . . . a mighty sham.[33]

The *Christian Examiner* dismissed Knox as "a boastful dogmatist, eaten up with German nonsense and his own conceit, uttering in snatches and riddles a theory of materialism and despair."[34] A more cogent criticism was that he treated man "simply as an animal", as if humans were "creatures of instinct" rather than "highly intelligent being[s]", "in a state of constant progress".[35]

Progress from the "savage" (from the Latin *Sylva*, those who dwelt in the woods) towards "civilization" (an eighteenth-century word for the social state or process), with its implications of racial transformism, was not something that Knox assumed. Despite writing of racial characteristics "receding towards the black" or "advancing to the white", and describing the face of the "Hottentot" as "like a baboon's", Knox envisaged the scale of races, like the *scala naturae*, as a fixed order with no suggestion of transformation or progress. Each race was fitted for its environment, and so Europeans could never colonize the tropics, nor the "dark races" become "civilized". The latter assertion has become notorious, though in common with some later anthropologists Knox made no claim that "the artificial existence" Europeans "choose to call 'civilization'", in which man was at "perpetual war" with nature, was superior to the life of the "coloured man, in harmony with all around him". Nor was his concept of such harmony rooted in romantic idealism: the reason the Native American did not exterminate the bison, or the Eskimo the seal, was that they were "unequal to their destruction".

That the European was "antagonistic of nature" had been amply demonstrated by his conduct in the Cape: "The wild acacia he wastes as firewood; the Chumie forests he utterly destroys, converting the timbers thereof into rafters for barracks and other hovels, for men to congregate in like pigs." Knox was also critical of English aggression in Hindustan, Afghanistan and China, and opposed colonization that robbed natives of their lands or enslaved them. According to his theory of racial fitness, empire building was in any case doomed to fail, as immigrants were invariably the "weaker", *i.e.* the less suited, race. He argued that "no Europeans can colonize a tropical country", and that "no Saxon race can ever hold a colony long", because "none but those whom Nature placed there can live there".[36]

The "disorganized" presentation of *The Races of Men*, whose subtitle proclaimed it "a fragment", has subsequently been blamed for providing unintended succour for the pro-slavery cause.[37] "A fragment of what, we wonder[?]", asked one exasperated reviewer, who found the text so "incoherent" that he understood Knox's thesis to be that "the several races of men are all originally distinct".[38] As writing and lecturing provided Knox's only income, he had been obliged to hurry into print (the same reviewer found ten errors on one page) and to interest a wide audience, but though, as a consequence, he failed to express his ideas with proper scientific clarity, he could hardly have anticipated that a book with so strong an anti-colonial message would be interpreted by some as a paean to Saxon supremacy. The *Medical Times and Gazette* recognized that his impulsive and sarcastic tone was intended as "bitter and wholesome medicine" for those who despised other races, but lines such as "Can the black races become civilized? I should say not?" were grist to the mill of the anti-emancipation lobby,[39] which had no reservations about the superiority of Western civilization: extracts from *Races* were quoted approvingly by John Campbell in *Negro-mania: Being an Examination of the Falsely Assumed Equality of the Races of Men* . . . (1851).

Among Knox's modern critics is Alan T. Davies, who sees him as a "racist" promoter of the "Saxon race myth", for whom egalitarianism was a sign of "racial progress" and whose dream of "an earthly apotheosis of the Saxon race" gave the future "an optimistic cast".[40] The view that enlightened human reason and scientific advancement would lead to social progress and the defeat of superstition and ignorance, which Oken had characteristically romanticized with reference to Napoleon ("The hero is the god of mankind / Through the hero is mankind free,"[41]) was certainly held by many radicals, but it was not a position that Knox would ever bring himself to share. His assumption of the inevitability of racial conflict was the antithesis of optimism, and his vision, in the words of Richards, was "a doctrine of despair – of political nihilism", a kind of "deconsecrated Calvinism" (though he shunned Calvinist theology, which he blamed for having "extinguished science and literature in Scotland for more than 200 years"[42]) that utterly rejected the possibility of interracial cooperation or social improvement.[43]

Oliver Wendell Holmes was prescient, though not alone, in recognizing that *The Races of Men* was the work for which Knox would be remembered; his *Lancet* obituary made the same assumption, understandably so since *Races* had drawn more critical reaction than any of his other writings. While, as an anticolonialist text, *Races* missed its mark, largely due to its flippancies of style, Knox can hardly be blamed for, still less assumed to have concurred with, the uses to which it was put after his death, when, under James Hunt's leadership, the Anthropological Society of London, the inner circle of which called themselves the Cannibal Club in mockery of their social and scientific unacceptability,[44] hijacked his reputation to support their own agenda. In the Society's *Memoirs*, Hunt used "human nature" to justify the "natural subordination" of the Negro, and invoked Knox's theories to bolster his own support for imperialism and slavery and opposition to black suffrage and Irish home rule. "Let Dr. Knox instruct us from his grave", he wrote sententiously. Had Knox stopped spinning long enough to take up the offer he might have pointed out, amongst other things, that Wallace's address on the origin of the races of men from a single stock, which was coolly received by the Anthrolopologicals in 1864, endorsed his own monogenist teachings from as long ago as 1850.[45]

For Knox, the future of mankind held not progress but a series of Cuvierian extinctions of races that, like the indigenous peoples of the Cape, had "mysteriously run their course, reaching the time appointed for their destruction." His stoical consolation as he contemplated "the extermination of the dark races of men" was that extinction would be the eventual fate of all races: since each was "[d]estined . . . to run, like all other animals, a certain limited course of existence, it matters little how their extinction is brought about." Men might claim their own race as "the highest development", but "so would have reasoned the Saurians": only "nature dies not . . . she is eternal."[46] This fatalistic prophecy was far from the rallying call for social change that the Aborigines Protection Society had once hoped for, but nor was it a dream of Saxon supremacy. The *Medical Times* (hardly impartial as it had published Knox's lectures on race), called Knox a "man of genius", but thought his book marred by an "undercurrent" of "misanthropical sarcasm, of irreligion, and of the most forlorn aspect of humanity".[47] If, as Davies suggests, the true subject of Knox's racial musings was himself,[48] it appears he identified not with any supposedly triumphant race, but with those predestined to destruction.

CHAPTER FOURTEEN

The Great Scheme of Nature

The Lancet praised *The Races of Men* as the work of "a highly original, though very erratic, mind", and judged Knox "a most acute observer of race", though with an "overbearing manner" and prone to "transcendental rhapsodies".[1] This was one of a very few reviews to comment on the book's transcendentalist subtext, which was as subtle as its racial generalizations were crude. One audience that did appreciate the link between race and philosophical anatomy was the Ethnological Society, where in his presidential address of 1851 Charles Malcolm spoke of Knox abandoning his attempts to discover the "origin" of man through historical accounts and "calling in the aid of transcendental anatomy to trace his evolution, and that of all those beings which participate with him in the common attribute of animal life . . . in air or water", an approach condemned in some quarters as irreligious, because it seemed that "the transcendental anatomist, who thinks that he is in possession of the highest discovery to which human intellect has yet attained, would trace man to an inferior animal . . . ".[2]

For Knox, establishing the origin of human races was a step towards answering the greatest question of philosophical anatomy; that of how new species came into being. If races constituted different "species", then the origin of race was, at least in a limited sense, the origin of species. It must be borne in mind that Knox was not using the term *species* in its modern, biological sense: in the mid-nineteenth century, a species was a group that could "breed freely and continuously", *i.e.* whose unions were always fertile and gave rise to offspring *resembling both parents*. Different species within the same genus could interbreed, but not "continuously", and animals in different genera could not interbreed at all.[3] Different species did not interbreed "continuously" because their offspring did not preserve a resemblance to both parents over time: hybrids could breed only with one of the parent species (unions between hybrids were thought to be barren) and so successive generations would come to resemble one or other parent, but not both. Thus, dogs and wolves were separate species because, although they could interbreed, wolf dogs could reproduce only by mating with either dogs or wolves, so their descendents would in time revert to the characteristics of one of the original species.

According to Knox, the races into which he divided mankind were distinct species that could interbreed but not "amalgamate", since characteristics derived from both parents could not coexist for more than a few generations: "dark blood has been observed to hold its ground in the descendents [of mixed marriages] for a hundred and fifty years", he wrote, but eventually it will lose its "peculiar moral and physical nature", with "some of the offspring reverting to one species, others to the other."[4] There was no moral or prescriptive element to his claim that races remained distinct, a conclusion based largely on observations from colonized lands such as South America, where natives greatly outnumbered colonists and mixed marriages were infrequent. In these areas, it was white blood that was destined to disappear: the "new product" would be unable to "stand its ground" and "mulattos" (which, like all hybrids, he supposed were infertile if they intermarried) would either "perish or return to the original Indian". In time, any mixed population would "of necessity fall back upon the stronger race", while "the weaker race", the colonists less suited to the environment, would be "obliterated."[5] The persistence of minority racial groups over long periods of time was difficult to account for according to these principles, and some readers were offended by Knox's suggestion that European Jews had remained racially distinct because they did not marry outside their own race.[6]

In order to sustain his thesis that "[u]nquestionably a race means a species",[7] Knox emphasized physical differences between races as much as he could: "the object of this work", he wrote of *The Races of Men*, "is to show that the European races, so called, differ from each other as widely as the Negro does from the Bushman; the Caffre from the Hottentot; the Red Indian of America from the Esquimaux, the Esquimaux from the Basque". Since the interracial differences that he and others had so far described were minor, he predicted, and for the sake of his theories no doubt hoped, that "remarkable" anatomical variants would soon be discovered in, for example, the native Australian, who, he anticipated, "differed in an extraordinary manner from the European".[8]

Such exaggerated claims led to his work being mistakenly regarded as polygenist, though this was a position he consistently opposed: "Some idle, foolish, and, I might almost say, some wicked notions, have been spread about of [the dark races] being descended from Cain; such notions ought to be discountenanced: they give a colour for oppression."[9] In Knox's youth, polygenism had offered a fashionable alternative to the Christian monogenist orthodoxy – most of the thirteen papers on race read between 1785 and 1812 at Edinburgh's Royal Medical Society had been polygenist in tone – but he had always defended "the unity of human life", and never published in the polygenist *Ethnological Journal*.[10] By rejecting polygenism, he necessarily accepted transformation of races; according to the proselytizing monogenist Thomas Smyth, Knox considered them permanent only for as long as the existing order of things prevailed; new races could be brought into existence by episodes of "great change".[11]

Comparing "the highly civilized nations of Europe" with "a horde of filthy Hottentots", the controversial Barts surgeon Sir William Lawrence (1783–1867) asked: "[a]re these all brethren? Have they descended from one stock? Or must we trace them to more than one?— and if so, how many Adams must we admit?"[12] Lawrence admitted only one Adam, but his monogenism was not dogmatic: he denied the authority of the scriptures in scientific questions and determined to pursue the study of man as he would any other branch of natural history. This was a radical position, and Abernethy, his predecessor at Barts, accused him of "propagating dangerous opinions . . . in concert with the French physiologists".[13] *The Races of Men* followed a similar approach to Lawrence, treating mankind from an anatomical or "zoological" perspective and assuming nothing about his "origin".[14] Consequently, despite Knox's insistence on the "unity" of mankind, his work failed to win the support of Christian monogenists because his transcendentalist principles were "more disagreeable to theologians [sic] than even the establishment of *diversity* itself!"[15]

A stumbling block for scientific monogenists was the archaeological and artistic evidence that human appearances had remained unchanged "within the historic period": if they shared a common ancestor, the various races must have appeared a very long time ago. The most widely accepted theory, articulated in Buffon's *Natural History* (1749), was that, as men had spread to various parts of the earth, differences in climate, food, and modes of living had caused them to depart from the original type, and these adaptations had then been transmitted to their offspring. In the 1840s and 1850s, racial differences were still typically ascribed to what was later (inaptly) known as Lamarckian inheritance of acquired characteristics: Turks had round heads through wearing turbans, the Dutch were phlegmatic from living in marshes, and French women had "vigorous" calves because their cities lacked pavements.[16] Knox briskly rejected such explanations, noting sardonically that after hundreds of years of circumcision among the Jews and foot binding among the Chinese, none had yet been born circumcised, or with small feet.

In common with Immanuel Kant, whose work underpinned much of *Naturphilosophie*, Knox looked to the embryo for the origin of races and species. He had observed that hatchling salmon and trout showed far greater similarities than did adults of the two species,[17] a finding he used in 1855 as the basis of a rather disjointed account of species formation:

> Thus all the species [*of salmonidae*] start from a form of young which is generic, but not specific; and by those generic characters may be foretold most if not all of the specific forms afterwards to appear. This is the real affiliation which species have to each other; it resides in the generic character of the young. It alone is perfect as it embraces all. But if this view be correct, it places zoology upon a scientific basis, and explains why one form of life prevailed at one time,

and afterwards another; it provides for the extinction of one species, and the appearance of another, differing, it is true, from the extinct, but generically the same. It explains serial unity and the persistence for a period of specific forms; it renders even the reappearance of extinct forms not only not impossible, but even probable, since they depend, or seem to depend, on geological cataclysms, and the nature of the external media.[18]

In other words, "the forms of many species are included in each and all" and "new" species are "merely the development of specific forms which lay concealed in [embryos of] the genus or family."[19] "Were our observations sufficiently delicate", Knox ventured, "I have no doubt that the principal species composing any natural family might be determined *à priori* by an inspection of the embryo and young".[20] Since all possible species within a family were derived from the same, generic embryo, species change "d[id] not require the interposition of a new creative impulse . . . but merely an alteration of the physical circumstances in which the young may be placed."[21]

It had long been believed that, during development, the human embryo passed through a series of stages reminiscent of the animal series, from lower to higher: there was, for example, an early, "fish-like" stage, with gill slits that later disappeared. In terms of the Meckel–Serres law familiar to modern biologists, the development of the embryo (ontogeny) recapitulated the tree of life (phylogeny). Knox called this the second great law of anatomy (the first being "unity of type") – that "the embryonic forms of man shadow forth the range of the animal kingdom as it now exists"[22] – and he envisaged the human embryo:

> passing through forms which represent the permanent forms of other adult beings belonging to the organic world, not human, but bestial; of whom some belong to the existing world, whilst others may represent forms which once existed, but are now extinct; or, finally, forms which may be destined some day to appear. . . . Thus in the embryonic changes or metamorphoses of man and other animals, are shadowed forth, more or less completely, all other organic forms. . . . Thus is man linked by structure and by plan to all that has lived or may yet live. One plan, one grand scheme of nature; unity of organization; unity in time and space; hence, here also we see the past and the present, and we conjecture a future.[23]

His third law was that "a great plan or scheme of Nature exists, agreeably to which all organic forms are moulded"; if the development of the embryo was perturbed the result could be either a simple "arrest of development" or the formation of "some other form, or possible existence embraced in Nature's scheme. This form may represent the sub-type, when perfect, of a now existing animal (as in the instance recorded above [the tiger arm]), or it may resemble an animal form now extinct, or one not yet called into existence."[24] The idea was not original: the production of new types through alterations in embryonic development had been suggested previously by Geoffroy, with respect to animal development, and by Blumenbach, who ascribed human variety to embryonic "variation".[25]

In a thorough and perceptive analysis of Knox's science, Richards concluded that *The Races of Men* advocated "a common material origin of life and its evolution by a process of saltatory descent"; that is to say, new species arose not by gradual change but by sudden leaps due to shifts in embryonic development.[26] In the first (1850) edition Knox's claims were tentative; he saw no evidence for "alteration or change" of one species into another during the historical period, but speculated that this "law" might be "neutralized" on occasion:

> In time, there is probably no such thing as species: no absolutely new creations ever took place.... So far back as [human] history goes, the species of animals as we call them have not changed; the races of men have been absolutely the same.... Are they commutable into each other? Are these causes in constant operation, slowly yet surely altering and changing everything? Or does this happen by sudden cataclysms or geological epochs?[27]

Having put forward the idea "that every embryo contains within itself elements sufficient to assume any other form, and to retain it, provided that it be insulated and put under circumstances calculated to bring them forth; to exaggerate certain qualities, and give them permanency", Knox immediately dismissed it as "untenable". This was, however, the essence of his claim, made in the second edition twelve years later, that "as the embryo of every individual of any species belonging to the natural family contains within itself the characters of the adults of all the species, it is then but a question of time and circumstances which species is to die out, and which to take its place."[28]

Knox's use of analogy between human races and animal species, and his emphasis on the unity of all that lived, raised the question of the affiliation of humans and other primates. Camper, Blumenbach and others had been content to observe that humans, uniquely, possessed a soul (and an upright posture), but later anatomists, like Knox, who were committed to a "zoological" study of mankind, were obliged to rely on anatomy to separate man from ape, which could be problematic, as even the great taxonomist Carl Linnaeus (1707–78) had professed himself unable to discover "the difference between man and the orangoutang, although all of my attention was brought to bear on this point . . . ".[29] So many anatomists tried to find a solution to the problem that in 1846 the satirical magazine *Punch* poked fun at the "siantificle" vogue for dissecting monkeys "to see . . . wether like our own specius inside as well as out".[30]

In a post-Darwinian world, the graded sequence of primate skulls from ape to Apollo calls to mind evolutionary progress, but for Knox and his contemporaries it was a static series familiar to all philosophers as the great chain of being. Nevertheless, the serial affinity between ape and man was a cause for concern. William Lawrence complained that those "writers, who expatiate with vast delight on what they call the regular gradation or chain of beings, and discover great wisdom of the Creator, and great beauty of the creation, in the circumstance, that nature makes no leaps, but has connected the various objects of the three kingdoms together like the steps of a staircase, or the links of a chain, represent man only as a more perfect kind of monkey; and condemn the poor African to the degrading situation of a connecting link between the superior races of mankind and the orangutang."[31]

If the whole of animal creation could be arranged in a continuous series, "it was but natural to suppose that man formed the last link", but this "grand doctrine of Unity" did not imply that man had ascended from species lower in the chain. Despite his scorn for the claims of the "Bridgewater school" that man's bipedal stance and erect, heavenward-gazing, attitude were unique, God-given features, Knox cherished the particular dignity of mankind, hence his aversion to the ugly, infantile transitional state between human and "brute". Despite all the anatomical similarities between man and ape (they were, after all, *simians*), the ape was no more than a caricature: they were "painfully" alike, but, he told Lonsdale, "man is man, after all".[32]

The hypothesis that change was abrupt and discontinuous allowed Knox to maintain the seemingly paradoxical position of emphasizing the unity of man with nature while asserting his uniqueness: man was "one of nature's material manifestations", but "[t]he human family stands profoundly apart from all others, implying that in the great chain of beings constituting nature's plan, some natural family filling up the link has disappeared", though in remarking that "[b]etween a gorilla and man, several intermediate links have been lost . . . " he rather disingenuously ignored the well-known anatomical similarities between human and orangutan.[33] In attempting to reconcile human uniqueness with the principle of plenitude, which required all possible forms in the chain of being to be represented at some point in time, Knox's logic, or his ability to express himself, for once proved unequal to the task:

> In nothing I have said do I mean to deny the great *serial* unity of all that ever lived; what I mean is, that the human family as it exists is one quite apart from the highest four-handed animals . . . at no time could I ever perceive any *serial affiliation* between the human family and the highest apes existing. I do not mean by this that man stands apart from the living world, and that a gap exists between him and all that lives; no such gap exists in Nature's works. But what I mean is this, that the *seeming* gap must not be offered as proof that such really exists. Apes are not convertible into men, and for this simple reason, they do

not belong to the same natural family. The species forming the natural family of man are numerous, and some may be extinct.[34]

Although he accepted both the transcendental principle that "man [is] linked by structure and by plan to all that has lived or may yet live", and Cuvier's opinion that "[t]he animals now existing on the surface of the globe may, after all, be the direct descendants of the animal and vegetable fossil world", Knox remained reluctant fully to commit himself to the logical conclusion, tentatively expressed in *The Races of Men*, that "simple animals . . . may have produced by continuous generation the more complex animals of after ages . . . the fish of the early world may have produced reptiles, then again birds and quadrupeds; lastly, man himself?"[35]

Meanwhile, London's two leading philosophical anatomists, the impoverished radical Robert Grant, and the gaunt, dandified, well-connected Richard Owen, were pursuing lines that Knox had previously abandoned. The early careers of all three men had been remarkably similar: Grant graduated from Edinburgh in the same year as Knox, studied under Cuvier and Geoffroy in France, joined the council of the Wernerian Society and, after losing out to Knox in the election for the Conservatorship of the College of Surgeons museum, accepted a chair in comparative anatomy in London, where he remained for the rest of his life.[36] Owen's interest in "Zootomical pursuits" had, like Knox's, been whetted by Barclay's "earnest" teaching, and he too had moved on to Barts, where Abernethy's patronage freed him from a not very eagerly anticipated career as a naval surgeon. As Assistant Conservator of London's Hunterian museum, Owen visited Paris in 1831 as the guest of Cuvier, whom he had welcomed to the Hunterian the previous year, and on his return to London a series of detailed papers on comparative anatomy earned him a reputation as the English Cuvier, a soubriquet originally bestowed by the *Lancet* on Grant. The two became rivals, and as Owen's reputation grew he managed to exclude Grant from the council of the Zoological Society of London, thereby denying him access to the corpses of zoo animals for his researches.

Grant's troubles were exacerbated by his stubborn but principled refusal to sit the licensing examination of the Royal College of Physicians, which left him unable to practise medicine and dependent for his income on a heavy teaching load, while Owen enjoyed a lucrative career.[37] Though they shared an obstinate nature, caustic wit and love of argument, Grant and Knox seem not to have met or corresponded whilst in London. Grant's enthusiasm for Lamarck's theory of transmutation of adult species in response to environmental changes, which was derided by Owen, held scant appeal for Knox, who saw external conditions not as the driving force for species change but merely as "potent checks to an infinite variety of forms".[38]

The Great Scheme of Nature

Owen's reputation as "England's Cuvier" was an allusion to his status rather than his views, and his approach was distinctly Geoffroyan: he was an enthusiast for the transcendental doctrine that the basic structural element was a modified vertebra, and in his monograph *On the Nature of Limbs* (1849) he set out what Steven Jay Gould considered the strongest version of that theory of any British anatomist.[39] Cross-species homologies – such as the similarities of bone structure between the limbs of different animals regardless of their function – were expressions of a universal archetype, common to all animals and man, and especially apparent in arrests of development. The similarity between ape and Aztec, with their "arrested brain-growth", was, Owen claimed, so striking, that "I cannot shut my eyes to the significance of that all-pervading similitude of structure – every tooth, every bone, strictly homologous – which makes the determination of the difference between *Homo* and *Pithecus* [the orangutan] the anatomist's difficulty."[40]

As the ideal archetype was compatible with, and perhaps even suggestive of, intelligent design, it allowed Owen to discuss comparative anatomy, especially with regard to man, within a politically and theologically neutral framework. Despite its ambitious scope, his work on homologies of structure and form was relatively uncontroversial, as it left open the questions of whence the archetype was derived and how its action was exerted. Richards has argued that Owen was a "closet evolutionist", who presented his theories in such a manner as to evade the politically unacceptable possibility (unacceptable because it smelled of radicalism) that new species came into being as a reaction to changes in the environment.[41] Like Knox, "transmutation of species in the ascending course" – a constant striving for progress – was not a model he favoured, and he too looked to the embryo as the source of new species, privately suggesting atrophy and hypertrophy, premature birth and prolonged foetation, developmental deformations and metagenetic change[42] as possible mechanisms for speciation. He accepted in principle Oken's claim that man had originated from the sea, and speculated that the Creation had been restricted to the smallest creatures, such as *infusoria*.[43] In public, however, Owen was diplomatically reticent when it came to ideas likely to alienate his conservative supporters. Though he admitted he could not rule out, in theory, the development of a "Hottentot" from a chimpanzee, he ruled it out in practice by drawing attention to supposed anatomical differences between them – particularly that "cerebral barrier between man and the apes", a small area of the brain known as the hippocampus minor.[44]

Knox took "every opportunity of denouncing the hippocampus minor controversy as a 'silly dispute'", and counted Owen among "the low transcendentalists of England ... who nibble at a question they cannot refute, yet dare not adopt".[45] Owen's public version of the appearance of new species ("ordained continuous becoming") was too redolent of the

Creator's grand plan for Knox, who eschewed such concessions to the *primum movens*, and argued that species change must result from the blind operation of the "secondary laws which regulate all material things".[46] In some respects, however, notably his rejection of Lamarckism and his Barcleian reverence for the uniqueness of humankind, Knox's position was closer to Owen's than either might have wished to acknowledge.

Knox's view that, as Darwin was to put it, "organisation progresses by sudden leaps", might have been expected to appeal to fellow radicals stirred by the analogy between social revolution and change in the natural world.[47] In Britain, species change had been a talking point since the publication, in 1844, of *Vestiges of the Natural History of Creation*, an influential presentation of the development of the cosmos, the Earth, its rocks, plants and animals as a series of successive improvements, which had been a scandalous best seller for its anonymous author, the Scottish journalist Robert Chambers. Knox, however, dismissed its allusions to the working out of a divine plan through the operation of natural laws as the work of "a nibbler at philosophy" – an "unconscious" Paleyite who saw man as the crown of creation – and repudiated the suggestion that "the development of new species" embodied "any kind of successive perfectability [*sic*]".[48] Instead, he looked forward to a time when "[t]he boast about the higher characters of the present organic races will be abandoned, and the law of development and progress simply stated as it is, without a reference to successive *improvement*; for *successive improvement* implies a final purpose [which is] a final cause."[49]

CHAPTER FIFTEEN

Distrust Your Genius, 1851–1855

The Great Exhibition of 1851 attracted over a hundred thousand people to "brick-built, filthy, common-place London". Knox paid his shilling but found the statuary lifeless, and the Crystal Palace unimpressive: "[t]his glass-house or monster glazed cast-metal case is not a building. . . . It is merely a national mistake, not at all unusual with the race to which the nation belongs".[1] His enjoyment of its contents may well have been marred by the presence, among many examples of French craftsmanship, of two thousand models of pathological anatomy, the collection of the late Dr Thibert, which had at last found an audience.[2] At least the influx of visitors to the capital, which finally made public anatomy museums a viable proposition (Kahn's in Oxford Street remained open until 1872),[3] allowed Knox to indulge his fancy for observing different races.

He caught the rising tide of public interest in anatomy with a second "popular" book on transcendentalism, *Great Artists and Great Anatomists* (1852), a six-shilling "great men" history that portrayed Cuvier and Geoffroy as an anatomical Caesar and Alexander, and anatomy as a quest for truth about "the origin of life". Cuvier's description of the whole animal kingdom and his demonstration of extinction were presented as epoch-making events in the history of knowledge that, along with Geoffroy's "great plan of the creation of living forms", had brought the organic world under the rule of natural laws and relegated the Creator to a remote first cause.[4]

Great Artists and Great Anatomists was evidently hurried into print, and it would be difficult to gainsay the opinion of the *Monthly Journal of Medical Science* that "It is hardly possible from such a jumbled, confused, unconsecutive string of sentences, to gather what Dr Knox would really be at", though the reviewer thought he understood enough to presume the book "sneered", or even "laughed outright" at the "First Great Cause".[5] Knox sneered at a good many things, though his pose that "all men are asses except Dr. R. Knox, and a few of 'my illustrious friends,'— that no living being understands any thing of anatomy, descriptive or transcendental, except Dr. R. Knox,— and that this science is about to receive a sudden illumination in these pages" was so exaggerated that the overall effect was "too amusing to be offensive".[6] The *Weekly News* perceptively wrote of Knox that:

He would probably take it no great compliment to be called one of the most vigorous and picturesque writers upon scientific subjects living; the higher claim to *making* science rather than *writing about it* being, more probably, his ambition. . . . The book before us is smart, pungent, racy, and inconsecutive, beginning everywhere, ending nowhere, and flying off on all occasions, and at all manner of tangents, everywhither. . . . Yet a better book might easily have been a worse one.[7]

Despite his extravagant literary style – it was, in the words of the *Weekly News*, what champagne was to effervescence – Knox's paean to anatomy was little more than rhetoric, and the thinly written concluding chapters on Leonardo, Michelangelo and Raphael were unlikely to have given the committee that turned him down for the lectureship at the Scottish Academy cause for regret. He no doubt relished the description of his book as "a tissue of rampant heterodoxy", whose "obnoxious tenets" were "repellent" to the reader, though he must have despaired at being called "a partisan of the school of Lamarck, and of the author of the 'Vestiges of Creation'".[8] These were typical, however, of the misapprehensions that plagued his hastily written popular works.

Knox completed two other books in 1852: *Manual of Artistic Anatomy*, which combined practical information for artists with a transcendental theory of beauty, and *Manual of Human Anatomy*, a six-hundred-page textbook that had obviously cost him much time and labour. It was a reminder of just how good a descriptive anatomist he was, for despite his preoccupation with philosophical anatomy in his later years, he never lost sight of the importance of these practical studies, however distasteful, and advised his readers to "Distrust your genius, and follow the example of Bichat and Cuvier" by dissecting the human body.[9] He sent a copy of the *Manual of Human Anatomy* to Goodsir, who had succeeded Monro in the Edinburgh chair, with a proposal that they co-edit a "quarterly fasciculus" on the latest discoveries in British anatomical science, but though his former pupil replied with a polite expression of gratitude and esteem, nothing came of his idea.[10] *Manual of Human Anatomy* did not attract much critical notice, though there were favourable reviews in the *Medical Times* and the *Lancet*, but of all Knox's works it came closest to fulfilling his stated aim of teaching anatomy "through the medium of the Press".[11]

The year 1853 brought a final opportunity for him to revive his lost career, when he was appointed lecturer in anatomy to the new Royal Free School of Medicine, which had been hastily organized during the summer by William Marsden, Frederick James Gant and T.H. Wakley, surgeons at the Royal Free Hospital. In the expectation that the school would be recognized by the Royal College of Surgeons of England, the *Lancet* optimistically announced the "great fact" that "every requirement of the licensing bodies has been conscientiously fulfilled", but the rival *Medical*

Circular retorted that the "*Lancet* clique" had failed to produce "either a museum, drawings, or brains" for their new school.[12] When it was announced that Knox was to teach anatomy, the *Medical Circular* made mocking reference to the West Port murders: "[t]here are two other gentlemen well known in the anatomical, surgical, or resurrectional – we hardly know which – annals of Edinburgh, which Dr. Knox might very appropriately introduce to aid him in the anatomical department".[13] The taunt was less remarkable for its wit than for being one of the first examples in print of the latterly ubiquitous misapprehension that Burke and Hare had been resurrection men.

Despite the "unfavourable" weather, the "spacious" new lecture theatre in Gray's Inn Lane was crowded on the evening of Tuesday 4 October 1853 for the official opening of the school.[14] The same was not true of the inaugural lecture of the anatomy course, which Knox delivered at 7 p.m. the following Monday.[15] The plan was for him to offer descriptive and surgical anatomy classes every morning at 9.30 for five guineas a session, but few students enrolled, which was just as well, as on 11 November the Royal College of Surgeons of England informed the school that they would refuse any certificates signed by Knox.[16] The students were given two weeks to transfer to a recognized school, and fourteen, presumably the majority, did so.[17]

The London College of Surgeons had acted in response to a letter from their opposite number in Edinburgh reminding them of Knox's interdiction. Not content with this, the Secretary of the Edinburgh College of Surgeons wrote again in November and requested that the facts be passed on to the other professors at the Royal Free School, in order that "the students attending it may be on their guard with respect to Dr Knox's lectures".[18] Clearly, there were still those in Edinburgh who wished him harm. Of all the Knoxian scandals, the Royal Free *débâcle* was perhaps the one in which he was least culpable. He had sensibly not volunteered the information that his certificates would not be recognized (though he might have expected Wakley, whose father had stirred up the Osborne affair, to have been aware of it), but there is no reason to suppose he deliberately deceived the school's founders, whose attitude to licensing requirements was cavalier. Frederick Gant, the school's would-be lecturer in anatomy and physiology, had been denied subjects for dissection at the Hunterian School of Anatomy as recently as November 1852 because he did not hold a license under the Anatomy Act, and since Knox too was unlicensed, the Royal Free School could not possibly have obtained bodies from legal sources.[19] The School had applied to the English College of Surgeons for recognition of certificates granted by Knox and Gant only after they had opened for business, and when representatives of the College paid a visit they found the museum – with which Knox had not been involved – inadequate, a deficiency that itself precluded the premises being licensed for teaching anatomy.[20] Frustrated of his last chance at an academic career, Knox was mocked by the *Medical Circular*, which suggested that the cholera fly (the subject of a recent paper in the *Lancet*) might be the cause of his choler.[21]

However bitterly he regretted the lost income from the failed school, he cannot have been altogether sorry to avoid the "charnel-house, called a dissecting room" and the "frequent contemplation" there of "the emblems of destruction and death" and "all that is detestable".[22] As the *British and Foreign Medico-chirurgical Review* put it: "Dr Knox . . . has evidently a taste for the artistic and the beautiful; and to such a man nothing can be more hideous and repugnant than the dissected human carcase."[23] The heyday of anatomy teaching was over: it would long remain the foundation of the undergraduate medical syllabus but it was no longer the summit of medical science, and had come to be seen by schools and pupils alike as something of an educational nuisance, a "mass of facts" to be learned by rote with the help of "crammers", and soon forgotten.[24] Few now burned with the zeal that the pupils of Barclay and Knox had shown; students were more likely to regret being compelled to spend their "best days" in "the loathsome atmosphere of the dissecting-room", whose "purulent abominations" were, like the "foul and gory liquid from slaughter-houses" and other "excrementitious matters", a potent source of "contamination" and a menace to health.[25] Medical schools did what little they could to ameliorate the risks – at St Bartholomew's and St Mary's hospitals they used charcoal traps to purify the air – but dissecting-rooms were still "liable to abound in putrescent gases and noxious odours".[26]

Frustrated as a teacher, Knox continued to scrape a living from writing: Longman issued a prospectus for his collected papers, "in the style and size of Lardner's Encyclopaedia", but they were never published, presumably for want of subscribers.[27] *Fish and Fishing in the Lone Glens of Scotland* (1854) was a labour of love whose reception was mixed: William Wright, in his marvellously titled *Fishes and Fishing: Artificial Breeding of Fish, Anatomy of Their Senses, Their Loves, Passions, and Intellects* called it an "excellent little work", but *Cambridge Essays* dismissed it as "a very tiresome book".[28] It is certainly imbued with unfeigned enthusiasm, and it is doubtful Knox was ever happier than during those holidays in the Scottish glens that he recalled with such nostalgia.

When he left Edinburgh, his children had remained behind at 15 Clerk Street in the care of the indispensable Mary Knox, who worked as an accountant until well into her sixties. Thomas Birnie, the orphaned nephew whom Knox had taken in at Newington Place, and whose education he had paid for, moved with them and practised as a surgeon under the name Thomas Knox Birnie before embarking on an army career in which he rose to the rank of deputy surgeon general.[29] The rest of household had more modest aspirations: when they were old enough, Susan was apprenticed to a milliner and Robert to a grocer.[30] In May 1854, young

Robert, then aged 20 or 21, died of heart disease. Two years before, his father had written that a child "best satisfies the craving of the soul for eternal life. All one's hopes are there; our hopes of to-morrow, perhaps our hopes of an hereafter".[31] The bereavement was a blow from which he did not recover for months: without the hope of life that the "healthy, lovely child" symbolized there were only the "emblems of approaching dissolution" and "the fear to die, to go we know not where, and to sink into nothing."[32]

Still in good physical health, Knox tried to have himself posted to the Crimea, but though Fergusson supplied a testimonial that he was "as full of energy as ever", there was no opening for the sixty-three-year-old surgeon.[33] In his London lodgings at Meissen House, Upper Clapton, he wrote magazine articles on sea bathing and sanitary reform – his remarks on the "most dangerous 'of all the classes,' the brutal, savage, but shrewd and powerful navvy"[34] show that his anti-Celtic feelings still rankled – while former pupils continued to distinguish themselves. In December 1855, *The Times* announced the appointment of William Fergusson, FRS, as Surgeon Extraordinary to the Queen. The only biographical information provided for readers who may not have heard of Fergusson was that he had been "a considerable time assistant to Dr Knox".[35]

Knox's spirits, and fortunes, were revived by the return to London in 1855 of the sensational "Aztecque" children, Bartola and Maximo. In contrast to other ethnological shows, which made the best of relatively unpromising material such as a boy and girl "belong[ing] to the yellow race of Southern Africa", the Aztecques were allegedly the sole survivors of a lost people, "the Last of the Ancient Aztecs of Mexico", brought from the "idolatrous city" of Iximaya in Central America, a place almost unknown to "civilized man", by one Pedro Velasquez. The "bright-eyed, olive-complexioned" boy and girl, aged about eighteen and twelve respectively, spoke no language, but their "peculiar" physiognomy and "playful" dispositions made them "interesting objects" in the eyes of the public.[36] To medical observers keen to substantiate their pet theories, these "dwarfed and idiotic Central American children" were a "wonderful" illustration of the "laws of Nature": Richard Owen examined them and pronounced them examples of "arrested development", James W. Redfield, MD, author of *Comparative Physiognomy or Resemblances Between Men and Animals*, was struck by "their resemblance to mice", *Buchanan's Journal of Man* thought them an excellent demonstration of phrenological principals, and Knox identified them as throwbacks to an extinct race.[37]

By delivering a public lecture on the children, Knox allied himself with a spectacle that, though it fascinated professionals and public alike, had already been heavily assailed as an imposture. A photograph shows Maximo wearing a shirt with a smiling sun embroidered on it and Bartola in a sun-ray pattern dress, looking like fairground entertainers (which in the 1890s, courtesy of Barnum and Bailey's circus, they became).[38] The New York press was particularly sceptical, and the children's American exhibitor had been forced to re-advertise them as Earthmen, "a well-known Indian tribe", in order to avoid a fine.[39] British commentators were also unconvinced: the Belfast Natural History and Philosophical Society noted that similar children had been born in Ireland, and the periodical *Notes and Queries* dismissed the Aztecs as a play on public gullibility.[40] The whole Aztec story was finally "refuted" when the children's father appeared and regained custody of them after taking legal action.[41] Of course, none of this controversy deterred Knox: in a paper in the *Lancet*, he called it "almost incredible" that the features of men represented in ancient South American bas-reliefs should be seen in the children currently exhibiting in London, and he proposed that Aztec blood, which like "Negro" or "Jewish blood", when "mingled with another race, seems never to disappear", had re-emerged after an interval of "some hundred years" by the law of "interrupted descent".[42]

In an advertisement for the "little folk" during a previous visit to London in 1853, Professor Owen, by then one of the most famous anatomists in Europe, had attributed the children's "remarkable" appearance to "arrested development".[43] If this was indeed Owen's opinion, rather than just a "crafty puff" by their exhibitor, he quickly changed his mind, and at a special meeting of the Ethnological Society on 6 July 1853 he stated that the nearest thing anatomically to the Aztec children was the skull of an "idiot" preserved at St Bartholomew's Hospital.[44] Whatever misleading claims may have been made in subsequent advertisements, Knox never supposed the children were literally long-lost Aztecs: they were throwbacks, about whom he observed "it does not follow that any number of such could reproduce the race, the necessary conditions for its existence having long ceased to be". His position was in fact similar to Owen's, though he replaced arrest of development ("no such law exists") with "retrogressive development towards other races of animals whose forms are included in the embryo or young, and are common to all the races of men." Although he explicitly denied that such retrogressive development demonstrated "a regular constant permanent affiliation with a lower animality", his comment that the retrogression was "not towards any lower animality now existing" hinted at the possible existence at some past or future time of what the *Anthropological Review* would later call a "missing link".[45] In a paper on the Aztec children in the *Lancet*, Knox reaffirmed his convictions that mankind was a single family, in which all races/species shared a common origin. Though he was obliged to admit that "[t]he originating or determining cause of species is not known", he speculated that "the species composing [the human family] are not formed by external circumstances alone, but by the development of *a form* in unison with the existing state of things, to the exclusion of others."[46]

At the time of his involvement with the Aztecs, Knox tried to rejoin the

Ethnological Society, but despite its "dying condition" he was apparently blackballed, perhaps by Quakers offended by his unscriptural views on species change, though *The Races of Men* had been favourably mentioned by Admiral Sir Charles Malcolm in his last address to the Society as its president in 1851. Knox's participation in public ethnological shows may also have prejudiced some members against him.[47] Although the Society would later reverse its decision and welcome him back into the fold, his theories on the Aztec children never gained widespread acceptance, and soon after his death the *Anthropological Review* bluntly declared the Aztecs to have been "idiot" microcephalics that transmutationists had misinterpreted as a missing link.[48] As in the case of the tiger arm, Knox had relied on a rare anomaly to support his arguments for retrogressive development. The Aztec children were scant data from which to posit the operation of a general law, but Knox avidly seized on any suggestion that lost races could reappear through altered embryonic development as this could explain "the appearance on Earth of new species", the one challenge at which even the great Cuvier had baulked, because the solution was to be found "in that form of philosophy which he disliked and rejected – the transcendental."[49]

CHAPTER SIXTEEN

The Hideous Interior

Knox's *Manual of Artistic Anatomy* was a mix of practical anatomical information for artists and a "theory of the beautiful" that bore comparison with Ruskin's *Modern Painters* (1843). For both men, awareness of natural beauty was intuitive, but only the trained philosophical mind could recognize beautiful things as types of the "Divine attributes".[1] Knox did not go so far as to claim he was "looking through Nature up to Nature's God", but he did see Nature's works as "emblems of a divine mind",[2] and it was this acute awareness of natural beauty, so intensely experienced as he wandered the veldt, that provided much of the inspiration for his studies in philosophical anatomy.

There was an obvious pragmatism to Knox's interest in artistic anatomy – in Edinburgh, lecturing to the Scottish Academy would have been a rewarding occupation for a struggling private teacher, and in London the one professional group, other than medics, who were likely to purchase books on anatomy were artists – but an understanding of beauty was fundamental to transcendentalism, which was a kind of "nature mysticism", an aesthetic rather than a purely scientific system that required the student to respond to the natural order of things rather than merely observing it.[3] Goethe, one of transcendentalism's founding fathers, had argued that aesthetic intuition was indispensable to understanding nature, and no-one, according to Knox, could grasp transcendental theories without an appreciation of the perfect and the beautiful. While this intuitive element may have increased transcendentalism's appeal to those who were not primarily scientists, it provoked criticism that its doctrines were no more than unsubstantiated flights of fancy: "rhapsodies", one reviewer called them,[4] though such objections carried little weight with transcendentalists, who made a virtue of their "mind over matter" approach. Knox saw beauty of form as an indication of conformity with the ideal type of a species, an aesthetic judgement that could be rendered more scientifically acceptable if it were shown not to be merely subjective, and so his work on artistic anatomy was primarily directed towards rationalizing perceptions of physical beauty.

He first referred to a theory of the Beautiful in the lengthy appendix to his translation of Julien Fau's *Anatomy of the External Forms of Man* (1849):

> The longer I taught anatomy, the more I became convinced that the true signification of external forms was unknown to anatomists and physiologists; now in the discovery of this, is mysteriously wrapped up the whole theory of Art; the knowledge of the Perfect, the Beautiful. I was quite aware that no true theory of the beautiful had ever been submitted to mankind; and that as a consequence the discovery of "Nature in Art" as manifested to us in the antique marbles, was still to be made.[5]

Representations of the human form in "antique marbles" had long occupied a privileged place in the borderland between anatomy and art: Bernardino Genga's *Anatomia* (1691) included illustrations of *écorché* versions of familiar classical statues, William Hunter commissioned a plaster cast of the flayed corpse of an executed smuggler, posed as a "dying Gaul", for London's Royal Academy (where it was given the title "smugglerius"), and the surgeon William Cheselden's *Osteographia or the Anatomy of the Bones* (1733), intended for artists, contained engravings of a skeletal Venus de' Medici and Apollo Belvedere.

Aesthetically, Knox considered the antique superior to the modern, the female to the male, and the adult to the infant. Take, for example, the thigh: "[t]he thigh slopes gently inwards in every well-formed limb, male or female, but most in woman. Straight thighs are an unsightly deformity; the thighs of the foetus and of some quadrupeds are straight."[6] The most faultless of all forms was that of Venus, whose matchless beauty made her "the perfect human figure": in modelling her, Knox argued, classical artists had unknowingly represented the ideal type of the Caucasian race, the "perfection of all Nature's works", and indeed "the only absolutely beautiful object on earth", whose contemplation moved the discerning observer to "ecstasy". Of course, such raptures did not mean that humanity was truly the summit of Nature's achievement: if fossil fishes had left records, Knox observed, they too would probably have thought themselves the finest of all Nature's works.[7]

He was not the first nineteenth-century medical man to attempt "a scientific knowledge of female beauty": the Scottish practitioner John Roberton (1776–1840), writing under the pseudonym T. Bell, MD, had pursued the same goal in *Kalogynomia, or the Laws of Female Beauty* (1821), in which he provided a helpful summary of general anatomy and physiology in order to enable the "gentleman" reader to "purify his taste", and so choose true beauty rather than following his own "selfish" desires. Roberton's brief observations lent a veneer of scholarly respectability to a work that may have been primarily purchased for its risqué plates. Like Knox, he found his ideal beauty in the Venus of classical sculpture – "an object finer, Alas! than nature seems even capable of producing", who would, had she existed, have been "even to herself, a source of indescribable pleasure"[8] – thus apparently anticipating the theory that Knox claimed was "first *enounced* by myself, that in *woman alone* resides the perfect and the beautiful". Another medical votary of Venus was Alexander Walker (1779–1852), who had impeccable transcendentalist credentials, having edited *The European Review*, to which Goethe, Cuvier and Geoffroy contributed, and studied under Barclay in Edinburgh and Abernethy in London, where he was expelled for publicly pointing out an error in dissection: Knox called him "a human anatomist second to none".[9] In *Beauty*, published in 1836, Walker treated the subject as "a branch of science, which is strictly founded on anatomy and physiology" and described techniques for "judging" female beauty with a view to improving male choices, since "the form of woman . . . is best calculated to ensure attention from men, and because it is men who, exercising the power of selection, have alone the ability thus to insure individual happiness and to ameliorate the species, which are the objects of this work". In the context of "sexual association", an informed appreciation of female beauty constituted man's "sole protection against low and degrading connexions."[10]

As Lucy Hartley has observed, Walker was following a physiognomical tradition that linked outward beauty with "moral symmetry": an informed choice of partner on the basis of beauty was expected to secure those moral qualities conducive to conjugal satisfaction.[11] To a modern reader, Walker's notion of beauty as an agency for improving the species is reminiscent of Darwin's theory of sexual selection in *The Descent of Man*, but Walker envisaged not *natural* selection but deliberate choices based on men's knowledge of the signification of beauty. Furthermore, he was chiefly concerned with moral rather than physical improvement in humans, though he did link beauty in the animal world to a Cuvierian fitness for purpose: the parts of an animal most pleasing to human eyes were those best suited to their proper functions.[12] He was aware that his account of beauty in terms of fitness was neither new nor universally accepted: Edmund Burke had written that a swine's snout, a pelican's bill, and a monkey's hands were all highly functional yet singularly unattractive, while a "well-fashioned" human mouth or a "well-turned leg" were certainly not those best suited for eating or running. Walker, however, replied that the snout did indeed possess the beauty of fitness for its purpose, and though a woman's mouth was not judged by its fitness for *eating*, it could "never be seen without suggesting ideas of fitness of some kind or other."[13]

Knox dismissed the "Saxon" theory that beauty lay in utility with arguments that paralleled Burke's: "why may not a wheelbarrow [be] beautiful? or a pigsty? or a pair of Jack-boots?" As for the human body, a "large, firm, hard, spatula-fingered hand" was, he supposed, far more serviceable than the slender hand of Venus.[14] Human beauty was not, however, a vague, ethereal quality that "genius" perceived through "inspiration";[15] in *The Races of Men*, Knox rationalized it in the following terms: "In proportion as any figure, whether human or bestial, displays through the exterior, that unseemly interior, which has no form that sense comprehends, or desires, so in the same proportion is that figure beautiful or the opposite."

Beauty was literally skin deep: the body's interior was "frightening and appalling to human sense – never beautiful, but the reverse; always horrible",[16] and so would mar any aesthetic pleasure unless it were utterly concealed from view. The soft integument that clothed the voluptuous back of Venus hid any trace of "the frightful chain of osseous nodosities" supporting it.[17] The most displeasing human forms, according to Knox, were those of old age and infirmity, because they exposed *"the interior; that dreaded interior, sure emblem of dissolution and death"* that awoke in the observer "an unknown dread of something that must happen to him, although he were never told it – a dread of dissolution, that most dreaded of all events." In the truly "beautiful figure", nature, or the artist, concealed these emblems of death, and the observer could forget his own mortality as he contemplated an unblemished image of "ever-returning youth".[18] Of the Townley Venus, Knox wrote: "not a trace of anatomy, of muscle, tendon, or vein, is to be seen in this charming face."[19] She was an anatomist's dream.

Knox confessed that, in his "younger days" he had supposed "anatomy as taught to the surgeon" to be "essential" to the artist, a view he later repudiated. Indeed, since the interior of the body consisted of "shapes without form or colour, frightful, hideous, shocking to behold", he came to the conclusion that artists who spent too long in the dissecting-room, exposed to things "which Nature intended should never be presented to human sight", would be blighted by their knowledge of the dead anatomy that lay beneath the living surface: their figures would become "corses" and their work would take on "a charnel-house look". It was only by harmonizing with Nature and seeking her true meaning that they could hope to produce "a figure embodying within it noble suggestions".[20]

In the days when Knox still encouraged artists into his dissecting-room, he had allowed John Oliphant to sketch the body of Mary Paterson, whom he drew in the attitude of the Medici Venus. Oliphant may have been inspired by the reclining "anatomical Venuses" that were a commonplace of anatomical waxwork shows, and his options were in any case limited by a model who was unable to sit or stand, but there was a peculiar appositeness in his choice of a figure praised by Roberton for her "voluptuous characteristics ... indicating at once her fitness for the office of generation and that of parturition".[21] In Knox's eyes, Mary's beauty would have been ample justification for preserving her, both corporeally and in art: in life, perfection was rare and imperfection common, and in death, in an Edinburgh dissecting-room, the voluptuous Mary became the ideal type of her species.[22]

Nature, according to Knox, "attained perfection" in the adult European woman aged "from seventeen to twenty-seven" and in full health: "above all, the adipose cellular layer interposed between the integuments and the aponeurotic and cellular sheaths of the muscles must be full, strong, and juicy", so that "all traces of the *interior* are concealed, and every emblem of dissolution and death removed from view". Mary Paterson might have been the inspiration for Knox's description, more than twenty years later, of the perfect type of a "finely-formed woman", whose bones are "most carefully concealed" by a "dense, firm integument", with its "grooves, furrows, and depressions of exquisite beauty" and "singular grace", whose "scapulae are perceptible only as rounded eminences" and whose thighs are "fleshy and rounded" and "meet or touch each other above."[23] Sickly Europeans, and some entire races, could never attain such perfection because "want of flesh" revealed the underlying anatomy so they resembled nothing more than "a skeleton, over which has been drawn a blackened skin."[24]

From a modern perspective, Knox's thesis that beauty lay in the effectual concealment of "that hideous machinery, which nature intended should never be seen, never suspected to exist . . . " invites psychological analysis, and there is much in his later writings to serve as grist for the psychoanalytical mill. Even those inclined to dismiss psychoanalysis as pseudoscience may wonder if the aversion to exposure of the body's interior that Knox expressed so forcefully in the 1850s represents a profound and perhaps unconscious reaction to his experiences in the dissecting-room; if his observations that the outline of the bones ought not to be visible in life, lest a person resemble "A living skeleton walking abroad in open day", or that ancient sculptors created beauty by "wrapping up the hideous interior" to "conceal from the eye . . . the horrible existence of bones and muscles, tendons and cartilages," reflect the private fears of someone with skeletons of his own to hide.[25] We may even wonder if he was troubled by the same grotesque waking nightmare that Robert Louis Stevenson contrived for his fictional anatomist in *The Body Snatcher*, that of being brought face to face with a reanimated corpse.

On the other hand, the expressions of distaste towards anatomy in Knox's later works seem unduly exaggerated, and it may be that he became an ardent critic of the dissecting-room because he had been forbidden to teach there: another example of Knoxian sour grapes. Like most anatomists, he taught human dissection in order to earn his living, and probably accepted it as a necessary evil, a tiresome chore by means of which he financed his true interests in comparative anatomy and race. It is possible he had always loathed it, but concealed his distaste, as doctors are so often required to do, for the sake of his career. That anatomists do not dissect bodies for pleasure is, however, a fact the public find difficult to accept, and even those who acknowledged Knox's aversion to this unpleasant work still made mock of his feelings: "Such are the notions of a professional anatomist", sneered a reviewer of *The Anatomy of the External Forms of Man*, "to whom the play of a muscle in the graceful attitudes of youth, or the course of a blue vein over a virgin bosom, recalls the horrible mysteries of the dissecting table!"[26]

The antithesis of the horrors of the dissecting-room was the transcendental search for beauty. For Knox, "the essentially beautiful must be in nature" and not in the "monstrous fictions" of the imagination, because no-one could imagine beauty greater than nature had already achieved, or at least "contemplated". However far above commonplace reality Venus appeared to be, artists had not created her, but had drawn her from nature: the "ideals" at which they aimed were transcendental realities, and the work of the anatomist was to search out, among the great "scheme of nature", that ideal form of a race or species, which artists perceived as beauty.[27] Knox did not rule out a mathematical basis for this ideal beauty – "a deep geometry, which the correct mind searches for" – though he did not seek it out. He had not the reductionist mind of Frankfurt anatomist Johann Lucae (1814–1885), who dissected a beautiful woman in order to establish the correct anatomical proportions, and he left it to others to determine whether such perfect figures "delight the eye in consequence of their relation to certain harmonic numbers".[28]

For Knox, the goal of philosophical anatomy – to discover "the true signification of external forms" – was not a matter of numbers. Transcendentalism was "mysteriously wrapt up" in the history of art, because the ideal archetype was glimpsed, as beauty, throughout nature by those whose minds were equipped to perceive it. Hence the discovery of the "Perfect" and the "Beautiful" had to be accomplished before one could offer theories of the "nature of Man", the "origin of race", or the "unity of organic structures", because these all depended upon the ability to see beyond the superficial to that "which must ever be transcendental and abstract; the eternal truth, the unchangeably true".[29]

CHAPTER SEVENTEEN

Organic Harmonies, 1855–1862

Knox's involvement with the Aztec children seems to have rekindled his transcendental enthusiasm: after a few years of comparatively scant literary activity, he published fourteen articles in the *Lancet* and *Zoologist* in 1855 alone, mostly on the "philosophy of zoology". A series of papers on "organic harmonies" followed, but this burst of scientific activity abruptly came to an end in 1858, the year in which Darwin and Wallace gave their papers on evolution at the Linnaean Society, and from that time onwards Knox never again published on philosophical anatomy. Though his public reaction to the theory of natural selection was muted, it is difficult to see the correspondence between the end of his attempts to solve the species question and the publication of the theory as fortuitous, especially since he continued to write on other subjects. Perhaps the realization that so much progress had been made along different lines from his own caused him to lose heart, though even after the publication of *On the Origin of Species* in 1859 he never repudiated his transcendental theories, and maintained that the question of how new species arose was still unanswered. How, therefore, did his mature work on transcendentalism stand in relation to Darwinian natural selection?

Over the course of an irregular career, Knox's writings on race and species had appeared piecemeal in various books and journals, and their fragmentary and disorganized presentation made it difficult to comprehend his theories in their entirety. As a result, his opinions on species change were little noticed in his lifetime, and quickly slipped into a posthumous obscurity so deep that even the apparently straightforward question of whether he was a transmutationist became moot: some commentators thought he was, some called him an "antitransmutationist", and some saw his conclusions as similar to those of Darwin.[1] By the time of Evelleen Richards's influential re-evaluation of his "moral anatomy" in 1989, his contributions to the debate had been largely forgotten.

Knox's contemporaries apparently entertained no doubts over where he stood: the liberal theologian Baden Powell, writing in 1855, called him one of transmutation's most "zealous supporters", and the *Church Review* criticized him for positing "unlimited formation and transformation of species in unknown time".[2] Richards has attributed the subsequent confusion to misinterpretation of passages such as "[t]he development of any species depends on its position in time and space, and not on the transmutation of one species into another", in which Knox ruled out species change at the adult level.[3] This did not, however, apply to the embryo, which he claimed had the potential to develop not only into any species presently in the genus, but also into any extinct or future forms: "[i]n the fullness of time, all will be developed" until no "gaps" remained, and the "grand scheme" of creation would become apparent. "[T]ransmutation theory", he wrote, "is a stumbling block in the way only of those who will not see the truth."[4]

In 1855, in a series of controversial articles in the *Lancet*, Knox accepted "generic creation" but described species as "accidental", in other words they were "instituted", and perished, over time.[5] He had already touched on how they might be instituted when he wrote in *The Races of Men* that "certain deviations, are not viable in the existing order of things; but they may become so".[6] In the words of Richards, Knox's hypothesis was that "'deformations' are constantly generated: those which are not 'viable' are unable to survive and reproduce, but those which are suited to the prevailing geographical and geological conditions flourish and increase in number, and so a new species is established."[7] Whether a newly minted species encountered favourable or unfavourable conditions depended on blind chance: there was no plan, no final purpose, no progress, and no ascent of the ladder of perfection. Unlike most theorists, from Geoffroy to the author of *Vestiges*, Knox refused to surrender Nature's independence to the sovereignty of "the Great First Cause".[8] For one contemporary reviewer, his claim that "Species is the product of external circumstances, acting through millions of years" was nothing less than a "contradiction of the Word of God": "bold, disgusting, and gratuitous atheism".[9]

The concept that, of the huge variety of animals within each natural family, only those suited to the prevailing conditions thrived and reproduced was an ancient one, which until exalted by Darwin as the pre-eminent cause of evolutionary change – natural selection – was merely a means by which the unfit were weeded out. When Knox attributed the formation and extinction of species to "geographical" effects, he presumably envisaged a Cuvierian cycle of terrestrial revolutions: sudden environmental upheavals that created suitable milieux for some of the countless new varieties churned out by the relentless operation of transcendental laws. In modern parlance, he proposed a theory of saltatory evolution, in which "deformations" in embryonic development produced "hopeful monsters" that, if fortuitously suited to the prevailing environmental conditions, could give rise to new species in a single, macroevolutionary leap.[10]

The fount of new species was the embryo, yet Knox, who took others to task for their "ignorance of embryology", showed little interest in the complexities of animal development.[11] He was essentially a vitalist: the embryo contained within it "all the forms or species which that natural family can assume, or has assumed in past time", and these were expressed as development proceeded through a sequence of "mysterious metamorphoses".[12] Quite how the embryo contained all forms was unclear, though it was evidently, in Aristotelian terms, *in potentio*, rather than preformed in some miracle of miniaturization. In the most complete expression of his theory of species change, published in 1857, Knox placed embryogenesis under the control of three transcendental "laws": "tendency to variety", "tendency to *hérédité*", and "tendency to return to the type of the race, or to perish altogether".

His third law, tendency to return to type, prefigured Galton's "typical law of heredity", which explicitly excluded species change by gradual adaptation – because variations in one generation would revert to the mean in the next – or by selective breeding from extreme variants, which were thought to be infertile: "[w]hen the variety proceeds to a certain point, the individual becomes either non-viable or ceases to be productive."[13] In effect, this law ruled out continuous environmental influences as the driving force for speciation. Instead, Knox proposed that new species were produced from the embryo by the interaction of the first two, opposing, laws: tendency to variety, also called the law of unity of organization or the law of deformation, which gave rise to generic (*i.e.* non-specific) forms, and tendency to *hérédité*, also known as the law of specialization or the law of formation, which yielded structures characteristic of the parent species. So with regard, for example, to cervical ribs (an extra pair of ribs in the neck), "[t]he law of species (individuality) gives to man twenty-four ribs . . . the transcendental law, or of unity and general formations, adds two more . . . " to give twenty-six, the number found in many other primates.[14]

Generic forms could be seen in deformities that resulted from so-called "retrogressive development", a term that Knox preferred to "arrested development" as it did not imply that development was a progressive, linear process, though the distinction was rather loose, and he retained the Geoffroyan concept of arrested development in some circumstances, for example when comparing human infants to mature apes:

> These peculiarities and disproportions [of the foetal skeleton] gradually give way with years, being succeeded by the *adult forms*, the specific attributes of the individual. When this does not take place the infantile forms remain, at least to a certain extent; they are of course *abnormal* as regards the adult individual; they are, in fact, *deformities* as regards the human adult form, but they are *normal* as regards the infant and the inferior forms of creation, recent and fossil. . . . In the pelvic or inferior extremities the thigh bones are short and straight, and with the legs and feet recall strongly to the mind the forms of the oran and chimpanzee, the two animals hitherto found which approach nearest to man's structure.[15]

This phenomenon explained why it was that:

> great artists avoided painting or sculpting new-born children, or even those a few days old. They were aware, although they knew not the reason, that such forms were not strictly human, out of all proportion, and displeasing to the eye. They avoided them therefore... although they knew not that such imperfectly-developed forms, in accordance with the laws of unity of the organization, represent more or less other lower forms of the organic world.

Such "infantile forms" were always "unpleasing" and "occasionally frightful", because they showed "no proper development", but represented a "transition state" between adult and "brute forms", or between the adult and "a world which has ceased to be".[16]

When writing of the Aztec children, Knox had speculated that, if all species that had ever lived or could live were arranged in series, the gaps between them would disappear.[17] Even the apparent gulf between man and the rest of creation, which he saw as evidence that a "class or natural family between man and animals is wanting [extinct], or they never have appeared", was theoretically amenable to being filled: "Anthropomorphous apes there are none, nor pithecian men; but as there unquestionably exists a *serial unity* of all that lives, or has lived, or may hereafter, so no such gap can be as that alluded to."[18]

The axiom that all species within a genus could interbreed necessarily consigned man to a separate natural family, since after reviewing some lurid tales of miscegenation Knox concluded that humans could not breed with any other animal. He seems to have regarded the "serial unity" of man and ape as essentially theoretical, and despite his philosophical differences with Owen he defended human uniqueness just as keenly: he rejected popular claims that "Bushmen" were "half human and half brute", and rebuffed attempts to link the Papuan and Australian races with chimpanzees and orangutans, or to set up the "Hottentots" as missing links in the "generic affiliation" between apes and men.[19] In 1857, he claimed to be the only anatomist:

> who denies the existence of any anthropomorphous apes, that is, who asserts that the supposed resemblance between man and apes arises merely from an incorrect appreciation of human anatomy, and that, in point of fact, no such resemblance really exists... but... as in Nature's scheme there can be no deficient link, that the *scale* must be perfect, so this gap will be filled up in time by fossil discoveries or by the further development of life on the globe. Close consanguinity, then, between the human kind and any other animal is thus denied... on the fact of infecundity of union between the different species or genera... that is there is no common parentage, either specific or generic... And so the question must be allowed to remain where it is; science offers no aid to its solution.[20]

Yet in the same paper that debarred consanguinity between man and ape in these apparently emphatic terms, Knox, by speculating on the common origin of genera, invited the reader to consider just such a possibility:

> The conversion of one of these species [of the same genus] into another cannot be so difficult a matter with Nature, especially when all or most of the specific characters are already present in the young. Thus a given species may perish, but another of the same *consanguinité* takes its place in space: it is a question of time, not of new creations: it is but the successive developments of species from one great family. How that family or genus stands with others has not yet been explained, and can only be by Paleontology, which gives us the matured, specific and individualized forms of what, in the living embryo, we can only guess at. The vertebra[t]e[s] have the most positive relations to each other in the unity of their organization, and especially of their skeleton. Thus *parenté* extends from species to genus and from genus to class and order, in characters not to be misunderstood.

Readers of *The Zoologist* (motto: "Wisdom of God in creation") were left with a final unsettling thought: "Is man an episode in creation? At first sight he seems to be so, for he is the only animal directly antagonistic of all that lives, adverse to his own interests."[21]

When, in this his last paper on the "species question", Knox predicted a "renaissance" of transcendentalism, he could not have been more wrong. After the reading of Darwin and Wallace's papers at the Linnaean Society the following year, unity of type, whose laws transcendentalists had wrestled with for decades, became "unity of descent".[22] In contrast to the highly speculative "evolutionistic" schemes of the philosophical anatomists, the *Origin of Species*, a précis of Darwin's projected work, set out his arguments for species change driven by natural selection, and for a branching tree of life rather than a chain, in meticulous detail, with numerous examples. The thoroughness and confidence with which Darwin explained evolutionary mechanisms and addressed possible objections, and the range of his evidence, drawn from geology, palaeontology, botany, taxonomy, and the breeding of domestic animals, gave his work an authoritative tone that was difficult to ignore.[23]

The combative Owen responded by questioning Darwin's scientific credentials. It was indeed ironic that a man who had scarcely entered a dissecting-room should have answered anatomy's greatest question, but the attack ultimately rebounded against Owen, who was posthumously dismissed as a doctrinaire anti-Darwinian who had "lied for God and for malice".[24] Grant, who had encouraged Darwin as a young man, praised the *Origin of Species*, but published his own alternative form of evolution, in which multiple evolutionary trees arose separately from spontaneously generated stock.

Knox and Darwin were not personally acquainted, and probably never met, though they were familiar with one another's works.[25] Given Knox's predilection for controversy, his own reaction to the *Origin of Species* was remarkably subdued: he all but ignored it, writing that it left the problem more or less where it had been before, and describing Darwin's "modern philosophies as to the origin of species" as "an ingenious hypothesis, [that] has great claims on our attention as a new philosophic reading of the phenomena of life, but – it is not science."[26]

The truism that Darwin's evolutionary theory could not be proven in strict scientific terms, which has formed the basis of relentless subsequent debate, was a curious objection for a transcendentalist to make, since Darwinism required just the kind of intuitive leap that Knox had readily accepted in *Naturphilosophie*. *On the Origin of Species* contained some details with which he could not possibly have agreed, for example the claim that acquired characteristics could be inherited, and he cannot have relished its overtones of Malthusianism, but these aspects were peripheral to its main argument.[27] The most serious difficulty for Knox is likely to have been Darwin's insistence that "Natura non facit saltum",[28] on which point he was uncharacteristically dogmatic:

> Why should not Nature have taken a leap from structure to structure? On the theory of natural selection, we can clearly understand why she should not; for natural selection can only act by taking advantage of slight successive variations; she can never take a leap, but must advance by the shortest and slowest steps.[29]

Though prepared to compromise on some contentious points (for example partheneogenesis) in the second edition, Darwin remained implacably opposed to saltation. Even Huxley, "Darwin's bulldog", thought that his insistence on gradual change (later known as evolutionary gradualism) created "unnecessary difficulty", and many distinguished biologists since have agreed with him.[30] To those outside this specialist field, the acrimonious, ongoing gradualism *versus* saltationism debate ("evolution by creeps" *versus* "evolution by jerks") seems to engender stronger reactions than are warranted by a difference of opinion over evolutionary mechanisms, which suggests that for some participants the perceived virtues of the rival theories extend beyond their capacity to explain the natural world. This was so from the beginning, for though Darwin presented his work far more clearly and cogently than had Knox, its reception was undoubtedly aided by the average reader's preference for unobstructed competition and gradual progress rather than sudden, radical leaps: for the Victorian reader, progress by revolution was perhaps even less desirable than ascent from lower species by a process of gradual improvement.[31]

Knox's failure to engage more fully with the questions raised by the *Origin of Species* may have been due in part to competing pressures on his time. On 18 October 1856, at the age of sixty-five, he was appointed pathological anatomist to the Cancer Hospital in Brompton, a free hospital founded in 1851 by William Marsden, another former pupil of Abernethy's, for "the exclusive treatment of cancer". This novel development was (like most novel developments) opposed by the British Medical Association, which claimed that its specialist ethos would destroy the "unity of disease", but by 1857 some 1,800 patients a year were being cared for, a fifth as inpatients, and a site in Fulham road had been earmarked for expansion.[32] As an Edinburgh graduate, Knox was not entitled to practise medicine or surgery in London, and was therefore restricted to a non-clinical rôle: his duties included examining tumours removed at operation and attending autopsies performed by the surgeons, who included his "friend" the pioneering ovariotomist Thomas Spencer Wells (1818–1897).[33] There is no record of the salary he received for this unusual post, though it is unlikely to have been generous, as the hospital relied on voluntary contributions and was chronically under funded, with fewer than half its beds occupied until Queen Victoria made a substantial donation in 1864, but the job did provide a degree of financial security that Knox had not enjoyed since his move to London.[34]

When the 1858 Medical Act levelled the profession by creating a single, national register of doctors regardless of their place and type of qualification, Knox applied for and was granted registration, which enabled him to take on some poorly-paid obstetric work in the neighbourhood of his modest lodgings at 9 Lambe Terrace, Hackney. He shared his digs with his son Edward, who was probably something of a liability, as he does not seem to have followed any trade or profession.[35] In the evenings, having made the tiresome six-mile return commute from his work, probably by 'bus and train,[36] Knox wrote popular articles on anatomy, physiology and art, and translated a French book on prostitution, which appeared, without its translator's name, as *The Greatest of our Social Evils*.[37] In an attempt to dissuade his "friend" Isidore Geoffroy St Hilaire from advocating the consumption of horsemeat, a diet Knox thought acceptable only in "savage" nations, he wrote to the *Lancet* to suggest that animals be imported from Africa until such time as French fish farming and cattle breeding programmes could be got under way. His ambitious proposal for "steam-vessels of great power" carrying "ample supplies of food" across the Mediterranean would have led to some exotic items on the menus of Paris, though his ulterior motive was to stir the French into founding colonies of their own before the Saxons, "bursting on Central Africa like an impetuous and irresistible torrent", overwhelmed it entirely.[38]

Writing is a lonely pastime, and Knox was increasingly in poor spirits: the death of his "beloved" eldest daughter Mary in 1858 "preyed very much on his mind and health", and he told his publisher Henry Renshaw "that he then, and only then, saw that he was mortal."[39] The transcendental doctrines of *The Races of Men*, which he revised for re-issue, seemed sadly old-fashioned, though he took the opportunity of a second edition to defend the "much maligned races" of the Cape against the cannibal libel, and to rebuke the Dutch for treating them like "wild beasts". "[N]o race ever possessed nobler qualities than the Caffre", he wrote, "whose degradation, if he really be degraded, is due to his contact with the intrusive European race." He defended his continuing preoccupation with race, "a tabooed subject, forbidden, interdicted", on the grounds that it was the one subject that Saxon colonialists, whose true intention was to "exterminate the heathen", particularly wished to avoid: "Look at Ireland and Australia; America, North and South; at Africa; at India. I was blamed for having first brought forward this dangerous topic, and for placing it so prominently before the reading public; but why conceal the truth?"[40]

On 27 November 1860 the Ethnological Society of London, meeting at the headquarters of the Royal Society of Literature in St Martin's Place, elected Knox an Honorary Fellow, apparently "to the indignation of the Quakers".[41] This belated recognition may have been prompted by the Society's dwindling numbers – in 1858 there were only thirty-eight paying members and just seven attended the annual general meeting – but it was still a significant honour and an indication that Knox's work was recognized in Britain as well as France, where he had recently been unanimously elected a Foreign Corresponding Member of the Anthropological Society of Paris.[42] In March 1861 he read papers on "human crania" and "some Early Forms of Civilisation", in which he drew attention to the fact that "many" civilized races of the past had disappeared, though in the discussion which followed it was put to him that civilization might be determined by circumstances, rather than by race.[43] Knox's racially deterministic views were, however, congenial to the Society's ascendant anthropological faction, who in June 1862 appointed him Honorary Curator of their "Museum of Crania", though there is no record of him undertaking any duties in connection with this office.[44]

In old age, Knox appeared less intimidating to his professional colleagues, and his manner was kinder, even "affectionate and cheerful".[45] He remained on friendly terms with some of his former students, including Fergusson and (Sir) Benjamin Ward Richardson, with whom he enjoyed chatting about science, but when he visited Richardson's home he avoided meeting his other guests, declined all offers of refreshment, and never revealed where he lived.[46] Hackney was not a place to which he wished to invite colleagues, and he could not accept hospitality that he was unable to return. At a meeting of the Ethnological Society on 1 July 1862 he spoke in public for the last time, the subject under discussion being the "simian affinity" of some archaeological human remains. Having heard the arguments at length, Knox rose and "with a gesture of eloquence, entirely put right the whole matter . . . The manner in which the great old man then spoke", recalled Carter Blake, "will never be forgotten by those who heard him."[47]

Several months later, he is said to have told Henry Renshaw: "I would rather discover one fact in science, than have a fortune bestowed upon me".[48] Mindful of his own mortality, and burdened by his duties at the Cancer Hospital (there was no old-age pension, and no prospect but continued labour), he was perhaps acutely aware that he would now never make the great discovery that would secure him lasting recognition. The last of his papers to appear during his lifetime was a nostalgic but inconsequential reminiscence of a patient wounded at Waterloo, forty-seven years previously, who had been treated by his "esteemed friend", the imperial surgeon Baron Larrey.[49]

On Tuesday 9 December 1862, Knox worked as usual at the Cancer Hospital, which had reopened in the Fulham Road, but arrived home in the evening "much exhausted" and took to his bed. Three days later he suffered a "fit" that left the right side of his body paralyzed. He died at his lodgings in Lambe Terrace on 20 December 1862 at the age of seventy-one. His last illness had been mercifully short, and news of his death came as a shock to acquaintances who had seen him in "tolerable" health only a few weeks before. The only one of his seven children to survive him was his son Edward, then aged twenty-one.[50] On 29 December he was buried, in accordance with his instructions, in the newly opened London Necropolis in Surrey, in a spot "where the sun would shine oftenest". It was a final affirmation of harmony with nature and his "mother earth":

> in infancy [man] seeks the green fields, the forest, the river banks; in the tide of manhood, he rushes from the smoky haunts of man to the mountain-top . . . and when about to quit for ever its mortal abode, the mind sees in blissful visions green fields and running streams, the representation of that earth from which he sprung, and to which he is about to return.[51]

CHAPTER EIGHTEEN

Science Run Mad

The efforts of Knox's biographers, past, present and future, to put the record straight and set the facts in order are unlikely to have much impact on how he is popularly remembered. It is fictional Knox, in the setting of popular tales of the nineteenth-century dissecting-room, who evokes an emotional response that continues to sway public perceptions of anatomy. Fiction influences values and behaviours, but it is also influenced by them, and the changing presentation of Knox's story, founded as it is on limited primary sources, reflects changing public attitudes to dissection, and to the moral responsibilities of the profession of medicine. These sometimes lurid tales of the dissecting room deserve our attention, for they constitute, for better or worse, Knox's enduring legacy.

Perhaps the earliest occurrence in English fiction of the radical, atheistic and intellectually arrogant anatomist, probing nature's secrets in a room hidden from the public gaze, is Disraeli's Marmion Herbert: a precocious freethinker, a "noxious", mischievous, "conspirator against society", and an amateur anatomist who, being a wealthy English gentleman, "shut himself up in his magnificent castle" where "in his laboratory or his dissecting-room he occasionally flattered himself that he might discover the great secret which had perplexed generations."[1] Herbert was based on Percy Shelley, and his anatomical interests served to emphasize his aristocratic particularity, indifference to common sensibilities, and superiority over his fellow creatures.[2] In Victorian fiction, the anatomist characteristically enjoyed, and often abused, literal power over the bodies of his social inferiors, thus representing metaphorically the oppressive exercise of social authority.

Such authority, based as it was on status and knowledge, was by its nature undemocratic, and so the anatomist was something of a *bête noir* for social reformers. In the penny dreadful *Mysteries of London* the chartist writer and journalist George W.M. Reynolds portrayed resurrection men (in 1837) as entirely subservient to the will of the surgeon-anatomist: "You command – we obey", is their prompt response when he tells them where (in a church) to dig. Despite being also a blackmailer (prefiguring Gray in Stevenson's *The Body Snatcher*), the resurrection man appeals to the reader's sympathies: "We ain't born bad: something then must have made us bad. If I had been in the Duke of Wellington's place, I should be an honourable and upright man like him;

and if he had been in my place, he would be – what I am... *in nine cases out of ten the laws themselves make us take to bad ways, and then punish us for acting under their influence*".[3] The anatomist, on the other hand, is inherently cruel because for him dissection is not a professional duty but a perverse and passionately driven hobby: "I amuse myself here in my leisure hours", says one fictional anatomist with studied ambiguity while showing a horrified visitor into his dissecting-room.[4]

Nor was this the chaste, formal passion of cold intellect: the surgeon's contact with a female corpse in *Mysteries of London* reads like a distorted sexual encounter. Though ordinarily "a man of a naturally strong mind", he "could not control the strange feelings which crept upon him" while watching the "regular and systematic movements" of the resurrection men as they violated the tomb. "The Resurrection Man took one of the long flexible rods... and thrust it down into the vault. The point penetrated into the lid of a coffin. He drew it back, put the point to his tongue, and tasted it."[5] When the coffin was finally wrenched open, "[t]he polished marble limbs of the deceased were rudely grasped by the sacrilegious hands of the body-snatchers; and, having stripped the corpse stark naked, they tied its neck and heels together by means of a strong cord" and lifted it into the surgeon's carriage.

Resurrected bodies were conveyed in secret to the surgeon's house, where an ambiguous fate awaited them:

> The Resurrection Man and the Buffer conveyed the body into a species of out-house, which the surgeon, who was passionately attached to anatomical studies, devoted to purposes of dissection and physiological experiment.
>
> In the middle of this room, which was about ten feet long and six broad, stood a strong deal table, forming a slightly inclined plane. The stone pavement of the out-house was perforated with holes in the immediate vicinity of the table, so that the fluid which poured from subjects for dissection might escape into a drain communicating with the common sewer. To the ceiling, immediately above the head of the table, was attached a pulley with a strong cord, by means of which a body might be supported in any position that was most convenient to the anatomist.[6]

Reynolds further alludes to the unwholesome intent of the anatomist in a "body-snatcher's song" that might have been written for Mary Paterson:

> In the churchyard the body is laid,
> There they inter the beautiful maid:
> "Earth to earth" is the solemn sound!
> Over the sod where their daughter sleeps,
> The father prays, and the mother weeps:
> "Ashes to ashes" echoes around!

> Come with the axe, and come with the spade,
> Come where the beautiful virgin's laid:
> Earth from earth must we take back now!
> The sod is damp, and the grave is cold
> Lay the white corpse on the dark black mould.
> That the pale moonbeam may kiss its brow!
>
> Throw back the earth, and heap up the clay;
> This cold white corpse we will bear away,
> Now that the moonlight waxes dim;
> For the student doth his knife prepare
> To hack all over this form so fair,
> And sever the virgin limb from limb![7]

The sinister anatomist of early Victorian fiction was a stock character rather than a representation of any one person, though the popularity of this disreputable stereotype, and the public's "melancholy interest" in anatomy, had its roots in the sensational reports and rumours surrounding the West Port and Italian Boy murders, after which "appalling events" there was "not at the present moment a more interesting subject than anatomical study". Anatomical fiction satisfied the public's appetite for further revelations of the "secrets of the dissecting-room",[8] and penny dreadfuls served up dissecting-room mysteries[9] in which the subject ideally turned out to be a young woman "of perfect proportions". The reader's reaction to this melancholy twist of fate was anticipated, and perhaps encouraged, by the suggestion that even the medical gentlemen in the story had a preference for a handsome corpse: "[t]hat evening there were many more persons in the dissecting-room than usual", began one account of the dissection of "a perfect Venus!"[10]

Sally Powell's contention that "in penny fiction . . . the snatching and dissection of the female corpse constitutes a rape" is convincing, but it must be borne in mind that it is the author and his readers, not the characters, who are complicit in the action.[11] Anatomists were, however, sufficiently concerned by rumours about dissecting-room "secrets" to distance themselves from any hint of self-indulgence:

> To hear the declaimers on this theme, it might be imagined that the process [of dissection] is one of great amusement and agreeability; and that the surgeons and their apprentices addict themselves to a secret indulgence at the public expense, which is untested by the less luxurious part of mankind. . . . Seriously and honestly, I beg . . . to assure my worthy friends . . . that there is nothing in a dissecting-room from which the most hardened *habitué* does not retreat at the earliest moment, when he has obtained the information he requires. Practical anatomy, at best, is a loathsome, fatiguing, cold, monotonous, and tiresome piece of business. . . . It is only a select few who, influenced by . . . a

lofty ambition of professional distinction, bear up against the tedium and disgust of the operation, and continue their dissections after having obtained a license to practise.[12]

Burke and Hare, in no position to defend themselves, featured in two French melodramas, Jules Lacroix's *L'Étouffeur d'Edimbourg* (1844) and Frédéric de Mercey's *Burk l'étouffeur* (1858), as ready-made villains of the blackest dye. In the latter novella they are hired by the evil Lord Archibald Gordon to abduct the virtuous Nelly, for which nefarious deed they are promised far more than the five guineas a body that Knox pays them.[13] Neither story, however, is concerned with the West Port murders, and Knox himself does not appear. He is also absent from James G. Bertram's novel *The Story of a Stolen Heir* (1858), published in London, which painted an horrific picture of life before the Anatomy Act, when "it was a common practice for persons to sell their dead relatives to the doctors for the purposes of dissection!", a fate that the infant heir of the title, who is nursed by Burke's wife, narrowly escapes. No anatomist is mentioned by name, but it is observed that, as a class, their "great anxiety" to "get dead bodies" led them to deal profligately with the criminal underworld. Even Mrs Burke underestimates the lengths to which they were prepared to go: "but sure the docthers would never make any use of an infant like –" she asks innocently, and Bertram swiftly reassures the reader that "[a]ll this has now been reformed [by the Anatomy Act], and there is no lack of bodies to operate upon."[14] The West Port murders also featured on the Victorian stage: the earliest known example being *Burke and Hare*, a "startling drama" with "Terrific situations", the script of which was on sale from the late 1860s, though the pair probably appeared before this in grand guignol or burlesque, for which scripts and performance records have not survived.[15]

The first novel in which Knox appeared as a character, and the only one to pass moral judgement on him during his lifetime, was *The Court of Cacus* (1861), a semi-fictionalized account of the West Port murders by the writer of popular Scottish history Alexander Leighton. Its present scarcity and the lack of contemporary reviews suggest that it attracted little notice (though it did manage a second edition), and it is quite possible that Knox, preoccupied with his work in London, never even heard about it. The title is a quotation from Dryden's translation of the *Aeneid*, which tells how Hercules exposed the lair of the "brutal" monster Cacus, an ambiguous creature, "more than half a beast", who lived off human flesh and nailed the heads and limbs of his victims to the door of a cave "foul with human gore".

Having flaunted the prospect of anatomical cannibalism in the title, Leighton offered a comparatively restrained critique of Knox as a "complex" man, whose vanity proved his undoing: while Burke, like Alexander the Great, had "desecrated the temple for money", Knox, like his hero Napoleon, had done so out of "ambition". Leighton conceded that the purchase of corpses by anatomists had been "justified by the necessities of their profession", and he accepted their failure to ask questions as unsurprising, since they were dealing with "smuggled goods". He concluded, however, as the 1829 enquiry had, that the medical gentlemen of Surgeons' Square were culpable in not having entertained any suspicion of murder. Had they been more vigilant, he claimed, examination of the bodies would have revealed signs of violence. Given this allegation, it is significant that he judged the doorkeeper David Paterson, who was the first to see the bodies and would have stripped them for dissection, "the most free from blame", perhaps because Paterson, "still a respectable inhabitant of Edinburgh", had supplied him with information.[16]

Leighton's assessment of Knox as self-obsessed and "without a touch of pity" rings true, though rather less plausible is his claim that an urge to "subjugate all people to his will" led Knox to whip up enthusiasm for anatomy among his pupils until it became a "science run mad". According to Leighton, the teacher's fervour spread to his pupils "like an inoculation", and their craving for anatomical knowledge grew into a "frenzy" in which they encouraged body snatching and strove to outdo one another in obtaining "things" for dissection, thus unwittingly creating a market for murder. This view of the anatomist as the driving force behind mad science was almost flattering in its intensity, for the passion that usurped his judgement was scholarly zeal rather than the private perversions of the penny dreadful: when the body-snatcher, a "sleazy dog" with an "Irish nose", brought a corpse to the dissecting-room, a place of "choking air, thick with gases" that no freshening breeze could dissipate, Knox, "the monoculus himself" saw only "valuable tissues,– in the midst of which lay the secrets these students were so anxious to reveal, not for the purpose of filling their pockets in after-times, but for the benefit of mankind . . . ".[17]

In David Pae's *Mary Paterson* (1866) Knox is a less inspiring figure, a dull villain lacking common humanity. The story, which like much of Pae's work first appeared in serial form in the *People's Friend*, combines a fairly accurate account of the West Port murders with fictional embellishments featuring Mary Paterson's admirers. Burke and Hare are depicted as an utterly brutal and loutish pair, whose Irishness ("Begorra, I niver thought uv that") is emphasized with almost every utterance. Burke's trial and hanging follow the actual course of events, while, as fiction requires that the bad end unhappily, Hare meets a well-deserved death at the hands of a lynch mob. Knox is "a smart, fussy, self-consequential man, wearing spectacles" and devoid of decent feelings. "Upon my soul, I never saw a more beautiful body", he says of Mary Paterson, running his eye over her "slowly". Apart from this untoward interest in Mary, his examination of the murder victims is culpably brief: "and of these crimes we must consider the doctors *presumptively* guilty, inasmuch as they carefully abstained from satisfying themselves that they were not committed."[18]

Though few Victorian works of fiction made overt reference to the West Port murders, the modern reader may suspect Knox's presence in the quintessentially Gothic figure of the cold-blooded, rational, ruthless scientist whose ambition drives him to transgress conventional morality. Comparisons between Knox and Frankenstein are inevitable, though when Mary Shelley's novel was published, in 1818, Knox was an obscure hospital assistant in the Cape. Victor Frankenstein, moreover, was neither a doctor nor a professional anatomist (not until the twentieth century did he become *Doctor* Frankenstein), and though he obtains corpses from "vaults and charnel-houses" as well as "[t]he dissecting room and the slaughter-house . . . ", he claims no more than to be "acquainted with the science of anatomy".[19]

The *Lancet* called the Anatomy Bill, that abortive precursor of the Anatomy Act, a creation of Frankenstein, and Tim Marshall has argued that "history recasts Frankenstein after Burke and Hare", necessitating a reinterpretation of the novel in the light of the Anatomy Act, which he sees as "The historical monster in *Frankenstein*".[20] There is, however, no reference to the West Port murders in Shelley's revised text of 1831, or in her letters and journals.[21] This is not to deny an implicit medical subtext to the story – as early as 1826, an adaptation for the Parisian stage was entitled *Le Monstre et le physician* – but the link with Knox was not made until the mid-twentieth century, and the adaptations of *Frankenstein* that were almost continuously on the English stage throughout the nineteenth century make no reference to him, open or implied.[22] It has recently been suggested that *Frankenstein* was a critique not of the appropriation of bodies for dissection, or the monstrous legislation intended to prevent this, but of the exaggerated objectivity and clinical detachment of the scientific anatomist, under whose gaze, in Foucaultian terms, the body became the only object of enquiry, the ultimate source of all self-knowledge.[23]

Whatever their origins, the medical aspects of *Frankenstein* were increasingly emphasized in twentieth-century film adaptations, and as codes of censorship in the USA and Britain that restricted the on screen portrayal of medical doctors in an unflattering light were relaxed "Dr Frankenstein" was gradually brought into the medical fold. In Universal Studios' *Frankenstein* (1931), Henry Frankenstein and his hunchbacked assistant Fritz rob a graveyard and steal a corpse from a medical school; in *Son of Frankenstein* (1939), Wolf Frankenstein (surely an echo of Stevenson's Wolfe Macfarlane) is assisted by Igor, a broken-necked body snatcher who survived the gallows, and in *Frankenstein Meets the Wolf Man* (1943) and *House of Frankenstein* (1944), Frankenstein is referred to as a doctor, but does not appear, though in the latter film Boris Karlof plays an unnamed "Mad Doctor".[24] The first film, and indeed the first work of any kind, in which the character of Frankenstein, by then ennobled as Baron Victor, was identified with Knox is Hammer Films' *The Curse of Frankenstein* (1957), in which Peter Cushing based his characterization of the title rôle on Knox, whom he went on to play in the 1959 film *The Flesh and the Fiends*.[25]

Perhaps the creation of Victorian fiction with the strongest claim to have been inspired by Knox is/are the title characters in Robert Louis Stevenson's *Dr Jekyll and Mr Hyde* (1886), though here too the earliest unmistakable connection between Hyde and Knox is a Hammer film, *Dr. Jekyll and Sister Hyde*, in which Burke and Hare make an appearance. Jekyll is not Knox's double – his medical researches are "rather chemical than anatomical" – but he seems to share something of his circumstances: his house with its attached laboratory once belonged to a "celebrated surgeon", and it incorporates an "old dissecting room." Stevenson may have had Knox in mind as the former owner of the house, but there is nothing in the text to identify him with Jekyll.[26] It is not out of the question that Stevenson intended the two-faced Jekyll to represent Knoxian duplicity, but the theme of concealment of a personal secret or vice was a common one in his storytelling, and Edinburgh's Old Town, where dark, noisome closes led off elegant thoroughfares and grand houses had doors opening onto both, where rich and destitute were perhaps more closely approximated than in any other British city, and where the turn of a corner could take the pedestrian from a fashionable street to a slum, was surely inspiration enough for a tale of a divided and hypocritical society where vice lay barely concealed beneath a respectable surface.

In any case, a veiled allusion to Knox would have been superfluous, as Stevenson had already aired his views in *The Body-Snatcher*, published two years earlier, in which Knox appeared as "Mr K_____". The narrator of the story is a failed medico named Fettes, one of Knox's former assistants and a man of dissolute character, who justifies his "blackguardly enjoyment" in the evenings by his success as a student of anatomy. As Knox's subordinate, one of his duties is to receive bodies from the resurrection men, while under instructions from his employer to "Ask no questions . . . for conscience' sake." This he duly does, until two Irishmen bring the body of Jane Galbraith, whom he knew to have been "alive and hearty yesterday" when he "jested" with her. Suspecting murder, Fettes seeks the advice of his immediate superior, the "clever, dissipated, and unscrupulous" class assistant, Wolfe Macfarlane, who decides for Knox's sake and their own to keep silent about the terrible revelation that "all our subjects have been murdered." The whole class is complicit in the conspiracy, and when the unfortunate girl is dissected, no-one appears to recognize her.[27]

Fettes's experiences thus far are based on the West Port case, but events subsequently take an even more dramatic turn: Macfarlane murders "a very loathsome rogue" called Gray (the name of the man who had alerted the police to the West Port murders) who has some unspecified hold over him from the past, and he too is dissected. When Knox runs short of subjects, Fettes and Macfarlane go grave robbing, only to discover that the body they have sacked up is not the grave's expected occupant but the reanimated and "long-dissected" Gray. At least, Macfarlane imagines it to be Gray, for he can no more lay his nemesis to rest than murder his own conscience.

Macfarlane differs too much from any real person to be libellous, though the "great rich London doctor" who as Knox's former assistant "jested" with Jane Galbraith/Mary Paterson is strongly reminiscent of Sir William Fergusson. However, as Goodsir pointed out in his former teacher's defence, in writing "K_____", Stevenson "might just as well have written KNOX".[28] Stevenson showed no sympathy for Knox, who, he wrote, had "skulked through the streets of Edinburgh in disguise" in fear of the mob, though he apparently had some misgivings about publishing a story "blood-curdling enough – and ugly enough – to chill the blood of a grenadier", and after completing it in 1881 he "laid [it] aside in a justifiable disgust, the tale being horrid" until 1884, when it was printed in the *Pall Mall Christmas Extra*, which advertised it on "ghoulish" posters and coffin shaped placards carried by men dressed in shrouds.[29]

Stevenson's depiction of anatomists was as damaging as any ever written, extending as it did beyond criticism of individuals to suggest that anatomy itself served no purpose beyond self-advancement and that it demoralized the character, a concern that was already being voiced within the medical profession. So entrenched had this notion become by the late 1880s that it was suspected the Whitechapel murders must be the work of a "scientific anatomist", someone "accustomed to the post-mortem room", who removed one victim's uterus to sell as a "specimen".[30] Though Jack the Ripper's medical connection was pure speculation, the profession was impotently indignant in the face of such "gross and unjustifiable" calumnies, which seemed "calculated to exert an injurious influence on the public mind".[31]

For the average reader the most unsettling aspect of *The Body-Snatcher* was probably not its evocation of the murder for anatomy scandals of fifty years ago but the appearance of Gray's reanimated corpse. Stevenson had used a similar plot device in *The Suicide Club*, in which a strong-willed doctor persuades a younger man to cover up a murder, and it seems that concealment or misplacement of a corpse had some significance for him, since he employed variations on the theme in *Treasure Island, Kidnapped, The Master of Ballantrae*, and *The Wrong Box*. Buckton has argued that the corpse that turns up in the young man's bed in *The Suicide Club* symbolizes "a homoerotic secret between the two men", and that the hidden corpses in Stevenson's later writing represent "the 'unspeakable' vice of sodomy".[32] The basis of Gray's hold over Macfarlane was blackmail, an omnipresent fear for homosexual men in Victorian Britain, and it may be that Stevenson's preoccupation with buried secrets and dual personalities reflected his own anxieties, or that he intended these themes to stir up his readers' private fears.

By the end of the nineteenth century, almost no-one remembered Knox's work or the scandals associated with his name. The taste for dissecting-room drama had passed, and Knox's story had slipped into obscurity, where it might have remained had not the Scottish playwright James Bridie revived it, a century after the West Port murders, in his tragicomedy *The Anatomist*. The play opened on 3 July 1930 at Edinburgh's Lyceum theatre and transferred to London the following year, where its reception was helped by fine performances from Henry Hinchliffe Ainley as Knox, "a compound of Dr Johnson and Long John Silver, with an eye missing instead of a leg", and Flora Robson as Mary Paterson, a rôle she later considered her finest.[33]

Bridie's Knox was a far more charismatic figure than his dissipated and cruel Victorian predecessors: a pragmatical bully and braggart in the dissecting-room, a dazzling, if somewhat overbearing, wit in Edinburgh society, and an articulate, compelling and earnest advocate of anatomical science in the lecture room, he emerges as "a wayward and capricious hero with a touch of real nobility".[34] Bridie (Osborne Henry Mavor, 1888–1951) was a Glasgow-trained doctor and professor of medicine, and the *Lancet* thought *The Anatomist* likely to appeal to medical men. It drew no conclusions regarding Knox's motives, though Bridie's notes on the published text suggest that one character's dismissal of him as a "vain, hysterical, talented, stupid man . . . wickedly blind and careless when [his] mind is fixed on something" most nearly represented the author's own opinion.[35]

Despite making Knox complicit in murder, rather than just culpably reckless, Bridie portrayed him in a favourable light, as a zealous and committed advocate of the benefits of science. In some respects, this partial moral rehabilitation reflected a shift in public and professional attitudes since the nineteenth century. When Knox began his career, a medical practitioner's actions had been judged according to his personal integrity; hence the emphasis on what Knox and others had known or believed about the supply of cadavers, and the concerns about the damage done by the dissecting-room and vivisection to students' morals and manners. The indispensable characteristic of a medical gentleman was "rectitude of principle",[36] and so the unreliability of Knox's certificates and his inconsistent dealings with the funeratory system proved more damaging to his career than the source of the bodies in his dissecting-room. In the twentieth century, however, Bridie's generation of medical men were a more homogenized professional group, reliant on paper qualifications rather than social standing, and with the General Medical Council in place to strike rogue doctors from the register, public concerns shifted to the responsibilities incumbent on the profession as a whole, some of which were adumbrated in Shaw's well-known preface to *The Doctor's Dilemma* (1909). Society's expectations of the state-regulated profession had changed, and in particular the rise of the eugenics movement fostered the notion that the physician had a greater duty to the whole population or "race" than to the individual patient. It was an acrimonious debate – saving the life of a "crippled" child or allowing it to die could both be seen as crimes against the human race[37] – but it made Knox's fictional justification of the dissection of Edinburgh's outcasts for the public good seem neither as callous nor as outlandish as it once had.

The Anatomist sparked a revival of interest in the anatomy scandals of a bygone age, which were an ideal subject for the Victorian-style melodramas that were then undergoing a revival. Theatregoers disinclined to dwell on the ethical problems of the anatomist's calling were entertained by *The Wolves of Tanner's Close or, The Crimes of Burke and Hare*, an "old-fashioned", "rip-roaring" melodrama with Tod Slaughter, famous for his rôle as demon barber Sweeney Todd, as Hare.[38] The play promised "Blood and bloodshed! Murder and butchery!", and opened in time for Christmas 1931 – "good fun provided you had a strong stomach".[39] "[B]lood satisfactorily flows!", announced *The Times* gleefully: "[y]ou have only to sit down for a minute in Burke's room and take a few gulps of laudanum and whisky to find yourself being strangled, packed in a box, wheeled away on a trolley and punctually delivered to the dissecting table under the single, fishy eye of Dr Knox", who was played by George M. Slater.[40]

Unsurprisingly, it was Bridie's more cerebral treatment of the story that was adapted for the more closely regulated medium of television. On 2 June 1939 the BBC broadcast a production of *The Anatomist* that *The Times*'s critic found "far more impressive" than the stage play, with Andrew Cruikshank in the rôle of Knox: "a provocative figure, a pioneer in medical science, a man to be reckoned with, a portent, a personality."[41] *The Anatomist* returned to the London stage in 1948 with the distinguished Scottish actor Alastair Sim, then Rector of Edinburgh University, as an "unexpectedly innocent" Knox, a man of science driven to depend on rogues for material vital to his research and courageously accepting moral responsibility for the death of his victims.[42] Though it has been criticized for presenting an unduly sympathetic picture of its subject, who one recent critic saw as "little more than a fantasy wish fulfilment figure for its author", the play proved to be Bridie's most durable work, and its popularity re-established Knox as an ambiguous and attractive dramatic character.[43]

"[I]t seems strange", wrote a reviewer of the 1939 television play, that the story had not yet been made into a film.[44] Murder for dissection was a difficult subject to bring to the cinema screen, and censorship issues ensured that the first attempt, Robert Wise's film of *Robert Louis Stevenson's "The Body Snatcher"* (RKO Radio Pictures 1945), was far more restrained in tone than the story on which it was based. Ostensibly, Knox does not appear in the film, which is set in Edinburgh in 1831, but the anatomist Dr Macfarlane, who is introduced as Knox's former "assistant", resembles him in dress and domestic circumstances (his devoted wife poses as a maid to avoid compromising his career), as well as in the single-minded arrogance with which he carries on his work: "I need these lifeless subjects for my students' enlightenment and my own knowledge." Macfarlane is a technically proficient surgeon who has shunned a career in surgery for teaching, and his nemesis, the resurrection man Gray, provokes him by emphasizing his failings as a practitioner, a rôle he claims Macfarlane is "afraid" to take on. According to Gray, the dissecting-room studies that furnished Macfarlane's "knowledge" have paradoxically disqualified him from practice: "Could you be a doctor, a healing man, with the things those eyes have seen?"

There had been no previous consideration of why Knox seldom practised surgery after his return from the Cape, despite being well trained and qualified to do so: there does not seem to have been any professional reason, and the answer presumably lay in his character. A more sympathetic hypothesis would have been that he was too sensitive to operate on living, conscious patients, rather than too unfeeling, though the latter explanation was preferred in 1945, when anatomy was considered so repugnant a subject that the Breen Office, responsible for film censorship in the USA, forbad any overt depiction of it, "because of the repellent nature of such matter, which has to do with grave-robbing, dissecting bodies, and pickling bodies".[45] Although *The Body Snatcher* complied with these restrictions, it was still deemed unsuitable for screening in the United Kingdom, where the British Board of Film Censors ordered the scenes showing Gray's corpse and a demonstration of the method of Burking to be cut, leaving the story all but unintelligible.[46]

Once it had been established, on both sides of the Atlantic, that the West Port murders could be alluded to, however obliquely, on film, the way was open for Tod Slaughter to reprise his larger-than-life performance as Burke in *The Greed of William Hart* (1948), a melodrama in the spirit of his company's pre-war productions at the Elephant Theatre. "By thunder, what an interesting specimen" cries Dr Cox – the British censors refused to allow references to Burke, Hare and Knox, and the names were changed on the soundtrack to Hart, Moore, and Cox – at the sight of the then still living daft Jamie. When it is suggested to Cox that Hart and Moore are murderers, he replies: "Impetuous young fool, can a man who has once tasted the fruit of the tree of knowledge lay it aside to be bound by the petty laws and trammels of blinkered mortals?" Cox, the autocratic, autonomous mad scientist, needs cadavers not to run a successful school but for his own researches, and while it is not clear what knowledge he hopes to obtain from human dissection, his scientific zeal at least has the nobility of being free of pecuniary ambition or immoral desire.

Thereafter, Knox was typically portrayed in film as a persuasive, if bombastic, advocate of utilitarian science, whose enthusiasm for anatomy is driven not by some private and misdirected passion, but by an altruistic and laudable desire to bring about scientific advancement for humanity's perceived good. In the 1959 film *The Flesh and the Fiends* he is an honourable figure, an enlightened opponent of medical ignorance and an independent, rational, scientific practitioner, who struggles to improve medical education in the face of opposition from the hidebound traditionalists of the Edinburgh establishment. His willingness to acquiesce to murder if needs must made him an ideal spokesman for moral relativism: in Dylan Thomas's 1953 screenplay *The Doctor and the Devils*, based on a story by Donald Taylor and first performed in Britain as a stage play in 1961,[47] Dr Rock (Knox) boldly argues that "the pursuit of the knowledge of Man . . . justifies any means. . . . Let no scruples stand in the way of the progress of medical science!"[48]

At the time, the idea of making "a choice between evils" was an important strategy for rationalizing non-consensual medical interventions such as leucotomy and electroconvulsive therapy – which were carried out paternalistically but "in good faith and in the patients' best interest" – as well as for justifying controversial techniques such as vivisection and organ transplantation.[49] With wartime atrocities fresh in their minds, many people, and some doctors, argued that "there must be a limit to the doctrine that the end justifies the means", and that some actions, for example "exceptionally painful" experiments on animals, could never be justified whatever the benefits.[50] Dr Rock articulated the alternative, consequentialist, viewpoint that even murder could be justified if knowledge so gained significantly alleviated future suffering: "what if she *was* murdered", he says of the Mary Paterson character, "[w]e are anatomists, not policemen. . . . She served no purpose in life save the cheapening of physical passion and the petty traffics of lust. Let her serve her purpose in death."[51] His musings prefigure a scenario subsequently introduced into discussions of transplantation ethics in which the transplanted organs from one murder victim could save five lives: while the intuitive response is that murder is always wrong whatever the consequences, there might be circumstances, for example if one's own life were one of those to be saved, where consequentialism would have its attractions.[52] By admitting that he knowingly deals with murderers to supply his anatomy school, Dr Rock, the successor of Bridie's urbane and articulate casuist, teases the audience out of their moral complacency: "Do you expect the dead to walk here . . . ?", he enquires, "[t]hey need assistance."[53]

Reviewing a production of *The Anatomist* in 1968, *The Times* noted the "temptation to make the play speak to us in contemporary terms, whether of heart transplants or the other contemporary medical dilemmas."[54] In recent years, whenever there has been public disapprobation of controversial medical procedures, such as recent proposals, backed by Scotland's Chief Medical Officer, to "harvest" organs for transplantation from brain-dead, beating heart donors who would be "presumed" to have given consent, the outraged response is that "Burke and Hare are alive and well".[55] Comparisons between modern medical practice and the misdeeds of nineteenth-century anatomists were particularly to the fore in the late 1990s after two well-publicized scandals at Alder Hey Children's Hospital and Bristol Royal Infirmary, both of which involved retention of organs and tissues from autopsies without proper consent from the next-of-kin.[56] According to one medical ethicist:

> Unlike their nineteenth-century peers, today's resurrectionists do not need to resort to murder. The moral outrage surrounding these "new" resurrectionists is equally strong as that regarding Burke and Hare in the nineteenth century, if not more so, since today we have developed rights-based culture and a clear expectation of consensual medical practices.[57]

The claim that public "outrage" at retention of tissue from autopsies could have been stronger than the reaction to a series of brutal murders is an indication of a deeply held and enduring distaste towards appropriation of body parts in scientific settings. Any failure of the medical profession to respect the sanctity of the dead appears "barbaric . . . like something out of Burke and Hare", a culpable disregard of decency that reduces the doctor to the level of a "butcher" and the body (in a phrase that harks back to the cannibal libel) to "a piece of meat".[58]

From a medical viewpoint these were unwelcome reminders, on the cusp of the twenty-first century, of the "chasm" in attitudes that still existed between professional and lay people, not least because the nineteenth-century view of morbid anatomy as a "perverse hobby" pursued by the medical profession seemed to be regaining currency.[59] In 2001, Nathan R. Francis and Wayne Lewis, a medical student and general practitioner respectively, revisited the debate over whether dissection was demoralizing to the dissector and detrimental to medicine as a profession. While not wishing "to call into question the value of dissection in medical education; [or] to charge dissection with being an inefficient or ineffective means of teaching", they questioned the "price" that might be paid for the knowledge so gained:

> Such hardening of medical students may irreparably sever them from their natural human response to death and human bodies, and replace it with a cold thirst for facts and observations from an inanimate "cadaver" object. This may

encourage and teach students to relate to their future patients in the same cold light, as teaching material, to be used as required.[60]

In the twenty-first century, the spread and development of transplant surgery has brought with it the renewed threat of a "market" in human organs, and once more there are fears that the corpse is set to become not just an "object of enquiry" but a commodity, from which tissues possessing "commercial and health value" might be "harvested" or "stolen".[61] In the face of such unease about the fate of unclaimed bodies, comparisons with the past are inevitable: "seldom . . . since Burke and Hare . . . had the focus on the human body and its parts been more intense".[62]

The Knoxian myth is now too well established to yield to facts, and nor, perhaps, should it, for it is a good story that adroitly sums up an important and unresolved ethical question: do we expect medical scientists to adhere to the same ethical and legal codes as the rest of society? Some clearly do not: it has recently been suggested for example, in a medical journal and by an "ethicist", that doctors should not allow "moral values" to "corrupt" their pursuit of the "public interest".[63] Many doctors were appalled by this, yet the public benefits of medical science such as new drugs, gene therapies and reductions in birth defects are often achieved through ethically contentious means such as animal experimentation, human cloning and stem cell research, responsibility for which is tacitly devolved upon the medical profession, with society's complicity. Of course, many lay persons, and some doctors, conscientiously object to the more controversial methods employed, but how often do critics of organ harvesting, animal testing, embryo research, animal–human hybridization, and all the morally questionable armamentarium of medical progress refuse, for themselves and their families, its benefits? As often, perhaps, as the citizens of Edinburgh, which boasted the highest-regarded schools of anatomy and the best trained doctors in Europe, asked how, with a legal supply of bodies in single figures, all this could have been achieved.

Notes

Introduction

1. Holmes 1887, 65. The meeting with Knox that Holmes describes took place in 1834.
2. *The Times* 31 Aug. 1908, 9e.
3. Malchow 1996, 111. Berlioz was writing in 1822.
4. *Ibid.*, 24, 102, 231.
5. Wilson 2001, 29; Richards 1989, 378–9; Richards 1994, 383.
6. RCP MS ALLCW/712/198, letter from Knox to Andrew Clark, 24 Mar. 1845, with later annotations by William Henry Allchin.
7. http://www.lib.ed.ac.uk/faqs/parqsutz.shtml#Staff2, viewed 17 Mar. 2009.
8. *MT* 1853; 6: 121.
9. Richards 1994, 405.
10. Lonsdale 1870, 235; *CE* 1851; 50: 503.
11. Knox 1846, 309; 1850, 277; 1852b, 140.
12. *MT* 1840; 1: 213; *MT* 1844; 10: 245–6.
13. *MT* 1844; 10: 245–6.
14. Knox 1854b, 393.
15. Cloquet 1836, I, 124.
16. Knox 1846, 307.
17. Charles Darwin, Robert Grant, Patrick Matthew and Lord Monboddo all studied in Edinburgh.
18. Jacyna 1983; Richards 1989, 1994.
19. Ruse 1996, 72.
20. Knox 1854b, 393.
21. Desmond 1992, especially pp. 25–100.
22. MacDonald 2006, 10.
23. Lonsdale 1870, 82.
24. Richardson 2001. The Human Tissue Act 2004, like its predecessor, looks set to become "a bureaucrat's bad dream".
25. NA HO 83/1, pp. 43–6, letter from S.M. Phillipps to David Craigie, 24 Jan. 1833.
26. Private anatomy schools continued long after the formation of the General Medical Council and the last, Cooke's in London, closed shortly after the Great War: Morton 1991.
27. Altick 1978, 339; Bates 2008.
28. Report from the select committee on medical education: with the minutes of evidence and appendices. *House of Commons Sessional Papers* 1834, XIII, 112–13.

29 Malchow 1996, 45–55.
30 Lonsdale 1870, 354.
31 Knox 1852a, 39.
32 Lonsdale 1870, viii.
33 RCP ALLCW/713/192, postcard from Sir John Struthers to W.H. Allchin, 1895.
34 *Ibid.*
35 *Lancet* 1847; 1: 567–71.
36 Stephen 1981; Kaufman 1997; 2001; 2003.
37 Macnee 1829; Roughead 1921; Douglas 1973; Mackay 1988; Edwards 1980.
38 Knox 1854b, 396.
39 Richardson 2000; 2001.
40 *The Scotsman* 25 Apr. 2005, http://news.scotsman.com/organ removalscandals/The-mother-of-all-battles.2621217.jp, viewed 17 Mar. 2009; Garwood-Gowers, Tingle and Wheat 2005, 7.
41 Foucault 1973; 1981, 92–102; MacDonald 2006, 10.
42 *The Leader* 1856; 7: 257–8.
43 Richards 1994; Dietrich 2003.
44 Bates 2006.

CHAPTER ONE The Darling Boy of the Family, 1791–1810

1 Brims 1990, 31.
2 Heron 1799, 358; Cosh 2003, 76–7.
3 Edwards 1980, 150.
4 *The Stranger's Guide to Edinburgh . . .* Edinburgh: T. Brown, 1817, 42.
5 Lonsdale 1870, 3.
6 Briggs 1959, 132.
7 Cobbett 1801, VII, 266.
8 *The Stranger's Guide to Edinburgh . . .* Edinburgh: T. Brown, 1817, 43.
9 *Parliamentary Register* 1794; 39: 432.
10 These words attributed to Braxfield were probably an invention; see *Law Magazine and Law Review* 1856; 1: 246.
11 SP OPR marriages 685/0010 500 0226 Edinburgh, 29 Oct. 1775; OPR births 578/0040 0181 Ayr, 8 Sept. 1776.
12 SP OPR births: 871/0010 0136 Kirkcudbright, 14 Dec. 1777; 871/0010 0141 Kirkcudbright, 22 Aug. 1779; 871/0010 0151 Kirkcudbright, 14 July 1781; 685/001 0380 0052 Edinburgh, 14 July 1787; 685/001 0380 0150 Edinburgh, 7 Aug. 1789.
13 SP OPR births 685/002 0120 0090 St Cuthbert's, 19 Apr. 1794. Knox was born on 4 September 1791 and baptized twenty days later: SP OPR births 685/002 0110 0414 St Cuthbert's, 24 Sept. 1791.
14 Lonsdale, 1870, 4, lists Robert and Mary's children in birth order as John, William, Archibald, Mary, Isabella, Paxton, Janet, Robert and Frederick. He apparently took the names from the Knox family bible. No birth or baptismal record has been identified for Paxton Knox.
15 Steven 1859, 183, 192.

16 *Edinburgh Directory* 1797–8; *Edinburgh and Leith Directory* 1800–1801; *Post Office Annual Directory* 1804–13: Ancestry.com., U.K. and U.S. Directories, 1680–1830 [database on-line].
17 Lonsdale 1870, 3.
18 Wallace 2007, 156–66.
19 Knox 1850, 206.
20 Lonsdale 1870, 2.
21 Callo 2006, 47.
22 Lonsdale 1870, 2.
23 *MTG* 1862; 2: 683–5.
24 Lonsdale 1870, 4; *MT* 1840; 1: 213.
25 *Idem.*
26 Stocking 1987, 30.
27 Knox 1850, 282
28 *The Parliamentary History of England (Hansard)* 1812, X, 284.
29 The average age of matriculation was 10 years: Steven 1849, 274.
30 Steven 1849, 160.
31 *The Stranger's Guide to Edinburgh* . . . Edinburgh: T. Brown, 1817, 102; Steven 1849, 155–6.
32 Bentham 1816, 93–4, 97.
33 Steven 1849, 276.
34 Hall 1807, II, 589.
35 Creech 1791, 82.
36 Bentham 1816, 87–8; Chambers 1830, 376–8; Steven 1849, 159, 270.
37 *The Stranger's Guide to Edinburgh* . . . Edinburgh: T. Brown, 1817, 102; Steven 1849, 280.
38 Steven 1849, 168, 177.
39 *MT* 1840; 1: 213.
40 Lonsdale 1870, 5.

CHAPTER TWO   A Beautiful but Seductive Science, 1810–1814

1 Rosner 1991, 166–8; Silliman 1812, II, 313–14.
2 Report made to His Majesty by a Royal Commission of Inquiry into the State of the Universities of Scotland. *PP* 1831, XII, 167; *List of the Graduates of the University of Edinburgh from MDCCV to MDCCCLXVI.* Edinburgh: Neill and Co., 1867, iv; Rosner 1991, 23.
3 Sketch of the life and doctrines of the late Dr John Brown of Edinburgh. *EMSJ* 1807; 3: 499–502; Bonner 2000, 65.
4 Silliman 1812, II, 313–14; *New Monthly Magazine* 1823; 7: 255.
5 *LPNR* 1817; 6: col. 1023–4.
6 UE, Lists of Medical Matriculations.
7 Rosner 1991, 44–5.
8 Sketch of the life and doctrines of the late Dr John Brown of Edinburgh. *EMSJ* 1807; 3: 499–502.
9 "Modern Greek" 1825, 220.
10 *European Magazine* 1824–5; 86: 134–5; "Modern Greek" 1825, 284–7, 302, 312.

11 *AR* 1808: 270–80.
12 "Modern Greek" 1825, 286–7.
13 *Pamphleteer* 1814; 3: 419.
14 "Aesculapius" 1818, 38.
15 Hancock 1824, 158.
16 Coleridge 1816, xvi.
17 Richards 1851, II, 163–4.
18 MacFarlane 1853, 99.
19 "Aesculapius" 1818, 39; Knox 1850, 284. For Chaplin on stoicism, see http://www.rcpe.ac.uk/library/history/chaplin/chaplin.php, viewed 11 Oct. 2008.
20 The music girl of the rue de la harpe. *Russell's Magazine* 1857; 1: 27–36.
21 "Aesculapius" 1818, 39; Bates 2005, 207.
22 "Graduate of Medicine" 1861, 26–7.
23 Hey 1822, 440.
24 Paley 1824, 122.
25 "Aesculapius" 1818, 48.
26 Report from the Select Committee on Anatomy. *Commons Sessional Papers* 1828, VII, 125.
27 Knox 1850, 119; 1855b. He claimed to have met Oken once: Knox 1844b, 242.
28 Darwin 1861, 184.
29 Cole 1944, 467.
30 Knox 1855b, 46.
31 Oken 1847, 641; Rehbock 1990, 147; Breidbach and Ghiselin 2002.
32 Parkinson 1804–11, III, 308; Knox 1844b.
33 Knox 1855b.
34 Knox 1852a, 52; 1852b, 140–1.
35 Knox 1850, 285.
36 Knox 1854b.
37 Arnot 1816, 551; UE Da 67 Phys, Royal Physical Society dissertations, 1806–13; 28: 249–65, 441–65, 539–50, 566–72.
38 UE Da 67 Phys, 1806–13; 28: 572.
39 Knox 1854b, 393.
40 UE Da 67 Phys, 1806–13; 28: 560.
41 Knox 1836d.
42 Guthrie 1965, 10.
43 *LMG* 1827–8; 1: 168.
44 Rosner 1991, 48–9.
45 Lonsdale 1870, 5–7.
46 Knox 1854b.
47 Silliman 1812, II, 314.
48 Walls 1964, 65.
49 Has execution by hanging been survived. *N&Q* 1854; 9: 453–5.
50 Bondeson 2001, 35–50.
51 Leighton 1861, 38–41.
52 Ure 1819; MacDonald 2006, 14–17; Whiter 1819, 446.
53 Knox 1836b.

54 *EJMS* 1826; 2: 496.
55 Barclay 1822, 400–1, 520, 530.
56 Dr. Knox, of Edinburgh. *MT* 1844; 10: 245–6.
57 "New'un" 1819, 5. Monro received a salary of £100 as professor of clinical surgery. The chair of anatomy carried no salary, though he received lecture and examination fees: Report made to His Majesty by a Royal Commission of Inquiry into the State of the Universities of Scotland. *PP* 1831, XII, 167.
58 Christison 1885, 70.
59 *The Stranger's Guide to Edinburgh* . . . Edinburgh: T. Brown, 1817, 188; Cosh 2003, 521.
60 Knox 1815, 52. This paper was based on Knox's MD thesis *De Viribus Stimulantium et Narcoticorum in Corpore Sano Continens*. Edinburgh: J. Ballantyne and Co., 1814.
61 *Ibid.*, 60.
62 *Ibid.*, 54–6.
63 *List of the Graduates of the University of Edinburgh from MDCCV to MDCCCLXVI*. Edinburgh: Neill and Co., 1867, IV, 48; *New Monthly Magazine* 1823; 7: 258.
64 "Aesculapius" 1818, 51; Rosner 1991, 170.
65 "New'un" 1824, 17.
66 Changes in the London hospitals. *Lancet* 1832–3; 1: 286–7.
67 Lonsdale 1870, 289; Knox 1850, 212.
68 *New Monthly Magazine* 1823; 7: 257.
69 Christison 1885, 199; *The Metropolitan* 1831; 1: 182–6; Knox 1854b.

CHAPTER THREE   Hospital Assistant, 1815–1820

1 "Modern Greek" 1825, 259; Rosner 1991, 22, 168–9.
2 *Pamphleteer* 1814; 3: 420.
3 Knox 1822.
4 Kaufman 2000, 112.
5 *LMRR* 1817, 81–2; Cantlie 1974, I, 426; Van Heyningen 2004, 175.
6 Knox 1852b, 149.
7 *Army List* 1816, 132.
8 Ladd 1825, 76–7.
9 Anglesey 1955, 118–19.
10 Knox 1856a.
11 "A Physician". *The Greatest of our Social Evils* . . . London: H. Baillière, 1857, 217.
12 Knox 1848a.
13 Eve 1857, 54–5.
14 Knox 1850, 219.
15 Knox 1862b.
16 Knox 1851.
17 *Living Age* 1846, 446.
18 Abercrombie 1830, 267.
19 Bacot 1828, 293.

Notes to pp. 32–40

20 Knox 1822.
21 *MT* 1840; 1: 225.
22 Knox 1856a.
23 Napier 1849, I, 207.
24 Cory 1910–30, I, 312.
25 Knox 1839b.
26 Knox 1850, 99; 1821b.
27 Knox 1836b; 1848b.
28 Campbell 1815, 110; Knox 1836a.
29 Knox 1855b, 45–6; Lonsdale 1870, 11, 13.
30 Pringle 1835, 170.
31 Knox 1821a, 282; Knox 1852b, 148–9.
32 Knox 1850, 310.
33 Knox 1852b, 153–4.
34 Knox 1850, 274–5, 321; 1852b, 155.
35 Knox 1852b, 154–5.
36 Lonsdale 1870, 14, 16.
37 Knox 1850, 10, 11, 155–62.
38 Knox 1852a, 6–7.
39 Knox 1839b.
40 *The Times* 12 Dec. 1811, 3b: see also Holmes 2007; Smith 1810, 223.
41 Campbell 1815, 88.
42 Napier 1849, I, 56–60, 63.
43 Knox 1850, 39, 50, 99.
44 Knox 1855a; 1850, 156.
45 Hutton 1887, I, 119.
46 *Ibid.*, I, 98.
47 Rae 1958.
48 Hutton 1887, I, 119.
49 *Ibid.*, I, vi; Knox 1853c, 233.
50 These were widely held views in Britain; in 1814 a petition against French slave traders raised 1,500,000 signatures: Malchow 1996, 11.
51 Knox 1850, 210.
52 Knox 1853c, 233.
53 Pringle 1835, 299–306.
54 Hutton 1887, I, 135–6.
55 NAS GD16/34/388/15(1), letter from Andries Stockenström to Capt. Drummond, 13 Mar. 1820.
56 NAS GD16/34/388/15(7), letter from Stockenström to Drummond, *c.* Mar. 1820
57 Hutton 1887, I, 161–2.
58 NAS GD16/34/388/15(4), copy of letter from Knox to Capt. Andrews, 22 Jan. 1820. Roodewal is in the Western Cape near Oudtshoorn.
59 NAS GD16/34/388/8(2), letter from Stockenström to Capt. Henry Somerset, 5 July 1820.
60 NAS GD16/34/388/15(8), letter from Stockenström to Somerset, 16 Apr. 1820.
61 NAS GD16/34/388/15(1), letter from Stockenström to Drummond, 13 Mar. 1820.

62 NAS GD16/34/388/1, copy of opinion of Court Martial; Hutton 1887, I, 165.
63 Hutton 1887, I, 129–30.
64 NAS GD16/34/388/10(3), letter from Stockenström to Drummond, 6 July 1820.
65 Cory 1910–30, II, 246. Bishop was an unusual Christian name, not an ecclesiastical title.
66 NAS GD16/34/388/14, copy of letter from Bishop Burnett to Mr Eaton, 4 July 1820.
67 Hutton 1887, I, 135–6. Knox had been appointed Assistant Surgeon in the 72nd Regiment of Foot, the Seaforth Highlanders, on 20 Apr. 1820: *Army List* 1821, 244.
68 It appears that no copy of the proceedings was sent to London: PRO WO 93/1A, records of the Judge Advocate General's Office.
69 Hutton 1887, I, 138, 162, 165; Cory 1910–30, II, 246.
70 Knox 1821a.

CHAPTER FOUR **Parisian Anatomy, 1821–1822**

1 *Caledonian Mercury* 10 Mar. 1821, 3; 17 May 1821, 3; Knox 1840c, 292; 1850, 181.
2 Mentioned in *EPJ* 1821–2; 6: 172.
3 Lonsdale 1870, 17.
4 *GM* 1830, 103.
5 Knox 1850, 217.
6 Knox 1852a.
7 Knox 1857a.
8 Taine 1881, 291.
9 Goncourt 1862, 373; *Mémoires inédits de Madame la Comtesse de Genlis* ... Paris: Librairie de le Duc de Chartres, 1825, 308.
10 Gould 1977, 35.
11 Guyader 2004, 5–6; Appel 1987, 11.
12 Guyader 2004, 3; Gould 2002, 282–3.
13 Knox 1852a, 32.
14 The *discours préliminaire* of Cuvier's *Recherches sur les ossemens fossiles des quadrupèdes* became *Essay on the Theory of the Earth* (London: W. Blackwood, 1813). Cuvier later sanctioned its separate publication as *Discours sur les revolutions de la surface du globe* ... (1825): see also Knox 1850, 291–2.
15 Knox 1852a, 73.
16 *The Leader* 1856; 7: 257–8.
17 Outram 1984, 180–1.
18 *GM* 1832; 102: 641–3.
19 Cuvier and his cabinet. *The Museum of Foreign Literature and Science* 1832; 21: 171–2; *DSB*, III, 524; Knox 1852a, 23.
20 History of the Garden of Plants. *Blackwood's* 1823; 14: 577–90.
21 Outram 1984, 183–4.
22 *Ibid.*, 123.

23 Knox 1852a, 56.
24 Knox 1855b, 626.
25 Cuvier 1825.
26 Knox 1850, 294.
27 Geoffroy 1818, xxxi; Gould 2002, 302.
28 Guyader 2004, 43–4; Knox 1856b.
29 Knox 1852a, 19–20; 1850, 129; 1856b.
30 Knox 1852a, 75.
31 Knox 1855b, 25
32 *Ibid.*, 626.
33 Knox 1852a, 73; Appel 1980; 1987, 119–20.
34 Knox 1855b, 162; Knox 1857a, 5480.
35 Swainson 1835, 197; Lovejoy 1964, 244; Cuvier 1831, I, xvii; Knox 1844b, 242; 1855b, 218.
36 Liste des auditeurs du cours de Lamarck au Museum d'Histoire Naturelle (1795–1823): http://www.lamarck.cnrs.fr/auditeurs/liste.php?lang=fr, viewed 17 Mar. 2009.
37 Outram 1984, 124, 127–8; Gould 2002, 171.
38 See Burkhardt 1977, 201–2; Desmond 1992, 45–52; Gould 2002, 172–81.
39 Knox 1850, 295–6; 1857a, 5494; 1855b, 218.
40 Knox 1855b, 626.
41 Outram 1984, 119.
42 Knox 1852a, 18–20.
43 WL AMS/MF/3/1, letter from Thomas Hodgkin to John Hodgkin, Oct. 1821. *La Pitié* was regarded as the better of the two dissecting establishments: *MCR* 1841; 15: 176.
44 Combe 1846, 20.
45 Kass and Kass 1988, 92; Knox 1845a, 156; WL AMS/MF/3/4, letter from Thomas Hodgkin to his father, 15 Apr. 1822.
46 WL AMS/MF/3/1, letter from Thomas Hodgkin to his brother, Dec. 1821. Hodgkin graduated MD Edinburgh in 1823 with a thesis entitled *De Absorbendi Functione*.
47 Kass and Kass 1988, 71; Hodgkin, 1829.
48 WL AMS/MF/3/1, letter from Thomas Hodgkin to his father, 13 Jan. 1822.
49 Knox, 1850, 320.
50 On 22 April 1822: Lonsdale 1870, 18.
51 Knox 1837b, 7; 1856a, 66, 535–7.
52 Knox 1854b, 395. Knox subsequently translated Béclard's work: Béclard 1830.
53 Knox 1853a, ix–x; Knox 1852a, 2–3; 1856a, 35.
54 Knox 1854b, 396.
55 Knox 1852a, 37.

CHAPTER FIVE   **Museum Medicine, 1821–1822**

1 UE GB 237 Dc 2 55, Wernerian Society minutes, 15 Nov. 1832; Knox 1823b; Lonsdale 1870, 21, 27.
2 UE GB 237 Dc 2 55, Wernerian Society minutes, 19 Apr. 1823, 26 Apr.

Notes to pp. 51–5

1823, 17 May 1823, 21 Feb. 1824, 17 Apr. 1824; *MWNHS* 1823–4: 5: 569.
3   Knox 1824b, 28.
4   Knox 1824a, 218–19.
5   Lawrence 1822, 289; *A Prodromus of a Synopsis Animalium, Comprising a Catalogue Raisonnée of the Zootomical Collection of Joshua Brookes, Esq. F.R.S* . . . n.p. [1828], 89: see also Blumenbach 1865, 146–276.
6   Holmes 2007, 28–9.
7   Urry 1989, 11.
8   Magubane 2003, 111–12. The *Caledonian Mercury*, 10 Mar. 1821, reported that Knox presented "skulls of the native tribes" to the University museum, but this probably refers to those he gave to Jameson and Monro.
9   Bank 1996, 393; Hutton 1887, I, 119.
10 Lonsdale 1870, 149.
11 "The Editor of the Cheap Magazine". *Popular Philosophy: or the Book of Nature Laid Open on Christian Principles* . . . Dunbar: G. Miller, 1826, 56.
12 *The Female Revolutionary Plutarch* . . . 3 vols. London: John Murray, 1805, III, 440–1.
13 Grégoire 1808, 33.
14 Knox 1850, 182.
15 Knox 1824a, 207.
16 In the first edition of *Races of Men* (1850, 123), Knox gave the date of his visit as 1822–3, but the second edition has 1821–2 (Knox 1862a, 181, 504), which was the correct date of Belzoni's exhibition; see Timbs 1855, 266. William Frédéric Edwards (1777–1842) was a physiologist and anthropologist whose work *De l'influence des agents physiques sur la vie* (1824) was translated into English by Hodgkin in 1832.
17 Knox 1824a, 210, 213.
18 Wilsone 1863. William Syme Wilsone, a teacher of music, married Mary Knox, then living at 15 Clerk Street, on 3 August 1849: OPR marriages 685/001 0690 0247 Edinburgh. The obituary gave the year of Knox's marriage as 1832.
19 Lonsdale 1870, 36.
20 Knox 1852a, 21, 39, 81.
21 History of the Garden of Plants. *Blackwood's* 1823; 14: 577–90, 586–9; Knox 1852a, 32.
22 *TRSE* 1826; 10: 459.
23 RCSEd Minute Book, Apr. 1824, p. 149; Lonsdale 1870, 37.
24 Knox 1855b, 626.
25 RCSEd Minute Book, 13 Jan. 1825, p. 205; Knox 1852a, 95.
26 Knox 1823a, 211; Tansey and Mekie 1982, 1; Knox 1846, 309.
27 Tansey and Mekie 1982, 5; *MT* 1840; 1: 213; Knox 1854a, 12.
28 RCSEd Minute Book, 13 Jan. 1825, pp. 207, 210, 215; Tansey and Mekie 1982, 8.
29 RCSEd Minute Book 1825, p. 228.
30 Bower 1830, III, 365.
31 Desmond 1992, 162–3.
32 Hodgkin 1829, iv–vii; Kass and Kass 1988, 71.
33 Guthrie 1965, 14, 37.

Notes to pp. 55–60

34 "Modern Greek" 1825, 221–2.
35 RCSEd Minute Book, 19 Apr. 1825, p. 248; Rosner 1991, 101.
36 RCSEd Minute Book, 15 May 1826, p. 363; Knox 1852a, 79; Lonsdale 1870, 39.
37 Lonsdale 1870, 211.
38 *Ibid.*, 44; RCSEd Minute Book, 3 Oct. 1826, pp. 404–7.
39 The same year that Barclay's collection was finally displayed at the College: Waterhouse 1841, 42–4; Tansey and Mekie 1982, 11.
40 *Catalogue of the Museum of the Royal College of Surgeons of Edinburgh. Part I: Comprehending the Preparations Illustrative of Pathology.* Edinburgh: Neill and Co., 1836, 140, 172, 223–4; Knox 1824b, 26; Lonsdale 1870, 28.
41 Knox 1846, 309.

CHAPTER SIX   Knox Primus et Incomparabilis, 1825–1828

1 Lonsdale 1870, 46.
2 Johnson 2005, 408.
3 Wilson 1852, 10–11.
4 Secord 2002, 46.
5 UE Dc 2 53, Minutes of the Plinian Society, 6 June 1826.
6 *Ibid.*, 11 July 1826, 28 Nov. 1826.
7 WL AMS/MF/3/4, testimonial to the President and Governors of the London Dispensary, 15 Sept. 1825; *The Times* 17 Sept. 1825, 2a; WL AMS/MF/3/27, letter from Knox to Thomas Hodgkin, 22 Aug. 1825.
8 WL AMS/MF/3/27, letter from Knox to Thomas Hodgkin, 22 Aug. 1825.
9 *Ibid.*, letter from Knox to Hodgkin, 3 Sept. 1825.
10 Tyrrell 1826, 8.
11 Alcock 1823, 8; Somerville 1832, 11.
12 Tyrrell 1826, 8, 73; Douglas 1848, II, 86.
13 "Yorick" 1819.
14 "Friend to Humanity" 1819, 7; *The Monthly Gazette of Health* 1824; 9: 975–8.
15 *Lancet* 1826; 5: 870–1.
16 Leighton 1861, 22.
17 Johnson 2005.
18 Lansbury 1985, 57; Lonsdale 1870, 60, 70; Johnson 2005, 409.
19 Knox 1850, 272.
20 Lizars 1823, ix.
21 Wise 2004, 175.
22 Lizars 1823, ix–xi.
23 *Mechanic's Magazine* 1825; 3: 249–51.
24 Reynolds 1846 I, 169; Routh 1849, 35.
25 Dissection wounds. *Chambers's Encyclopaedia.* London: William and Robert Chambers, 1888–92, IV, 14; *Terrific Register* 1825; 1: 732–3; Report from the select committee appointed to consider the validity of the doctrine of contagion in the plague. *House of Commons Sessional Papers* 1819, II, 89.

26 Rosner 1991, 159; Kaufman 2004, 228.
27 Somerville 1832, 4.
28 Knox 1837b, 7.
29 *Caledonian Mercury* 12 July 1827, 3; Lonsdale 1870, 131, 161–2; Shapin and Schaffer 1985.
30 Roughead 1921, facing p. 80.
31 *Hansard* 1827, XVII (new series), col. 1350; "Edinensis". Study of anatomy in Edinburgh. *Lancet* 1837–8; 1: 589–90; Lonsdale 1870, 65, 68.
32 WL AMS/MF/3/7, letter from Knox to Thomas Hodgkin, undated.
33 Lonsdale 1870, 129, 134–6, 148, 151.
34 Blake 1870, 332–3.
35 Lonsdale 1870, 126, 148.
36 Wise 2004, 179–80.
37 *DNB* 2004, VII, 923–5; Altick 1978, 27.
38 *MT* 1844; 10: 245–6; Lonsdale 1870, 125.
39 *Journal of Psychological Medicine and Mental Pathology* 1854; 7: 504–11.
40 *University Maga* 1835; 1: 5–6.
41 "Beta" 1830, 205.
42 Leighton 1861, 17.
43 Cloquet 1828, vii.
44 *LMG* 1827–8; 1: 314–17.
45 Knox 1845b, 266; Lonsdale 1870, 138; *EJMS* 1826; 1: 342–7.
46 Lonsdale 1870, 144, 277–8.
47 Knox 1844b: 242, 278; Knox 1855b, 68.
48 Lonsdale 1870, 118, 154, 259; Cloquet 1828, v.
49 Leighton 1861, 21.
50 CRO D HUD 17/90/12, letter from Andrew Whelpdale to his father, 18 Nov. 1833.
51 Knox 1854a, 46.
52 His private collection also included pathological specimens from the Royal Infirmary (mostly kidney and bladder stones) and the crania of fourteen Europeans, a native of Van Diemen's Land, a Peruvian, and a "Caffre": Ross and Taylor 1955, 270–3.
53 Knox 1850, 106.
54 Blake 1870, 335.
55 Richards 1989, 433; Knox 1855a, 359.
56 Darwin 2004, 35, 39, 196.
57 Audubon 1899, 146, 152.
58 Lonsdale 1870, 97.
59 KCL KH/PP7, notes by Sir William Fergusson, undated.
60 *Zoist* 1846–7; 4: 575; *DNB* 2004, XXX, 656–7.
61 Lonsdale 1870, 279.
62 Wilson and Geikie 1861, 139; Knox 1855b, 45.
63 Knox 1855b, 163; Lonsdale 1870, 131, 159, 199; Ross and Taylor 1955, 273; *DNB* 2004, XLI, 917. Glenorchy (1796–1862) was Grand Master of the Scottish Freemasons from 1824 to 1826 and Rector of Glasgow University from 1840 to 1842: *DNB* 2004, IX, 832–3.
64 Lonsdale 1870, 275.

CHAPTER SEVEN   The West Port Murders, 1828–1829

1. Macnee 1829, 32–3; Edwards 1980, 80–2. I have retained the conventional form of "Burke", though the man himself wrote "Burk".
2. "Modern Greek" 1825, 149–50.
3. Sanitary Inquiry 1842, 10, 153–4.
4. Macnee 1829, viii-ix.
5. Sanitary Inquiry 1842, 155; Lonsdale 1870, xiii.
6. Macnee 1829, 33.
7. *Ibid.*, vii.
8. *EMSJ* 1834; 41: 207; Wardlaw 1843, 44–5.
9. Leighton 1861, 224.
10. Lonsdale 1870, 101; Malchow 1996, 79. For the cultural history of female bodies in the male preserve of the dissecting room see Showalter 1992 and Jordanova 1993.
11. Roughead 1921, 29.
12. Richardson 2001, 327; Lonsdale 1870, 101.
13. Richardson 2001, 96.
14. "Echo of Surgeons Square" 1829, 17; Edwards 1980, 129.
15. Lonsdale 1870, 92–3. In 1837, Knox had 71 enrolled students and was supplied with 15 bodies for the 1838–9 session; with a class of 400 he would have needed at least 85 bodies and probably more, as the 1838 allocation was regarded as inadequate: PRO MH 74/13, pp. 194, 259; MH 74/36.
16. Macnee 1829, xvii–xviii, 3, 67–8.
17. Macnee 1829, 18; MacGregor 1884, 157; Roughead 1929, 82.
18. *Caledonian Mercury* 3 Jan. 1829, 3.
19. Christison 1885, 310.
20. Report from the Select Committee on Anatomy. *Commons Sessional Papers* VII, 1828, 48; Leighton 1861, 53–5.
21. Christison 1885, 311.
22. Macnee 1829, 70.
23. *Ibid.*, v-vi, ix–x, 69, 200.
24. *Caledonian Mercury* 17 Jan. 1829, 2; 26 Jan. 1829, 3.
25. Kelly 1821, II, 25–30. For a similar episode see Johnson 2005.
26. *Caledonian Mercury* 24 Jan. 1829, 3; MacGregor 1884, 103.
27. *Caledonian Mercury* 17 Jan. 1829, 2; 26 Jan. 1829, 3; MacGregor 1884, 161, 163.
28. *Caledonian Mercury* 24 Jan. 1829, 3.
29. Roughead 1921, 89.
30. Pae 1866, 246.
31. Macnee 1829, 46–7. The laborious pun becomes more ominous if one remembers that in archaic usage, noxious meant guilty. This contemporary account suggests that Burke died without a struggle.
32. *Ibid.*, 48.
33. Somerville 1832, 8–9.
34. Edwards 1980, 94–8. For a contrary view, see Cole 1964.
35. Macnee 1829, 13, 32–7.
36. MacGregor 1884, 222.

Notes to pp. 72–9

37 Roughead 1921, 271–2.
38 *Belfast News-Letter* 17 Feb. 1829, 2; Lonsdale 1870, 79.
39 *Ibid.*, 111.
40 Spineto 1829, 145.
41 Lonsdale 1870, 115.
42 Macnee 1829, 23.
43 *Caledonian Mercury* 21 Mar. 1829, 4.
44 *Blackwood's* 1829; 41: 371–400.
45 *Ibid.*, 388; Lonsdale 1870, 83.
46 Johnson 2005, 408.
47 *Scotsman* 25 Mar. 1829; Lonsdale 1870, 132.
48 Turner 1868, I, 25–6.
49 Lonsdale 1870, 111; for Vesalius's pilgrimage, see O'Malley 1954.
50 *London Magazine* 1827; 7: 250–61.
51 Lonsdale 1870, 79.
52 Creswell 1914, 154–6; 1926, 205–6; Cosh 2003, 818.
53 Somerville 1832, 5–6.
54 *LMG* 1827–8; 1: 638.
55 Scott 1890, II, 217; Edwards 1980, 130.
56 *LMG* 1829; 3: 572–4. The committee's eight members were the advocates M.P. Brown and J. Shaw Stewart, James Russell, professor of clinical surgery, W.P. Alison, professor of medical jurisprudence, Sir George Ballingall, professor of military surgery, Sir William Hamilton, Bart, professor of history, George Sinclair, writer and member of parliament, and Thomas Allan, mineralogist.
57 Moir 1838, I, 122–3.
58 *CEJ* 5 Oct. 1839, 289–90; Johnson 2005, 408.
59 Macnee 1829, 6–7, 57–8.
60 *AR* 1815: 8.
61 Wise 2004, 174.
62 Somerville 1832, 13.
63 Leighton 1861, 223. Some Burkers and resurrection men allegedly escaped justice by joining the navy: Napier 1862, I, 274.
64 *Lancet* 1829–30; 2: 50.
65 Macnee 1829, x.

CHAPTER EIGHT   **A Nation of Cannibals**

1 Hodgkin 1841, 149–50.
2 *Punch* 1842; 2: 145–6.
3 *Lancet* 1832–3; 1: 245.
4 Lonsdale 1870, 78.
5 *Liverpool Mercury* 13 Mar. 1829, 6.
6 Fonblanque 1837, II, 336–7.
7 *The Times* 22 Sept. 1792, 2c; Malchow 1996, 67.
8 Malchow 1996, 68.
9 *The Times* 3 Sept. 1792, 2d.
10 Knox 1850, 189.

Notes to pp. 79–86

11 Malchow 1996, 11; Reynolds 1846, I, 202.
12 Ritvo 1997, 210; Boswell 1799, I, 506.
13 Napier 1849, I, 187.
14 Knox 1850, 316.
15 Malchow 1996, 53.
16 *Ibid.*, 47, 71, 97–8.
17 Macnee 1829, v.
18 *Punch* 1858; 34: 242.
19 *GM* 1834; 2: 14–22, 17.
20 Malchow 1996, 70.
21 Wilde 2005, 148; Douglas 1848, 86.
22 Gordon-Grube 1988, 405.
23 Gordon 1815, 124–5; Monro 1827, 6; Grainger 1829, 34, 54, 136, 160, 429.
24 *LMG* 1829–30; 5: 695–8.
25 "One in the Ranks" 1848, 59–60.
26 *Ibid.*, 60–1.
27 Cannibals. *Edinburgh Encyclopaedia* 1830, V, 381–5.
28 *The Fatal Effects of Gambling, as Exemplified in the Murder of William Weare.* London: Thos. Kelly, 1824, 58; *Terrific Register* 1825; 1: 787–8.
29 Hunt 1841, 47–8; Lansbury 1985, 56.
30 *Lancet* 1829–30; 2: 50; Knox 1852b, 138.
31 Knox 1854b, 394; Desmond 1992, 32.
32 Knox 1839a, 249; Lonsdale 1870, 215.
33 *LMG* 1836–7; 20: 807–8.
34 Lonsdale 1870, 12.
35 Lansbury 1985, 52–3.
36 Drummond 1838, 154.
37 *N&Q* ser. 7; 12: 128; Barilan 2006, 233.
38 WL iconographic collections, 652252i.
39 Malchow 1996, 76.
40 Cottom 2001, 1–2.
41 Taylor 1829, 51–2.
42 *LMG* 1831; 9: 270.
43 Taylor 1829, 45.

CHAPTER NINE   The Most Popular Teacher in Our Metropolis, 1830–1836

1 Ross and Taylor 1955, 275.
2 Knox 1829, 392.
3 Knox 1856b, 298.
4 Lonsdale 1870, 174–5.
5 Dingwall 2005, 134.
6 Tansey and Mekie 1982, 17–18.
7 Creswell 1926, 83.
8 RCSEd minute book, June 1831, p. 509.
9 MacLaren 2000; Tansey and Mekie 1982, 17.
10 RCSEd minute book, June 1831, p. 521.

Notes to pp. 86–92

11 MacLaren 2000.
12 Lonsdale 1870, 21. On army pay see Cantlie 1974, I, 435.
13 Lonsdale 1870, 212–13. £300 in 1830 was roughly equivalent to £25,000 today: see http://www.measuringworth.com/ukcompare/result.php.
14 Committee for the Society for the Sons and Daughters of the Clergy. *The New Statistical Account of Scotland*. 15 vols. Edinburgh: William Blackwood, 1845, II, 334; Lonsdale 1870, 166.
15 WL AMS/MF/3/2, letter from Knox to Thomas Hodgkin, 17 Jan. 1832.
16 F.J. Knox 1835; 1838; *Caledonian Mercury* 18 Aug. 1836, 3.
17 Knox 1831, 479.
18 *LMSJ* 1830; 5: 435–56, 447; *Lancet* 1829–30; 1: 749–53; *DNB* 2004, XLII, 114–15. For the political background to this affair, see Desmond 1992, 94–100.
19 Outram 1984, 200; Appel 1987; Gould 2002, 308–12.
20 Knox 1855f, 4840.
21 Knox 1831, 481–3, 486.
22 RCSEd GD100/3, prospectus for Knox's school, n.d.
23 KCL KH/PP7, prospectus for Knox's school, 1832.
24 WL AMS/MF/3/2, letter from Knox to Thomas Hodgkin, 17 Jan. 1832.
25 KCL KH/PP7, notes by Sir William Fergusson, n.d.
26 RCSEd GD100/3, prospectus.
27 NAS AD 14/29/16, precognition for the crime of violation of sepulchres, 1829.
28 Fergusson 1832, 81–2.
29 *AR* 1832, 304; Cosh 2003, 825.
30 Fergusson 1832, 81–2.
31 Knox 1853b.
32 *Hansard* 1831 ser. 3, V, col. 614.
33 *LMG* 1828–9; 3: 513; *A Key to Both Houses of Parliament* . . . London: Longman, Rees, Orme, Brown, Green and Longman, 1832, 723.
34 *London Medical and Physical Journal* 1828; 4: 554–7.
35 *LMG* 1828–9; 3: 514.
36 Peel 1853, I, 733; *CE* 1830; 8: 160–74.
37 Richardson 2001.
38 *LMG* 1832; 10: 617–19.
39 *GM* 1829; 99: 215–16, 279.
40 *Blackwood's* 1829; 25: 700–4.
41 *LMG* 1832–3; 11: 89–92, 91.
42 Knox 1855g.
43 NA MH 74/12, 16, records of the Anatomy Inspectorate, Scotland.
44 NA HO 83/3, Home Office register of anatomy licenses.
45 NA MH 74/14, letter from Somerville to Phillips, 12 Feb. 1842, p. 119.
46 *Lancet* 1834–5; 1: 362–3. From its style, this pseudonymous communication may have been from Knox.
47 NA HO 83/1, letter from S.M. Phillips to David Craigie, n.d., pp. 26–7.
48 NA MH 74/12, pp. 53–4.
49 NA MH 74/12, p. 27.
50 NA MH 74/12, p. 64.

51 NA HO 83/1, letter from Phillips to Craigie, 24 Jan. 1833, pp. 43–6.
52 *Ibid.*
53 NA HO 83/1, letter from Phillips to Craigie, 15 Feb. 1833, pp. 49–51.
54 NA HO 83/1, letters from Phillips to Craigie, 21 Feb. and 2 Mar. 1833, pp. 51–5.
55 GUL MS Gen 1476/A/8946, letter from J. Small, University of Edinburgh, to Allen Thomson, 2 June 1880.
56 NA HO 83/1, letter from Phillipps to David Craigie, 5 Nov. 1833, pp. 100–103.
57 NA HO 83/1, letter from Phillipps to Craigie, 22 Jan. 1834, p. 130.
58 NA HO 83/1, letter from Phillipps to Craigie, 23 Jan. 1834; *Lancet* 1836–7; 1: 645, pp. 131–2.
59 NA MH 74/36, minutes of the Teachers of Anatomy, 24 Mar. 1834.
60 NA HO 83/1, letter from Phillipps to Craigie, 13 June 1834, p. 153–5.
61 Wilson 1852, 35; Lonsdale 1870, 157.
62 KCL KH/PP7, letter from John Reid to Knox, *c.* 1831.
63 Lonsdale 1870, 209.
64 With the proviso that he paid his own expenses: HO 83/1, pp. 62, 80, 126, letters from Phillipps to Craigie, 1833.
65 *Maga* 29 Jan. 1835: 5–6.
66 *University Medical and Quizzical Journal* 1834; 1: 32.
67 *University Medical and Quizzical Journal* 1834; 1: 9–12, 20–3.
68 There were 460 university students and 186 extra collegiate ones in 1832–3: *Medical Quarterly Review* 1834; 2: 139–41.
69 The earliest claim in print that Knox was the pamphleteer is Miles 1918, 214; see also Rae 1964, 117.
70 CRO D HUD 17/90/11, letter of Andrew Whelpdale to his father, 10 Nov. 1833; *An Examination . . .* , quoted in *Medical Quarterly Review* 1834; 2: 139–41.
71 Knox 1855d, 4718–19; Knox 1837b, 5; Turner 1868, I, 20–24.
72 UE Dc 8 21, Anatomical Society minute book 1833–43; *DNB* 2004; XXXIV: 417
73 *Maga* 29 Jan. 1835: 5–6.
74 Turner 1868, I, 59, 104; *Report of the Trial of the Students . . .* Edinburgh: Andrew Shortrede, 1838, 40; Wilson 1860, 227.
75 Lonsdale 1870, xii.
76 CRO D HUD 17/90/17, 31, letters from Andrew Whelpdale to his father, 3 May 1834, April 1837.
77 *MT* 1840; 1: 225; *Journal of Psychological Medicine and Mental Pathology* 1854; 7: 504–11.
78 Jacyna 2001, 232.
79 Knox 1836c, 93; Knox 1838b, 395.
80 Jacyna 2001, 232.
81 *Medical Almanack* 1835, 49; 1837, 49.
82 Kaufman 2004, 231. The allocation of male and female bodies was roughly equal: *ibid.*, 233.
83 NA HO 83/1, letter from William Gregson to David J. Rae, 23 Mar. 1835, pp. 193–4.

Notes to pp. 97–102

84 NA HO 83/1, letter from J. Russell to Craigie, 15 Oct. 1836, pp. 233–8; *Lancet* 1836–7; 1: 645.
85 Wilson 1852, 42, 61. Fergusson was subsequently Professor of Anatomy and Surgery at the Royal College of Surgeons, Sergeant-Surgeon to the Queen, and was created baronet in 1866. Knox was wont to boast of having predicted his success.
86 *Lancet* 1835–6; 2: 681.

CHAPTER TEN   A Scandalous Monopoly, 1836–1840

1 NA MH 73/13, p. 100.
2 NA MH 74/13, pp. 100, 108, 109; NA MH 74/14, p. 119, letter from James Somerville to S.M. Phillipps, 12 Feb. 1842.
3 NA MH 74/13, p. 127.
4 *Ibid.*, 130.
5 NA HO 83/1, pp. 270–3, letter from the Anatomy Office to Monro, 23 Sept. 1837.
6 NAS CH2/718/259/23, Anatomy Teachers' accounts, 1843.
7 NA MH 74/36.
8 Lonsdale 1870, 195, 255; Wilson 1987, 351; Knox 1837b, 6.
9 Knox 1840a, 349.
10 Knox 1837b, 3.
11 *Ibid.*, 4.
12 Knox 1837c, 1.
13 *Ibid.*, 1; Syme 1837, 8.
14 Knox 1837c, 1.
15 Knox 1837b, 6, 8.
16 Knox 1837c, 7; *Lancet* 1834–5; 1: 362–3.
17 Knox 1837c, 5.
18 Syme 1837, 8.
19 Boyd 2005.
20 Lonsdale 1870, 190.
21 Campbell and Smellie 1983, 71–2.
22 *MT* 1840; 1: 213; Lonsdale 1870, 190–3.
23 *Ibid.*, 214
24 NA MH 74/13, pp. 192, 194.
25 Somerville 1832, 10.
26 Quain 1832, 100.
27 *LMG* 1839–40; 25: 759–62; 1829–30; 5: 695–8.
28 In 1838–9 the Edinburgh schools received 45 bodies, the English provincial schools together 125 bodies, and the London schools 322: NA MH 74/16, Anatomy Office statistical returns.
29 Lonsdale 1870, 196.
30 Denham 1837, 44; NA MH 74/13, p. 196.
31 Knox 1850, 130, 137; In 1838, Knox wrote of having visited the museum some two years before: Knox 1838a, 364.
32 NA HO 83/3.
33 GUL MS Gen 1476/A/9254, registration of students, 1839.

34 Blainville 1839, 138.
35 Knox 1840b.
36 Lonsdale 1870, 213; *MT* 1840; 1: 225.
37 Leighton 1861, 19.
38 NAS GD112/74/42/13–14, letter from Knox to Breadalbane, 11 Mar. 1838.
39 Knox 1838a, 364.
40 Turner 1868, I: 62.
41 GUL MS Gen 1476/A/9191, 9193, draft letter and regulations, Association of Teachers.
42 NA MH 74/36, copy of letter from James Hope to the Association of Teachers of Anatomy, 14 Nov. 1839; Quetelet 1842, 46. Mortality was high owing to the incidence of typhoid.
43 NA MH 74/36.
44 NA MH 74/14, pp. 122, 127–8, letter from Somerville to Phillipps, 12 Feb. 1842.
45 GUL MS Gen 1476/A/9193, draft regulations for distribution of bodies.
46 NA MH 74/14, pp. 119–20, letter from Somerville to Phillipps, 12 Feb. 1842.
47 NAS MH3/1, p. 13, letter from Andrew Wood to Mr Fraser, 17 Apr. 1843.
48 Malchow 1996, 71–3.
49 GUL MS Gen 1476/A/9191, draft letter from the Association of Teachers to the Home Secretary; NA MH 74/14, pp. 120–1, 123 letter from Somerville to Phillipps, 12 Feb. 1842.

CHAPTER ELEVEN **Nature's High Priest, 1840–1844**

1 RCP MS ALLCW/712/215, letter from Charles Alexander Lockhart to William Henry Allchin, 5 Mar. 1895.
2 *MT* 1839–40; 1: 225; Knox 1837a; Lonsdale 1870, 198, 251.
3 *MT* 1840; 1: 225.
4 *LMG* 1839–40; 25: 330–3.
5 *The Times* 8 Feb. 1843, 7a.
6 Greenhill 1843, 4, 61.
7 *MT* 1840; 1: 220.
8 Knox 1840a, 294.
9 Knox 1840d.
10 *MT* 1840; 1: 225
11 Brett 1924, II, 24. Frederick married Margaret Russell, the daughter of an ironmonger from Peebles, on 12 Dec. 1825 at St Cuthbert's, Edinburgh: SP OPR marriages 685/002 0410 0068 St Cuthbert's. He arrived in New Zealand on 14 Nov. 1840: *New Zealand Gazette and Wellington Spectator* 21 Nov. 1840.
12 WL AMS/MF/3/17, letters from Hodgkin to Frederick Knox, 3 July 1840 and 30 Dec. 1841. Frederick Knox qualified LRCSEd in 1831, but when in New Zealand claimed an MD: Beasley 2001.
13 WL AMS/MF/3/18, letter from Hodgkin to Robert Knox, 4 Jan. 1844.
14 *Transactions and Proceedings of the Royal Society of New Zealand* 1863;

Notes to pp. 107–12

6: 368–9. Frederick died on 5 Aug. 1873 at Wellington Hospital and was buried in Bolton Street Memorial Park.
15 Lonsdale 1870, 217; *DNB* 2004; XXXIV: 417.
16 NA MH 74/13, p. 329.
17 NA MH 74/13, p. 330.
18 NA MH 74/13, p. 331; GUL MS Gen 1476/A/9187, letter from William Campbell to William Mackenzie, 2 Mar. 1842; NAS MH3/1, pp. 162–3, Anatomy Office statistics 1834–5; *WLHR* 1844; 3: 375.
19 NA MH 74/14, pp. 158–9, letter from James Somerville to S.M. Phillipps, 30 July 1842.
20 *Medical Almanack* 1841, 53; Lonsdale 1870, 217; Guthrie 1965, 19.
21 Knox 1838a, 364.
22 *MT* 1840; 1: 213.
23 Knox 1841a, 211.
24 Lonsdale 1870, 210; *LMG* 1840–1; 27: 333–6* (page numbers out of sequence).
25 *Idem*.
26 Lonsdale 1870, 220.
27 "Modern Greek" 1825, 213; Lonsdale 1870, 261.
28 *Proceedings of the Royal Society of London* 1887; 42: xv.
29 Lonsdale 1870, 220–1.
30 WL AMS/MF/3/9, letter from Hodgkin to the President [*sic*] and Town Council of Edinburgh [1841]. William Henderson was appointed to the chair.
31 Knox 1845b, 266.
32 Lonsdale 1870, 222.
33 GROS 1841 census data 685/02 222/02 007.
34 GROS 1841 census data 692/01 016/01 007.
35 Lonsdale 1870, 222–33.
36 *Ibid*., 241.
37 Sir David Monro. *DNB* 2004; XXXVIII: 645–6.
38 *MT* 1841; 4: 1.
39 Lonsdale 1870, 239, 241; Callanan 2006, 48.
40 Kaufman 2004, 228–9.
41 Richardson 2001, 250; PRO MH 74/14, p. 119, letter from Somerville to Phillipps, 12 Feb. 1842; NAS MH3/1, pp. 81–3, letter from Wood to Lonsdale, 1 Aug. 1844.
42 Knox 1853a, v.
43 NA MH 74/14, pp. 117–18, 157, Anatomy Office records of bodies supplied: Thomson received 8 bodies, Menzes at 1 Surgeons' Square 6, and Sir Charles Bell, Handyside and James Miller one each.
44 Cathcart 1882; Lonsdale was licensed in June 1842: NA MH 74/14, p. 154, letter to Phillipps, 8 June 1842; Lonsdale 1870, 257.
45 NAS MH3/1, pp. 81–3, letter from Wood to Lonsdale.
46 *Ibid*., 53.
47 *Caledonian Mercury* 13 May 1844, 3.
48 RCP MS ALLCW/713/192, postcard from Sir John Struthers to Allchin, 1895; 712/214, letter from Struthers to Allchin, 1 Feb. 1895.

49 RCP MS ALLCW 712/210, letter from William Richardson to Allchin, 11 Dec. 1894.
50 Lonsdale 1870, xiii.
51 Desmond 1992, 421.
52 Knox 1841b.
53 *LMG* 1842–3; 32: 500–1; Knox 1852b, 167.
54 Knox 1843, 501; 1844a, 137; 1844b, 279.
55 *Certificates of a Very Rare Specimen of Hermaphroditism*. London: Meggs [1836], 2.
56 Knox 1844b, 476.
57 *Ibid.*, 477, 512.
58 Blake 1870, 334; Knox 1843, 501; Fau 1849, 248–9.
59 WL AMS/MF/3/1-2, letters from Knox to Hodgkin, 30 June 1827 and 17 Jan. 1832.
60 Hodgkin 1845; Keith 1917, 17; WL AMS/MF/3/18, letter from Hodgkin to an unidentified correspondent, 5 Jan. 1844.
61 Lonsdale 1870, 237.
62 WL AMS/MF/3/18, letter from Hodgkin to an unidentified correspondent, 5 Jan. 1844.
63 WL AMS/MF/3/25, letter from Knox to Hodgkin [1844].
64 Rae 1964, 133.
65 He was licensed on 25 November 1844: NA HO 83/3; Lonsdale 1870, 258–9.
66 NAS MH3/1, pp. 147, 158, Anatomy Office statistics and letter from Andrew Wood to Dr Lyon, 14 Nov. 1845.
67 RCSEd GD100/32/1, letter from Knox to A. Maxwell Adams, 17 June [1845].
68 Knox 1846, 309; Kaufman 2001.
69 RAI Ethnological Society Council Minutes, 24 May 1845, p. 20.
70 RCP MS ALLCW 712/214, letter from Struthers to Allchin, 1 Feb. 1895.

CHAPTER TWELVE   **Popular Anatomy, 1845–1848**

1 Knox 1850, 20; Watson 1897, 344.
2 Knox 1852b, 158.
3 Knox 1850, 23; *MT* 1839; 1: 127.
4 Knox 1845b, 266.
5 Knox 1845a, 12: 22.
6 Knox 1845b, 266.
7 *Caledonian Mercury* 29 Dec. 1845, 3.
8 *MT* 1845–6; 13: 380; Knox 1852a, 80.
9 Lonsdale 1870, 284, 341.
10 BL 1880. b. 31, p. 1, programmes of London entertainments; *Living Age* 1846; 9: 401.
11 Knox 1846, 327–8.
12 *The Times* 12 Sept. 1846, 3c; *Living Age* 1846; 11: 310.
13 Denham 1837, 96.
14 *Glasgow Mechanics' Magazine* 1825; 3: 416.

15 RCSEd minute book, Oct. 1847, p. 87.
16 Skidmore 1829, 320.
17 *Eliza Cooke's Journal* 1853; 9: 325–6.
18 *LMG* 1846; 37: 797; *MT* 1845; 12: 380; *The Times* 18 Aug. 1846, 1d.
19 *The Times* 2 May 1848, 1b; 30 Oct. 1848, 8e; 1 Dec. 1848, 8f; 21 Dec. 1848, 12f; *A Catalogue of the Collection of Models of Pathological Anatomy, Forming the Museum of the late Dr Felix Thibert, of Paris . . .* London: Alfred Robbins, 1848.
20 Altick 1978, 340.
21 "Graduate of Medicine" 1861, 8, 90.
22 Kahn 1855, viii, 86, 109–15; Bates 2006.
23 Lonsdale 1870, 343–4.
24 *Bristol Mercury* 2 Oct. 1847, 6.
25 Hopkins 1977, 58–60, 73–4, 93, 180–1.
26 *The Times* 5 May 1847, 7f; 6 May 1847, 6f; 7 May 1847, 7d.
27 *Lancet* 1847; 1: 565–71, 630, 653–4, 685.
28 *MT* 1839; 1: 171–2.
29 *LMG* 1837–8; 22: 297–300.
30 RCP MS ALLCW/712/198, letter from Knox to Andrew Clark, 24 Mar. 1845, with later annotations by William Henry Allchin.
31 RCSEd minute book, Oct. 1847, pp. 85–6.
32 Campbell and Smellie 1983, 72.
33 Knox 1854a, 5, 11; 1852b, 150–1.

CHAPTER THIRTEEN **The Races of Men, 1848–1851**

1 Christison 1885, I, 311.
2 *Pictorial Times* 12 June 1847, 376, quoted in Lindfors 1996, 12–13; *Athenaeum* 15 May 1847; Timbs 1855, 267.
3 Lindfors 1996, 11–12.
4 *Bentley's Miscellany* 1850; 28: 393–5.
5 Blumenbach 1865, 236–7.
6 Hodgkin 1829.
7 Bindman 2002, 213–15. White claimed his theory was supported by anatomical observations, but he apparently examined only one Negro skeleton: see Stepan 1982, 29.
8 Bindman 2002, 203–5, 218–19.
9 Bindman 2002, 221.
10 "condamné à une éternelle infériorité": Cuvier, Joubert and Passard 1864: 221–2; Stocking 1987, 26.
11 Quetelet 1842, viii.
12 Knox 1845a, 55.
13 Knox 1850, 7, 11–13.
14 *MT* 1848; 18: 241–2.
15 Knox 1850, 318; 1862a, 568; Biddiss 1976, 248.
16 Richards 1994, 391.
17 Knox 1850, 65–6, 147.
18 Rupke 1994, 84.

19 Knox 1850, 39.
20 *Ibid.*, 150, 179.
21 Blake 1870, 333.
22 Callanan 2006, 22
23 Curtin 1964, 377; Lindqvist 2002, 124.
24 Callanan 2006, 44–75.
25 Knox 1850, 7.
26 Disraeli 1847, I, 303.
27 Knox 1850, 45, 108; Knox 1852b, 3.
28 Knox 1848c; 19: 1.
29 Knox 1850, 216, 226.
30 Blake 1870, 336.
31 Knox 1850, 7–8.
32 *GM* 1850: 528–9.
33 *BM* 1850: 393.
34 *CE* 1851; 50: 502–4.
35 *Eclectic Magazine* 1850; 19: 1–22.
36 Knox 1850, 11, 38, 56, 66, 79, 149, 157, 307–9, 311.
37 Richards 1989, 408.
38 *CE* 1851; 50: 502–4, p. 502
39 *MTG* 1862; 2: 226–7; Knox 1850, 162.
40 Davies 1988, 74–5.
41 Gould 1977, 44, his translation.
42 Knox 1862a, 518.
43 Richards 1989, 388.
44 Keith 1917, 20.
45 Richards 1989, 415, 418–27.
46 Knox 1850, 66, 302, 313–14.
47 *MT* 1850; 22: 259–60.
48 Davies 1988, 75.

CHAPTER FOURTEEN   **A Great Scheme of Nature**

1 *Lancet* 1850; 2: 392–3.
2 Malcolm 1854, 90. The term "evolution" signifies the development of diverse life forms, though not in a Darwinian sense.
3 Knox 1857a, 5484–6.
4 Knox 1862a, 491.
5 Knox 1850, 58, 66–7. Biologists may note the similarity between Knox's arguments and Francis Galton's objection to Darwinism: that hybrids would, by breeding with the rest of the population, produce offspring that would regress over a few generations to resemble one of the parent species. For Galton, and Knox, new species could arise only from discontinuous variants: Gould 2002, 343–7.
6 *MT* 1848, 242.
7 Knox 1857a, 5491.
8 Knox 1850, 10, 39.
9 Myres 1944; Stocking 1987, 65; Knox 1850, 163.

Notes to pp. 131–8

10 Knox 1850, 301; Kidd 2003, 879. N.C. Pitta, the president of Edinburgh's Royal Physical Society, published a *Treatise on the Influence of Climate on the Human Species* in 1812.
11 Smyth 1850, 100.
12 Lawrence 1822, 212–13.
13 *Ibid.*, 5.
14 Knox 1850, 9.
15 Maury *et al.* 1857, 448.
16 Knox 1850, 31, 130.
17 Knox 1854a, 8.
18 Knox 1855a, 358.
19 Knox 1862a, 503; Knox 1857a, 5482.
20 Knox 1855e, 4790.
21 Knox 1862a, 502.
22 Knox 1852a, 60–2.
23 Knox 1850, 29–30.
24 Knox 1852a, 63–4.
25 Bindman 2002, 195. *Abartung* is sometimes translated as "degeneration", but "variation" is more appropriate.
26 Richards 1994, 389.
27 Knox 1850, 34, 145.
28 Knox 1862a, 130, 489.
29 Stepan 1982, 7; Knox 1840c, 293.
30 *Comic Annual* 1842 ser. 2, 1: 323–36.
31 Lawrence 1822, 107.
32 Bischoff 1863, 55; Knox 1852a, 107; Lonsdale 1870, 256.
33 Knox 1852b, 156; 1850, 315; 1862a, 590.
34 Knox 1855a, 359.
35 Knox 1850, 29, 121.
36 Grant joined the council of the Wernerian Society in 1826, two years after Knox: Desmond 1992, 58, 65.
37 Richard Owen. *DNB* 2004; XLII: 245–54; Robert Grant. *DNB* 2004; XXIII: 337–40.
38 Knox 1855b, 45.
39 Gould 2002, 317.
40 Huxley 1863, 130.
41 Richards 1994, 400.
42 The alternate development of two different forms in the life cycle of an organism: the best-known example is the jellyfish, in which polyps reproduce asexually and medusae, sexually.
43 Rupke 1994, 225–6, 230–2.
44 Huxley 1863, 115; Rupke 1994, 259–60.
45 *ER* 1863; 117: 563; Knox 1850, 20.
46 Knox 1852a, x.
47 Knox 1855b, 627; Darwin 1861, xv.
48 Knox 1840c, 294.
49 Secord 2000, 449; Knox 1850, 129.

CHAPTER FIFTEEN Distrust Your Genius, 1851–1855
1. Knox 1852b, 7, 9, 149.
2. *Official Descriptive and Illustrative Catalogue of the Great Exhibition of the Works of Industry of All Nations.* London: W. Clowes and Sons, 1851, 1218.
3. Bates 2008.
4. Knox 1852a, viii-x, 1, 4, 12.
5. *MJMS* 1852; 15: 469–77.
6. *Leader* 1852; 3: 517.
7. *Weekly News* 1 May 1852.
8. *MJMS* 1852; 15: 469–77.
9. Knox 1852a, viii.
10. Turner 1868, I, 142.
11. *MT* 1853; 6: 121.
12. RFH 1/2/1/2, management committee minutes, 6 July 1853, p. 390; RFH 1/3/1/2, weekly board minutes, 6 July 1853, p. 649; *Lancet* 1853; 2: 342–3; *MC* 1853; 3: 120.
13. *MC* 1853; 3: 234.
14. *The Times* 5 Oct. 1853, p. 7c; *Lancet* 1853; 2: 269, 342–3.
15. *The Times* 8 Oct. 1853, p. 5a.
16. RFH 1/2/1/2, management committee minute book, 24 Nov. 1853, p. 420.
17. RCSEd GD100/76/1, copy of the Royal College of Surgeons of England Court of Examiners' minutes, 1853. The originals in London were not available for inspection when I visited the College archive in 2008.
18. *Ibid.*
19. NA MH 74/15, letter from John Bacot to Frederick James Gant, 20 Nov. 1852, p. 326.
20. RCSEd GD100/76/1, Court of Examiners' minutes.
21. *MC* 1853; 3: 409.
22. Knox 1852b, 10.
23. *BFMR* 1850; 5: 108–10.
24. Newman 1957, 285; Dungison 1846, 16.
25. Hayward 1855, 421; Normandy 1850, 584.
26. Bird 1857, 84.
27. Lonsdale 1870, 354–5.
28. Wright 1858, 73; *Cambridge Essays* 1856; 244.
29. *MTG* 1862; 2: 683–5; *United Service Magazine* 1853; 1: 315; *Bulletins and Other State Intelligence* 1861; 1: 381; *BMJ* 11 Jan. 1890, 111.
30. 1851 census data 685/02 161/02 010 and 011.
31. Knox 1852b, 168.
32. Lonsdale 1870, 355; Knox 1852b, 168.
33. Lonsdale 1870, 365; Rae 1964, 156.
34. Knox 1855g, 633.
35. *The Times* 27 Dec. 1855, 4b.
36. Knox 1855a, 359; *Student* 1851–2; 4: 167–8; Bogdan 1988, 127–30. See also Aguirre 2003.
37. *American Journal of the Medical Sciences* 1859; 37: 455; *Eclectic Medical*

Notes to pp. 144–50

    Journal 1852–3; 4: 55–67; Redfield 1857, 65; Warren 1851; Richards 1994, 402.
38 Bogdan 1988, 127–8, 132.
39 *New York Daily Times* 26 Feb. 1852; *New York Medical Times* 1856; 5: 54–5.
40 *Natural History Review* 1853–4; 1: 32; *N&Q* 1853; 8: 309.
41 Wilson 1859, 525.
42 Knox 1855a, 359.
43 *The Times* 19 July 1853, 8e.
44 Timbs 1854, 234–5; *JES* 1856; 4: 120–37.
45 Knox 1855a, 359–60.
46 *Ibid.*, 357–8.
47 Malcolm 1854, 89. Knox wrote to the Society early in 1855, presumably asking to rejoin: RAI Ethnological Society Council Minute Book, 7 Feb. 1855, p. 177. The minutes record only successful elections; the story of Knox being blackballed by the Quakers "headed by Dr Hodgkin" dates to 1868: On the origin of the Anthropological Review and its connection with the Ethnological Society. *AR* 1868; 6: 431–42; see also Richards 1939, 411. Keith (1917, 17) blamed the Society's leaders Benjamin Brodie and Sir James Clark, rather than Hodgkin, for opposing Knox.
48 *AR* 1863; 1: 188–9.
49 Knox 1855a, 360.

CHAPTER SIXTEEN   **The Hideous Interior**
1 *Blackwood's* 1851; 70: 326–48.
2 Read 1862, 218; Fau 1849, 313.
3 Bindman 2002, 191, 194–5.
4 *Lancet* 1850; 2: 392–3.
5 Fau 1849, x–xi.
6 Knox 1852b, 126.
7 Knox 1850, 34, 246; 1852b, 153.
8 Bell 1821, 5–6, 74; Knox 1852b, 169.
9 *DNB* 2004; LVI: 809–10; Knox 1863, 138.
10 Walker 1836, vii, 12–13, 17, 20, 150.
11 Hartley 2001.
12 Walker 1836, 59–61, 99–101.
13 Burke 1834, I, 52–3; Walker 1836, 99–101.
14 Knox 1850, 276.
15 Fau 1849, 285.
16 Knox 1850, 277.
17 Knox 1852b, 22.
18 Knox 1850, 278.
19 Fau 1849, 266.
20 Knox 1852b, 4, 10, 19.
21 Knox 1852b, 141; Bell 1821, 73; Bates 2006.
22 Knox 1852b, 203.
23 *Ibid.*, 78–9, 126, 170–1.

24 Knox 1850, 153.
25 Fau 1849, 283, 304.
26 Ritchie 1859, I, 142.
27 Fau 1849, 242, 245, 262, 286.
28 Bindman 2002, 201.
29 Knox 1862a, 48.

CHAPTER SEVENTEEN Organic Harmonies, 1855–1862

1 Richards 1989, 374–5.
2 *Idem.*; The unity of mankind. CR 1856–7; 9: 530–46.
3 Knox 1855c.
4 Richards 1989, 399–400; Knox 1852a, 110.
5 Knox 1855b, 70.
6 Knox 1850, 298.
7 Richards 1989, 403.
8 Knox 1850, 129.
9 CR 1856–7; 9: 530–43.
10 Gould 2002, 396–466; Richards 1989, 40.
11 Knox 1853a, 34.
12 Knox 1855b, 25; 1852a, 108.
13 Knox 1857a, 5492.
14 Knox 1844a, 137.
15 Knox 1853a, 106.
16 Knox 1852b, 58, 165, 167.
17 Knox 1855a, 357.
18 Knox 1855b, 627.
19 Wells 1856, 358; Knox 1855a, 359–60.
20 Knox 1857a, 5493–4.
21 *Ibid.*, 5486, 5493.
22 Gould 2002, 253.
23 Lovejoy 1959.
24 *DNB* 2004; XLII: 252.
25 They were both present at a meeting of the British Association in 1846, and spoke on different days: LA 1846; 9: 310.
26 Knox 1862a, 488.
27 For example, in his chapter on "Variation under Nature", Darwin wrote: "who can say that the dwarfed condition of shells in the brackish waters of the Baltic, or dwarfed plants on Alpine summits ... would not in some cases be inherited for at least some few generations?" and elsewhere he proposed that organs underwent a "gradual reduction from disuse", though "aided perhaps by natural selection": Darwin 1861, 46–7, 125.
28 The adage "Natura non facit saltus" (Nature does not make leaps) seems to have been proverbial since at least the seventeenth century. Sir Edward Coke applied it to law, "Natura non facit saltus, ita nec lex", see *N&Q* 1888 ser. 7; 6: 133. Darwin probably read it in Linnaeus's *Philosophia Botanica*.
29 Darwin 1861, 158.

30 Gould 2002, 151.
31 Desmond 1992, 2; Richards 1994, 411.
32 *The Times* 2 Aug. 1851, 1d; *Lancet* 1856; 2: 501; *BMJ* 4 June 1859, 452; *Cincinnati Medical Observer* 1857; 2: 470–2; Lonsdale 1870, 365
33 *Lancet* 1857; 2: 223; *MTG* 1862; 2: 104–5; Wells 1873, 119.
34 *The Royal Cancer Hospital Fulham Road, London 1851–1951: A Short History of the Royal Cancer Hospital Prepared for the Centenary 1851*. n.p. [1951], p. 5.
35 Lonsdale 1870, 389–90; PRO RG 9/162, 1861 census, pp. 45–6. The house belonged to chemist Robert Todman and his sister Charlotte; Edward Knox was still living there in 1881.
36 Horse buses ran from Brompton to Islington every five minutes; from there the North London Railway would have taken him to Hackney. The cost would have been around 12 pence a day, compared to about 12 shillings for a cab. See *Stanford's New London Guide*. London: Edward Stanford, 1860, 1–2, 6.
37 "A Physician". *The Greatest of our Social Evils: Prostitution, as it now exists in London, Liverpool, Manchester, Glasgow, Edinburgh and Dublin* . . . London: H. Baillière, 1857.
38 Knox 1857b.
39 Wilsone 1863.
40 Knox 1862a, 542, 546, 548, 549, 563.
41 Richards 1989, 411–12; *DNB* 2004; XLII: 245–54.
42 Keith 1917, 16.
43 RAI Ethnological Society Minute Book, Mar. 1861, p. 265; *GM* 1861, 10: 663–4.
44 RAI Ethnological Society Minute Book, 17 June 1862, pp. 188, 291.
45 *Lancet* 1863; 1: 19–20.
46 MacNalty 1950, 7; Rae 1964, 159.
47 Blake 1870, 337. Presumably Knox's last public pronouncement was against man's kinship with apes.
48 *Lancet* 1863; 1: 19–20.
49 Knox 1862b.
50 *Lancet* 1863; 1: 19–20; Wilsone 1863. Edward was still living in East London in the 1890s: he had no occupation.
51 Knox 1852b, 5. His grave is plot 100, Brookwood cemetery. It is sometimes said to have been an unmarked grave, though the original flat stone may have had an inscription. A new memorial was placed there by Fellows of the Royal College of Surgeons of Edinburgh in 1966.

CHAPTER EIGHTEEN Science Run Mad
1 Disraeli 1837, 121.
2 *N&Q* 1874 ser. 5; 2: 177.
3 Reynolds 1846, 126, 191.
4 Revenge of Leonard Rosier. *New Mirror* 1843; 1: 21–3.
5 Reynolds 1846, 126–7.
6 *Ibid.*, 331.

Notes to pp. 163–70

7 *Ibid.*, 125.
8 *Imperial Magazine* 1832 ser. 2; 2: 475–6.
9 A series of at least six, formerly in the Ono collection, now apparently lost, entitled "Secrets of the dissecting-room" appeared around 1840: *Collector's Miscellany* 1935; 10: 70; Summers 1941, 499.
10 Shortfield 1849, 224–7.
11 Powell 2004, 46. Showalter (1992) and Jordanova (1993) have addressed the symbolism of the female body in the male preserve of the dissecting-room.
12 *Metropolitan* 1832; 3: 131–7.
13 Mercey 1858, 100.
14 Bertram 1858, I, 255, 259, 288.
15 *Era* 24 Feb. 1867; 22 Mar. 1874.
16 Leighton 1861, 6, 17, 88, 220, 227.
17 *Ibid.*, 2,4, 15–16, 51, 86, 228–9.
18 Pae 1866, 57–8, 114, 134.
19 Shelley 1992, 53–4, 56.
20 *Lancet* 1830; 1: 921–2; Marshall 1995, 327–8.
21 See Ketterer 1997.
22 Forry 1990, 122.
23 Liggins 2000, 130–2.
24 Glut 1984, 200–7.
25 Cushing 1994, 11.
26 Stevenson 2002, xxxiii; Maynard 2000, 369.
27 Stevenson 2006, 73–5.
28 Rae 1964, 150.
29 Stevenson 2006, 71, 191; Prideaux and Livingstone 1917, 153–4.
30 Malchow 1996, 79; Walkowitz 2004, IV, 173; *The Times* 27 Sept. 1888, 5f.
31 *The Times* 28 Sept. 1888, 4c.
32 Buckton 2000, 43–5.
33 *The Times* 4 July 1930, 14b; Agate 1969, 300.
34 *Lancet* 1931; 2: 863–4.
35 Bridie 1931, xiii, 66–7.
36 "Aesculapius" 1818, 12.
37 *The Times* 18 Nov. 1915, 7e.
38 *Who Was Who in the Theatre 1912–1976*, IV, 2205; Wearing 1990, III, 274. *The Wolves*, which ran for 26 performances, was the work of Gladys Hastings-Walton, who also adapted *Frankenstein* for the stage.
39 *Era* 23 Dec. 1931, 10.
40 *The Times* 18 Dec. 1931, 10b.
41 The play was again filmed by the BBC in 1980, with Patrick Stewart as Knox: *The Times* 26 July 1980, 9a.
42 *The Times* 3 Nov. 1948, 6d; 21 Aug 1956, 4a.
43 *Sunday Herald* 21 Feb. 1999: http://findarticles.com/p/articles/ mi_qn4156/ is_19990221/ai_n13935970.
44 *The Times*, 12 June 1939, 20a. *The Anatomist* was filmed in 1961 with Alastair Sim as Knox.

45 Bansak 1994, 284.
46 This cut print was the only version available in the UK until 1998: http://imdb.com/title/tt0037549/alternateversions, viewed 17 Mar. 2007.
47 It opened at the Vanbrugh theatre, London and was staged at the Edinburgh International Festival in 1962 but not filmed until 1985: *The Times*, 14 Feb. 1961, 6d; 22 Aug. 1962, 5e.
48 Thomas 1953, 10.
49 *BMJ* 1952; 1: 909–10; *Canadian Medical Association Journal* 1985; 132: 1366–8.
50 *Lancet* 1949; 2: 259.
51 Thomas 1953, 70.
52 Foot 1967.
53 Thomas 1953, 105.
54 *The Times*, 15 Feb. 1968, 6f.
55 Chief medic backs our campaign for new organ donor law. *Scotland on Sunday* 7 Oct. 2007: http://scotlandonsunday.scotsman.com/health.cfm?id=1600822007.
56 Lawrence 2002.
57 Rodgers 2005, 152.
58 *Ibid.*, 156–7.
59 Brazier 2006, 191; Matthews 2006.
60 Francis and Lewis 2001.
61 Healy 2006, 110; Waldby and Mitchell 2006, 37–8.
62 McLean and Williamson 2005, 10.
63 Savulescu 2006; for responses see http://www.bmj.com/cgi/eletters/332/7536/294.

Bibliography

Abbreviations

Archives

BL	British Library, London.
CRO	Cumbria Record Office, Carlisle.
GU	Glasgow University Library.
KCL	King's College London Archives.
NA	National Archives, Kew.
NAS	National Archives of Scotland, Edinburgh.
RAI	Royal Anthropological Institute, London.
RCP	Royal College of Physicians, London.
RCSEd	Royal College of Surgeons of Edinburgh.
RFH	Royal Free Hospital Archives, London.
SP	Scotland's People (http://www.scotlandspeople.gov.uk).
UE	Edinburgh University Library Special Collections.
WL	Wellcome Library, London.

Periodicals

The place of publication is Edinburgh unless otherwise specified.

AR	*Annual Register* (London).
BFMR	*British and Foreign Medico-Chirurgical Review* (London).
Blackwood's	*Blackwood's Magazine*.
BMJ	*British Medical Journal* (London).
CE	*The Christian Examiner* (Boston).
CEJ	*Chambers' Edinburgh Journal*.
CR	*The Church Review and Ecclesiastical Register* (New York).
EJMS	*Edinburgh Journal of Medical Science*.
EJNGS	*Edinburgh Journal of Natural and Geographical Science*.
EJS	*Edinburgh Journal of Science*.
ELJ	*Edinburgh Literary Journal*.
EMSJ	*Edinburgh Medical and Surgical Journal*.
ENPJ	*Edinburgh New Philosophical Journal*.
EPJ	*Edinburgh Philosophical Journal*.
GM	*Gentleman's Magazine* (London).
JES	*Journal of the Ethnological Society of London* (London).
Living Age	*Littell's Living Age* (Boston).
LMG	*London Medical Gazette* (London).
LMRR	*London Medical Repository and Review* (London).

Bibliography

LPNR	*The Literary Panorama and National Register* (London).
MCR	*Medico-Chirurgical Review* (London).
MT	*Medical Times* (London).
MTG	*Medical Times and Gazette* (London).
MWNHS	*Memoirs of the Wernerian Natural History Society*.
N&Q	*Notes and Queries* (London).
PP	*Parliamentary Papers* (London).
PRSE	*Proceedings of the Royal Society of Edinburgh*.
TESL	*Transactions of the Ethnological Society of London* (London).
TMCSE	*Transactions of the Medico-Chirurgical Society of Edinburgh*
TRSE	*Transactions of the Royal Society of Edinburgh*.
WLHR	*Western Lancet and Hospital Reporter* (Cincinnati).

Works of reference
DNB   Oxford *Dictionary of National Biography*. 60 vols. Oxford: Oxford University Press, 2004.
DSB   *Dictionary of Scientific Biography*. 16 vols. New York: Scribner's, 1970–80.

Published Works
Works by Robert Knox

1815   On the relations subsisting between the time of the day, and various functions of the human body; and on the manner in which the pulsations of the heart and arteries are affected by muscular exertion. *EMSJ* 11: 52–65, 164–7.

1821a   On the climate of Southern Africa, with an abstract of a meteorological register kept at Graaf Reynet. *EPJ* 5: 279–87.

1821b   Observations on the *Taenia solium*; and on its removal from the human intestinal canal by spirits of turpentine. *EMSJ* 17: 384–93.

1822   Observations and cases, illustrative of the pathology and treatment of necrosis. *EMSJ* 18: 62–73.

1823a   Observations on the regeneration of bone, in cases of necrosis and caries, being a supplement to a memoir on the same subject, inserted in the Edinburgh Medical and Surgical Journal for January 1822. *EMSJ* 19: 210–20.

1823b   On the anatomy of the Ornithorynchus paradoxus of New South Wales. *EPJ* 9: 377–81.

1824a   Inquiry into the origin and characteristic differences of the native races inhabiting the extra-tropical part of Southern Africa. *MWNHS* 5: 206–19.

1824b   Observations on the anatomy of the lacteal system in the seal and cetacea. *EMSJ* 22: 23–31.

1829   Notice regarding the osteology and dentition of the dugong. *EJS* 1: 157–8.

1831   Observations on the structure of the stomach of the Peruvian lama; to which are prefixed remarks on the analogical reasoning of anatomists, in the determination à priori of unknown species and unknown structures. *TRSE* 11: 479–98.

1836a Observations on the statistics of hernia, and on the anatomical causes which determine its production. *EMSJ* 46: 76–89.

1836b Remarks on the lately discovered microscopic entozoa, infesting the muscles of the human body; with some observations on a similar animal found beneath the intestinal mucous membrane of the horse. *EMSJ* 46: 89–94.

1836c On the newly discovered microscopic entozoon infesting the muscles of the human body. *PRSE* 1: 133.

1836d On the haemorrhagic hepatization of the lungs, occasionally mistaken for pulmonary apoplexy, and on the origin of the "soft pulpy tubercle" of Bailie. *EMSJ* 46: 404–8.

1837a *The Edinburgh Dissector: or System of Practical Anatomy; for the use of students in the dissecting room.* Edinburgh: P. Rickard.

1837b *Letter to the Right Honourable the Lord Provost and Town-Council of Edinburgh.* Edinburgh, s.n.

1837c *Second Letter to the Right Honourable the Lord Provost and Town-Council of Edinburgh.* Edinburgh, s.n.

1838a Reply of Dr. Knox to passages in Meckel's "Comparative Anatomy". *Lancet* 2: 364–5.

1838b On the Cysticercus cellulosae inhabiting the human muscles. *Lancet* 2: 395–8.

1839a Some observations on the structure and physiology of the eye and its appendages. *Lancet* 1: 248–51.

1839b Some remarks on the treatment of wounds inflicted by poisonous snakes. *Lancet* 1: 199–203.

1840a Observations on the pathology of puerperal fever. *Lancet* 1: 349–50.

1840b Memoir on the gibbon varié, with a critical examination of M. de Blainville's account of the gibbon. *Lancet* 2: 265–8.

1840c Inquiry into the present state of our knowledge respecting the orang-outang & chimpanzee. *Lancet* 2: 289–96.

1840d Contributions to the history of the corpus luteum, human and comparative. *Lancet* 2: 226–9.

1841a Some remarks on the placental tufts described by Weber; and on their distribution and supposed functions. *LMG* 27: 209–13.

1841b On the occasional presence of a supra-condyloid process in the human humerus. *EMSJ* 56: 125–8.

1843 Contributions to anatomy and physiology: on some varieties in human structure, with remarks on the doctrine of "unity of organization". *LMG* 32: 499–502, 529–532, 554–6, 586–91, 637–40, 860–2.

1844a Contributions to anatomy and physiology: the cervical ribs in man: a memoir. *LMG* 33: 136–45, 166–72, 210–12.

1844b Contributions to anatomy and physiology: hermaphroditism; a memoir read to the Royal College of Surgeons of Edinburgh in 1827 and 1828. *LMG* 33: 241–3, 277–80, 293–300, 447–51, 472–7, 510–12.

1845a Lectures on the physiological anatomy, the special philosophy of man, and on the anatomy of tissues – morbid and healthy. *MT* 12: 7–8, 21–2, 33–4, 55–7, 74–5, 136–7, 156–7, 239–40.

1845b On the supposed advantages of a knowledge of anatomy to the artist. *MT* 12: 264–8, 285–7.

Bibliography

1846 Anatomical museums: their objects and present condition. *MT* 14: 307–9, 327–8.

1848a Wounds of the thoracic region or chest: superficial, penetrating, and complicated. *MT* 17: 477.

1848b Some remarks on the treatment of gunshot and other wounds of the thorax and extremities. *MT* 17: 503–5.

1848c The races of men. *MT* 18: 97–9, 114, 117–20, 133–5, 147–8, 163–5, 199–201, 231–3, 263–4, 283–5, 299–301, 315–16, 331–2, 365–6; 19: 1–3, 17–18, 33–4, 49–50, 69–70, 121–3, 175, 191–3, 247–8, 315–16.

1850 *The Races of Men: a Fragment.* London: Henry Renshaw.

1851 Some observations on excision of the pelvic extremity of the femur. *MT* 2: 689–93.

1852a *Great Artists and Great Anatomists.* London: John van Voorst.

1852b *A Manual of Artistic Anatomy, for the use of Sculptors, Painters and Amateurs.* London: Henry Renshaw.

1853a *A Manual of Human Anatomy: Descriptive, Practical, and General.* London: Henry Renshaw.

1853b The cholera fly. *Lancet* 2: 479–80.

1853c The Earthmen tribe of the Bosjieman and Hottentot races of Southern Africa. *Illustrated London Magazine* 1: 232–6.

1854a *Fish and Fishing in the Lone Glens of Scotland: with a History of the Propagation, Growth, and Metamorphoses of the Salmon.* London: G. Routledge and Co.

1854b Xavier Bichat: his life and labours; a biographical and philosophical study. *Lancet* 2: 393–6.

1855a Some remarks on the Aztecque and Bosjieman children, now being exhibited in London. *Lancet* 1: 357–60.

1855b Contributions to the philosophy of zoology, with special reference to the natural history of man. *Lancet* 1855; 1: 625–7; 2: 24–6, 45–6, 68–71, 162–4, 186–8, 216–18.

1855c Some observations on the Salmo estuarius, or estuary trout. *Zoologist* 13: 4662–73.

1855d On the food of certain gregarious fishes. *Zoologist* 13: 4709–24.

1855e Inquiries into the Philosophy of Zoology. *Zoologist* 13: 4777–92.

1855f Contributions to the philosophy of zoology. *Zoologist* 13: 4837–42.

1855g The sanatary [sic] movement. *The Empire* 1 Sept., 633.

1856a Contributions to surgical anatomy and operative surgery. *Lancet* 1: 35–6; 535–7; 2: 65–7.

1856b On organic harmonies: anatomical co-relations, and methods of zoology and paleontology. *Lancet* 2: 245–7, 270–1, 297–300.

1857a Zoology: its present phasis and future prospects. *Zoologist* 15: 5473–502.

1857b The food question in France. *Lancet* 1: 500–1.

1862a *The Races of Men: A Philosophical Enquiry into the Influence of Race over the Destinies of Nations.* 2nd ed. London: Henry Renshaw.

1862b On a case of gunshot wound of the cranium, followed by some remarkable psychological phenomena. *Lancet* 1: 539–40.

1863 Some additional observations on a collection of human crania and other human bones, at present preserved in the crypt of a church at Hythe, in Kent. *TESL* 2: 136–40.

Primary Sources

Abercrombie, John. 1830. *Pathological and Practical Researches on Diseases of the Stomach, the Intestinal Canal, the Liver, and Other Viscera of the Abdomen.* Edinburgh: Waugh and Innes.

"Aesculapius". 1818. *The Hospital Pupil's Guide* . . . 2nd ed. London: E. Cox and Sons.

Alcock, Thomas. 1823. An essay on the education and duties of the general practitioner in medicine and surgery. *Transactions of the Associates Apothecaries and Surgeon-Apothecaries* 1: 1–135.

Anglesey, Marquess of, ed. 1955. *The Capel Letters* . . . London: Jonathan Cape.

Arnot, Hugo. 1816. *The History of Edinburgh: From the Earliest Accounts, to the Year 1780.* Edinburgh: Thomas Turnbull.

Bacot, John. 1828. Essays on syphilis. *LMG* 2: 289–94.

Barclay, John. 1822. *An Inquiry Into the Opinions, Ancient and Modern, Concerning Life and Organization.* Edinburgh: Bell and Bradfute.

Béclard, P.A. 1830. *Elements of General Anatomy.* Transl. R. Knox. Edinburgh: Maclachlan and Stewart.

Bell, T. 1821. *Kalogynomia, or the Laws of Female Beauty: being the Elementary Principles of that Science.* London: J.J. Stockdale.

Bentham, Jeremy. 1816. *Chrestomathia* . . . London: Payne and Foss.

Bertram, James G. 1858. *The Story of a Stolen Heir: A Novel.* 3 vols. London: T.C. Newby.

"Beta". 1830. The University of Edinburgh: defence of the School of Medicine. *Lancet* 2: 204–6.

Bird, James. 1857. *Vegetable Charcoal, its Medicinal and Economic Properties* . . . London: John Churchill.

Bischoff, T. 1863. On the difference between man and brutes. *Anthropological Review* 1: 54–60.

Blainville, H.M.D. de. 1839. Comparative osteography. Ed. Robert Knox. *Lancet* 1: 137–45.

Blumenbach, Johann Friedrich. 1865. *The Anthropological Treatises of Johann Friedrich Blumenbach* . . . Ed. and transl. T. Bendyshe. London: Longman for the Anthropological Society.

Boswell, James. 1799. *The Life of Samuel Johnson, LL.D* . . . 3rd ed., 4 vols. London: H. Baldwin.

Bower, Alexander. 1830. *The History of the University of Edinburgh* . . . 3 vols. Edinburgh: Waugh and Innes.

Burke, Edmund. 1834. *The Works of the Right Hon. Edmund Burke.* 2 vols. London: Holdsworth and Ball.

Campbell, John. 1815. *Travels in South Africa, Undertaken at the Request of the Missionary Society.* London: Black and Parry.

Chambers, William. 1830. *The Book of Scotland.* Edinburgh: Robert Buchanan.

Cloquet, H. 1828. *A System of Human Anatomy.* Ed. and transl. R. Knox. 2nd ed., Edinburgh: Maclachlan and Stewart.

Bibliography

Cloquet, Jules. 1836. *Recollections of the Private Life of General Lafayette*. 2 vols. New York: Leavitt, Lord and Co.

Cobbett, William. 1801. *Porcupine's Works* . . . 12 vols. London: Cobbett and Morgan.

Coleridge, Samuel Taylor. 1816. *The Statesman's Manual* . . . London: Gale and Fenner.

Combe, George. 1846. *Moral Philosophy; or the Duties of Man Considered in His Individual, Domestic, and Social Capacities*. 3rd ed. Edinburgh: Maclachlan, Stewart and Co.

Creech, William. 1791. *Edinburgh Fugitive Pieces*. Edinburgh: printed for William Creech.

Cuvier, Georges. 1825. *Discours sur les révolutions de la surface du globe*. Paris: G. Dufour and E. d'Ocagne.

Cuvier, Georges. 1831. *The Animal Kingdom: Arranged in Conformity with its Organization*. Transl. H. M'Murtrie, 4 vols. New York: G. and C. and H. Carvill.

Cuvier, G., P.-Ch. Joubert, and F.-L. Passard. 1864. *Discours sur les révolutions du globe*. Paris: Passard.

Darwin, Charles. 1861. *On the Origin of Species* . . . 3rd ed. New York: D. Appleton and Co.

Darwin, Charles. 2004 [1871]. *The Descent of Man: and Selection in Relation to Sex*. London: Penguin.

Denham, William Hempson. 1837. *Verba Consilii; or, Hints to Parents Who Intend to Bring up their Sons to the Medical Profession*. London: John Churchill.

Disraeli, Benjamin. 1837. *Venetia*. 3 vols. London: Henry Colburn.

Disraeli, Benjamin. 1847. *Tancred: or, the New Crusade*. 3 vols. London: Henry Colburn.

Douglas, Robert. 1848. *Adventures of a Medical Student*. 2 vols. New York: Burgess, Stringer and Co.

Drummond, William H. 1838. *The Rights of Animals, and Man's Obligation to Treat them with Humanity*. London: John Mardon.

Dungison, Robley. 1846. *Medical Lexicon: A Dictionary of Medical Science* . . . Philadelphia: Lea and Blanchard.

"Echo of Surgeons Square, The". 1829. *A Letter to the Lord Advocate* . . . Edinburgh, *s.n.*

Eve, Paul F. 1857. *A Collection of Remarkable Cases in Surgery*. Philadelphia: J.B. Lippincott and Co.

Fau, J. 1849. *The Anatomy of the External Forms of Man; Intended for the Use of Artists, Painters and Sculptors*. Ed. R. Knox. London: Hippolyte Baillière.

Fergusson, William. 1832. Notes and observations upon the contagion of typhous fever, and contagion generally. *EMSJ* 38: 67–86.

Fonblanque, Albany. 1837. *England Under Seven Administrations*. 3 vols. London: Richard Bentley.

"Friend to Humanity, A". 1819. *Answer to a Pamphlet Entitled The Medical School of Edinburgh*. Edinburgh: for the booksellers.

Geoffroy Saint-Hilaire, Étienne. 1818. *Philosophie Anatomique*. Paris, *s.n.*

Goncourt, Edmond and Jules de. 1862. *La femme au dix-huitième siècle*. Paris: Firmin Didot, 1862.

Bibliography

Gordon, John. 1815. *A System of Human Anatomy*. Edinburgh: William Blackwood.

"Graduate of Medicine, A". 1861. *The Elements of Social Science: or Physical, Sexual, and Natural Religion*. 4th ed. London: E. Truelove.

Grainger, R.D. 1829. *Elements of General Anatomy* . . . London: S. Highley.

Greenhill, William A. 1843. *Address to a Medical Student*. London: Rivingtons, Churchill.

Grégoire, Henri. 1808. *De la littérature des Nègres, ou recherches sur leurs facultés intellectuelles, leures qualities morales et leur littérature* . . . Paris: Maradan.

Hall, James. 1807. *Travels in Scotland by an Unusual Route* . . . 2 vols. London: J. Johnson.

Hancock, Thomas. 1824. *Essay on Instinct, and its Physical and Moral Relations*. London: William Phillips.

Hayward, George. 1855. *Surgical Reports, and Miscellaneous Papers on Medical Subjects*. Boston: Phillips, Sampson and Co.

Heron, Robert. 1799. *Scotland Delineated* . . . 2nd ed. Edinburgh: Bell and Bradfute.

Hey, John. 1822. *Lectures in Divinity Delivered in the University of Cambridge*. Cambridge: J. Smith.

Hodgkin, Thomas. 1829. *A Catalogue of the Preparations in the Anatomical Museum of Guy's Hospital*. n.p.

Hodgkin, Thomas. 1841. *The Means of Promoting and Preserving Health*. 2nd ed. London: Simpkin, Marshall and Co.

Hodgkin, Thomas. 1845. On the ancient inhabitants of the Canary Islands. *ENPJ* 39: 372–85.

Holmes, Oliver Wendell. 1887. *Our Hundred Days in Europe*. Boston: Houghton, Mifflin and Co.

Hunt, Leigh. 1841. *Essays*. London: Edward Moxon.

Hutton, C.W., ed. 1887. *The Autobiography of the Late Sir Andries Stockenstrom, Bart., Sometime Lieutenant-Governor of the Eastern Province of the Colony of the Cape of Good Hope*. 2 vols. Cape Town: J.C. Juta and Co.

Huxley, T.H. 1863. *Evidence as to Man's Place in Nature*. New York: D. Appleton and Co.

Kahn, Joseph. 1855. *Men With Tails: Remarks on the Niam-Niams of Central Africa* . . . London: W. J. Golbourn.

Kelly, Mrs. 1821. *The Fatalists; or, Records of 1814 and 1815*. 5 vols. London: A.K. Newman.

Knox, F.J. 1835. *Account of the Rorqual, the Skeleton of Which is Now Exhibiting in the Great Rooms of the Royal Institution, Princes Street*. Edinburgh: A. Balfour and Co.

Knox, F.J. 1838. *Catalogue Of Anatomical Preparations Illustrative of the Whale, Particularly the Great Northern Rorqual (Balaena maximus borealis), Now Exhibiting in the Pavilion, North College Street*. Edinburgh: Neill and Co.

[Ladd, W.] 1825. *The Essays of Philanthropos on Peace and War*. Portland: Shirley and Edwards.

Bibliography

Lawrence, W. 1822. *Lectures on Physiology, Zoology, and the Natural History of Man, Delivered at the Royal College of Surgeons.* London: Benbow.

Leighton, Alexander. 1861. *The Court of Cacus; or, the Story of Burke and Hare.* 2nd ed. London: Houlston and Wright.

Lizars, John. 1823. *A System of Anatomical Plates; Accompanied with Descriptions, and Physiological, Pathological, and Surgical Observations. Part II – The Blood-Vessels and Nerves.* Edinburgh: Daniel Lizars.

MacFarlane, Charles. 1853. *Kismet, or The Doom of Turkey.* London: Thomas Bosworth.

Macnee, John. 1829. *Trial of William Burke and Helen M'Dougal, before the High Court of Justitiary, at Edinburgh . . .* Edinburgh: Robert Buchanan.

Malcolm, Charles. 1854. Address to the ethnological society of London, delivered at the anniversary, 14 May 1851. *JES* 3: 86–102.

Maury, Alfred, Francis Pulszky and J. Aitken Meigs, eds. 1857. *Indigenous Races of the Earth . . .* Philadelphia: J.B. Lippincott.

Mercey, Frédéric Bourgeois de. 1858. *Burke l'etouffeur.* Paris: P. Hachette.

"Modern Greek, A" [Robert Mudie] 1825. *The Modern Athens: a Dissection and Demonstration of Men and Things in the Scotch Capital.* London: Knight and Lacey.

Moir, D.M., ed. 1838. *The Modern Pythagorean: a Series of Tales, Essays, and Sketches by the late Robert Macnish, LL.D.* 2 vols. Edinburgh: William Blackwood and Sons.

Monro, Alexander [*tertius*]. 1827. *The Morbid Anatomy of the Brain.* Edinburgh: Maclachlan and Stewart.

Napier, E. Elers. 1849. *Excursions in Southern Africa, Including a History of the Cape Colony, an Account of the Native Tribes, &c.* 2 vols. London: William Shoberl.

"New'un, A". 1824. *More "Hints" and More to the Purpose, on . . . a Medical Degree in the University of Edinburgh.* Edinburgh: Adam Black.

Normandy, A. 1850. *The Commercial Hand-Book of Chemical Analysis.* London: George Knight and Sons.

Oken, Lorenz. 1847. *Elements of Physiophilosophy.* Transl. Alfred Tulk. London: The Ray Society.

"One in the Ranks" [M. Constable] 1848. *Othello in Hell, and The Infant: with A Branch of Olives.* Dublin: James McGlashan.

[Pae, David]. 1866. *Mary Paterson; or The Fatal Error: A Story of the Burke and Hare Murders.* London: Fred. Farrah.

Paley, William. 1824. *Natural Theology and Tracts.* New York: S. King.

Parkinson, James. 1804–11. *Organic Remains of a Former World . . .* 3 vols. London: Sherwood, Neely and Jones.

Peel, Robert. 1853. *The Speeches of the Late Right Honourable Sir Robert Peel, Bart . . .* 4 vols. London: George Routledge and Co.

Pringle, Thomas. 1835. *Narrative of a Residence in South Africa.* London: Edward Moxon.

Quain, Jones. 1832. Lecture, introductory to the course of anatomy and physiology, delivered at the opening of the session 1831–1832, at the university of London. *Monthly Review* 1: 91–104.

Bibliography

Quetelet, M.A. 1842. *Treatise on Man and the Development of His Faculties.* Ed. T. Smibert, transl. R. Knox. Edinburgh: William and Robert Chambers.

Read, Hollis. 1862. *The Hand of God in History* . . . Glasgow: W. Collins.

Redfield, James W. 1857. *Comparative Physiognomy or Resemblances Between Men and Animals.* New York: Redfield.

Reynolds, George W.M. [c. 1846] *The Mysteries of London.* London: John Dicks.

Richards, Alfred Bate. 1851. *Poems, Essays and Opinions.* London: Aylott and Jones.

Ritchie, Leitch. 1859. *Winter Evenings.* 2 vols. London: Hurst and Blackett.

Routh, C.H.F. 1849. On the causes of the endemic puerperal fever of Vienna. *Medico-Chirurgical Transactions* 32: 27–40.

Sanitary Inquiry – Scotland. 1842. *Reports on the Sanitary Condition of the Labouring Population of Scotland.* London: W. Clowes and Sons.

Scott, Walter. 1890. *The Journal of Sir Walter Scott: from the Original Manuscript at Abbotsford* . . . 2 vols. Edinburgh: D. Douglas.

Shelley, Mary Wollstonecraft. 1992 [1818]. *Frankenstein.* Ed. Johanna M. Smith. Boston: Bedford Books of St Martin's Press.

Shortfield, Luke. 1849. *Wild Western Scenes: a Narrative of Adventures in the Western Wilderness, the Nearest and Best California.* Philadelphia: Grigg, Elliot and Co.

Silliman, Benjamin. 1812. *Journal of Travels in England, Holland, and Scotland* . . . Boston: T.B. Wait.

Skidmore, Thomas. 1829. *The Rights of Man to Property* . . . New York: Alexander Ming.

Smith, Samuel Stanhope. 1810. *An Essay on the Causes of the Variety of Complexion and Figure in the Human Species* . . . New Brunswick: J. Simpson.

Smyth, Thomas. 1850. *The Unity of the Human Races* . . . New York: George P. Putnam.

Somerville, James C. 1832. *A Letter Addressed to the Lord Chancellor, on the Study of Anatomy, &c.* London: J. Hatchard and Son.

Spineto, Marquis. 1829. *Lectures on the Elements of Hieroglyphics and Egyptian Antiquities.* London: C.J.G. and F. Rivington.

Steven, William. 1849. *The History of the High School of Edinburgh.* Edinburgh: Maclachlan and Stewart.

Steven, William. 1859. *History of George Heriot's Hospital: With a Memoir of the Founder* . . . Edinburgh: Bell and Bradfute.

Swainson, W. 1835. *A Treatise on the Geography and Classification of Animals.* Longman, London.

Syme, James. 1837. *Letter to the Right Hon. The Lord Provost, Magistrates, and Town-Council of Edinburgh in Regard to the Chair of Pathology.* Edinburgh: John Carfrae and Son.

Taylor, Robert. 1829. Christianity, the cause of crime. *The Lion* 3: 49–54.

Timbs, John. 1854. *The Year-Book of Facts in Science and Art* . . . London: David Bogue.

Timbs, John. 1855. *Curiosities of London* . . . London: David Bogue.

Tyrrell, Frederick. 1826. *An Introductory Lecture on Anatomy, Delivered at the*

Bibliography

New Medical School, Aldersgate Street, October 2d 1826. London: Longman, Rees, Orme, Brown and Green.
Ure, Andrew. 1819. An account of some experiments made on the body of a criminal immediately after execution, with physiological and practical observations. *Journal of Science and the Arts* 6: 283–94.
Walker, Alexander. 1836. *Beauty: Illustrated Chiefly by an Analysis and Classification of Beauty in Woman.* London: Effingham Wilson.
Wardlaw, Ralph. 1843. *Lectures on Magdalenism: its Nature, Extent, Effects, Guilt, Causes and Remedy.* New York: J.S. Redfield.
Warren, J. Mason. 1851. An account of two remarkable Indian dwarfs exhibited in Boston under the name of the Aztec children. *American Journal of Medical Sciences* 42: 286–93.
Waterhouse, G.R. 1841. *The Naturalist's Library. Mammalia. IX. Marsupialia or Pouched Animals.* Edinburgh: W.H. Lizars.
Wells, David A., ed. 1856. *Annual of Scientific Discovery* . . . Boston: Gould and Lincoln.
Whiter, Walter. 1819. *A Dissertation on the Disorder of Death; or that State of the Frame Under the Signs of Death Called Suspended Animation* . . . London: Printed for the Author.
Wilson, George. 1852. *Life of Dr John Reid, late Chandos Professor of Anatomy and Medicine in the University of St. Andrews.* Edinburgh: Sutherland and Knox.
Wilson, George and Archibald Geikie. 1861. *Memoir of Edward Forbes.* London: MacMillan and Edmonston.
Wilson, Jessie Aitken. 1860. *Memoir of George Wilson, MD, FRSE* . . . Edinburgh: Edmonston and Douglas.
Wilson, Robert Anderson. 1859. *A New History of the Conquest of Mexico* . . . Philadelphia: James Challen and Son.
Wilsone, W. Syme. 1863. The late Dr Robert Knox. *Lancet* 1: 49.
Wright, William. 1858. *Fishes and Fishing: Artificial Breeding of Fish, Anatomy of Their Senses, Their Loves, Passions, and Intellects.* London: Thomas Cautley Newby.
"Yorick". 1819. *The Sadducee, or, a Review of Some Pamphlets Lately Published on Important Subjects.* Edinburgh: for the booksellers.

Secondary sources

Agate, James. 1969. *Red Letter Nights* . . . New York: Benjamin Blom.
Aguirre, Robert D. 2003. Exhibiting degeneracy: the Aztec children and the ruins of race. *Victorian Review* 29: 40–63.
Altick, Richard D. 1978. *The Shows of London.* Cambridge MA: Belknap.
Appel, Toby A. 1980. Henri de Blainville and the animal series: a nineteenth-century chain of being. *Journal of the History of Biology* 13: 291–320.
Appel, Toby A. 1987. *The Cuvier–Geoffroy Debate* . . . Oxford: Oxford University Press.
Audubon, Maria R. 1899. *Audubon and His Journals.* New York: C. Scribner.
Bank, Andrew. 1996. Of "native skulls" and "noble Caucasians": phrenology in colonial South Africa. *Journal of South African Studies* 22: 387–403.

Bibliography

Bansak, Edmund G. 1994. *Fearing the Dark: the Val Lewton Career.* Jefferson NC: McFarland and Co.

Barilan, Y. Michael. 2006. Bodyworlds and the ethics of using human remains: a preliminary discussion. *Bioethics* 20: 233–47.

Bates, A.W. 2005. *Emblematic Monsters: Unnatural Conceptions and Deformed Births in Early Modern Europe.* Amsterdam: Rodopi.

Bates, A.W. 2006. Dr Kahn's museum: obscene anatomy in Victorian London. *Journal of the Royal Society of Medicine* 99: 618–24.

Bates, A.W. 2008. "Indecent and demoralising representations": public anatomy museums in mid-Victorian England. *Medical History* 52: 1–22.

Beasley, A.W. 2001. The other brother – a brief account of the life and times of Frederick John Knox LRCSEd. *Journal of the Royal College of Surgeons of Edinburgh* 46: 119–23.

Biddiss, M.D. 1976. The politics of anatomy: Dr. Robert Knox and Victorian Racism. *Proceedings of the Royal Society of Medicine* 69: 245–50.

Bindman, David. 2002. *Ape to Apollo: Aesthetics and the Idea of Race in the 18th Century.* London: Reaktion.

Blake, C. Carter. 1870. The Life of Dr. Knox. *Journal of Anthropology* 1: 332–8.

Bogdan, Robert. 1988. *Freak Show: Presenting Human Oddities for Amusement and Profit.* Chicago: University of Chicago Press.

Bondeson, Jan. 2001. *Buried Alive: The Terrifying History of Our Most Primal Fear.* New York: W.W. Norton and Co.

Bonner, Thomas Neville. 2000. *Becoming a Physician: Medical Education in Britain, France, Germany, and the United States, 1750–1945.* Baltimore: Johns Hopkins University Press.

Boyd, D.H.A. 2005. William Henderson (1810–72) and homeopathy in Edinburgh. *Journal of the Royal College of Physicians of Edinburgh* 36: 170–8.

Brazier, Margot. 2006. Human(s) (as) medicine(s). In: Sheila A.M. McLean, ed. *First Do No Harm: Law, Ethics and Healthcare.* Aldershot: Ashgate, pp. 187–202.

Breidbach, O. and Ghiselin, M.T. 2002. Lorenz Oken and Naturphilosophie in Jena, Paris and London. *History and Philosophy of the Life Sciences* 24: 219–47.

Brett, Henry. 1924. *White Wings: Fifty Years of Sail in the New Zealand Trade, 1850 to 1900.* 2 vols. Auckland: Brett Printing Co.

Bridie, James. 1931. *The Anatomist.* London: Constable.

Briggs, Asa. 1959. *The Age of Improvement.* London: Longmans, Green and Co.

Brims, J. 1990. From Reformers to "Jacobins": The Scottish Association of the Friends of the People. In: T. M. Devine, ed. *Conflict and Stability in Scottish Society, 1700–1850.* Edinburgh: John Donald, pp. 31–50.

Buckton, Oliver S. 2000. Reanimating Stevenson's Corpus. *Nineteenth-Century Literature* 55: 22–58.

Burkhardt, R.W. 1977. *The Spirit of System: Lamarck and Evolutionary Biology.* Cambridge MA: Harvard University Press.

Callanan, Laura. 2006. *Deciphering Race: White Anxiety, Racial Conflict, and the Turn to Fiction in Mid-Victorian English Prose.* Columbus: Ohio State University Press.

Bibliography

Callo, Joseph. 2006. *John Paul Jones: America's First Sea Warrior*. Annapolis: Naval Institute Press.

Campbell, Neil and R. Martin S. Smellie. 1983. *The Royal Society of Edinburgh (1783–1983)* . . . Edinburgh: Royal Society of Edinburgh.

Cantlie, Neil. 1974. *A History of the Army Medical Department*. 2 vols. Edinburgh: Churchill Livingstone.

Cathcart, C.W. 1882. Some of the older schools of anatomy connected with the Royal College of Surgeons, Edinburgh. *Edinburgh Medical Journal* 27: 769–81.

Chambers, William. 1830. *The Book of Scotland*. Edinburgh: Robert Buchanan.

Christison, Robert. 1885. *Life of Sir Robert Christison*. Edinburgh: William Blackwood and Sons.

Cole, F.J. 1944. *A History of Comparative Anatomy*. London: Macmillan and Co.

Cole, Hubert. 1964. *Things for the Surgeon: a History of the Resurrection Men*. London: Heinemann.

Cory, G.E., 1910–30. *The Rise of South Africa: A History of the Origin of South African Colonisation and of its Development Towards the East from the Earliest Times to 1857*. 5 vols. London: Longmans, Green and Co.

Cosh, Mary. 2003. *Edinburgh: The Golden Age*. Edinburgh: John Donald.

Cottom, Daniel. 2001 *Cannibals and Philosophers: Bodies of Enlightenment*. Baltimore: Johns Hopkins University Press.

Creswell, Clarendon Hyde. 1914. The Royal College of Surgeons of Edinburgh: Anatomy in the early days. *Edinburgh Medical Journal* 12: 141–56.

Creswell, Clarendon Hyde. 1926. *The Royal College of Surgeons of Edinburgh: Historical Notes from 1505–1905*. Edinburgh: Oliver and Boyd.

Curtin, Philip. 1964. *The Image of Africa* . . . London: Macmillan and Co.

Cushing, Peter. 1994. How I became a monster hunter. In: Peter Haining, ed. *Peter Cushing's Monster Movies*. 2nd ed. London: Robert Hale, pp. 1–13.

Davies, Alan T. 1988. *Infected Christianity: A History of Modern Racism*. Montreal: McGill-Queen's University Press.

Desmond, Adrian. 1992. *The Politics of Evolution* . . . Chicago: University of Chicago Press.

Dietrich, Michael R. 2003. Richard Goldschmidt: hopeful monsters and other "heresies". *Nature Reviews Genetics* 4: 68–74.

Dingwall, Helen M. 2005. *"A Famous and Flourishing Society": The History of the Royal College of Surgeons of Edinburgh, 1505–2005*. Edinburgh: Edinburgh University Press.

Douglas, Hugh. 1973. *Burke and Hare: the True Story*. London: Hale.

Edwards, Owen Dudley. 1980. *Burke & Hare*. Edinburgh: Polygon Books.

Foot, P. 1967. Abortion and the doctrine of double effect. *Oxford Review* 5: 28–41.

Forry, Steven Earl. 1990. *Hideous Progenies* . . . Philadelphia: University of Pennsylvania Press.

Foucault, Michel. 1973. *The Birth of the Clinic: an Archaeology of Medical Perception*. Transl. A.M. Sheridan Smith. London: Tavistock.

Foucault, Michel. 1981. *History of Sexuality: an Introduction*. Transl. Robert Hurley. London: Penguin.

Bibliography

Francis, Nathan R. and Wayne Lewis. 2001. What price dissection? Dissection literally dissected. *Journal of Medical Ethics* 27: 2–9.

Garwood-Gowers, Austen, John Tingle and Kay Wheat. 2005. *Contemporary Issues in Healthcare Law and Ethics*. Edinburgh: Butterworth Heinemann.

Glut, Donald F. 1984. *The Frankenstein Catalogue . . .* Jefferson NC: Macfarland and Co.

Gordon-Grube, Karen. 1988. Anthropophagy in post-Renaissance Europe: the tradition of medicinal cannibalism. *American Anthropologist* 90: 405–8.

Gould, Stephen Jay. 1977. *Ontogeny and Phylogeny*. Cambridge MA: Belknap.

Gould, Stephen Jay. 2002. *The Structure of Evolutionary Theory*. Cambridge MA: Belknap.

Guthrie, Douglas. 1965. *Extramural Medical Education in Edinburgh and the School of Medicine of the Royal Colleges*. Edinburgh: E. and S. Livingstone.

Guyader, Herve le. 2004. *Geoffroy Saint-Hilaire: a Visionary Naturalist*. Chicago: University of Chicago Press.

Hartley, Lucy. 2001. A science of beauty? Femininity, fitness, and the nineteenth-century physiognomic tradition in mid-nineteenth century Britain. *Women: A Cultural Review* 12: 19–34.

Healy, Kieran. 2006. *Last Best Gifts: Altruism and the Market for Human Blood and Organs*. Chicago: University of Chicago Press.

Holmes, Rachel. 2007. *The Hottentot Venus. The Life and Death of Saartjie Baartman: Born 1789 – Buried 2002*. London: Bloomsbury.

Hopkins, Harry. 1977. *The Strange Death of Private White: A Victorian Scandal That Made History*. London: Weidenfeld and Nicolson.

Jacyna, L.S. 1983. Immanence or transcendence: theories of life and organization in Britain 1790–1835. *Isis* 74: 311–29.

Jacyna, L.S. 2001 "A host of experienced microscopists": the establishment of histology in nineteenth-century Edinburgh. *Bulletin of the History of Medicine* 75: 225–53.

Johnson, A. 2005. My friend Dr Knox: a pupil writes about the anatomist. *Surgeon* 3: 407–10.

Jordanova, Ludmilla. 1993. *Sexual Visions: Images of Gender in Science and Medicine Between the Eighteenth and the Twentieth Centuries*. Milwaukee: University of Wisconsin Press.

Kass, Amalie M. and Edward H. Kass. 1988. *Perfecting the World: The Life and Times of Dr. Thomas Hodgkin 1798–1866*. Boston: Harcourt Brace Jovanovich.

Kaufman, M.H. 1997. Another look at Burke Hare: the last day of Mary Paterson – a medical cover-up? *Proceedings of the Royal College of Physicians of Edinburgh* 27: 78–88.

Kaufman, Matthew H. 2000. *Surgeons at War: Medical Arrangements for the Treatment of the Sick and Wounded in the British Army During the Late 18th and 19th Centuries*. Westport: Greenwood Press.

Kaufman, M.H. 2001. Frederick Knox, younger brother and assistant of Dr Robert Knox: his contribution to "Knox's Catalogues". *Journal of the Royal College of Surgeons of Edinburgh* 46: 44–56.

Kaufman, M.H. 2003. *Medical Teaching in Edinburgh During the 18th and 19th Centuries*. Edinburgh: Royal College of Surgeons.

Bibliography

Kaufman, M.H. 2004. Transfer of bodies to the University of Edinburgh after the 1832 anatomy act. *Journal of the Royal College of Physicians of Edinburgh* 34: 228–36.

Keith, Arthur. 1917. How can the institute best serve the needs of anthropology? *Journal of the Royal Anthropological Institute* 47: 12–30.

Ketterer, David. 1997. "Furnished . . . materials": the surgical anatomy context of *Frankenstein*. *Science Fiction Studies* 24: 119–23.

Kidd, Colin. 2003. Race, empire, and the limits of nineteenth-century Scottish nationhood. *History Journal* 46: 873–92.

Lansbury, Coral. 1985. *The Old Brown Dog: Women, Workers, and Vivisection in Edwardian England*. Wisconsin: University of Wisconsin Press.

Lawrence, Christopher. 2002. Alder Hey. *Journal of Epidemiology and Community Health* 56: 4–5.

Liggins, Emma. 2000. The medical gaze and the female corpse: looking at bodies in Mary Shelley's *Frankenstein*. *Studies in the Novel* 32: 129–46.

Lindfors, Bernth. 1996. Hottentot, Bushman, Kaffir: taxonomic tendencies in nineteenth-century racial iconography. *Nordic Journal of African Studies* 5: 1–28.

Lindqvist, Sven. 2002. *Exterminate All the Brutes*. London: Granta.

Lonsdale, Henry. 1870. *A Sketch of the Life and Writings of Robert Knox, the Anatomist*. London: Macmillan and Co.

Lovejoy, Arthur O. 1959. The argument for organic evolution before *The Origin of Species*. In: Bentley Glass, Owsei Temkin and William L. Straus, eds. *Forerunners of Darwin*. Baltimore: Johns Hopkins Press.

Lovejoy, Arthur O. 1964. *The Great Chain of Being*. Cambridge MA: Harvard University Press.

MacDonald, Helen. 2006. *Human Remains: Dissection and its Histories*. New Haven: Yale University Press.

MacGregor, George. 1884. *The History of Burke and Hare and of the Resurrectionist Times*. Glasgow: Thomas D. Morison.

Mackay, John. 1988. *The True Story of Burke and Hare*. Glasgow: Lang Syne.

MacLaren, I. 2000. Robert Knox MD, FRCSEd, FRSEd 1791–1862: the first conservator of the college museum. *Journal of the Royal College of Surgeons of Edinburgh* 45: 392–7.

McLean, Sheila A.M. and Laura Williamson. 2005. *Xenotransplantation: Law and Ethics*. Aldershot: Ashgate.

MacNalty, Arthur Salusbury. 1950. *A Biography of Sir Benjamin Ward Richardson*. London: Harvey and Blythe.

Magubane, Zine. 2003. Simians, savages, skulls, and sex: science and colonial militarism in nineteenth-century South Africa. In: Donald S. Moore, Jake Kosek and Anand Pandian, eds. *Race, Nature and the Politics of Difference*. Durham: Duke University Press, pp. 99–121.

Malchow, H.L. 1996. *Gothic Images of Race in Nineteenth-Century Britain*. Stanford: Stanford University Press.

Marshall, Tim. 1995. *Murdering to Dissect: Grave-Robbing, Frankenstein and the Anatomy Literature*. Manchester: Manchester University Press.

Matthews, Tina. 2006. Review of *Human Remains: Dissection and its Histories*. *Bulletin of the Royal College of Pathologists* no. 136: 77.

Bibliography

Maynard, Katherine Kearney. 2000. The perils and pleasures of professionalism in Stevenson's *Strange Case of Dr. Jekyll and Mr. Hyde* and Doyle's *A Study in Scarlet* and other fictions. *The European Legacy* 5: 365–84.

Miles, Alexander. 1918. *The Edinburgh School of Surgery Before Lister*. London: A. and C. Black.

Morton, L.T. 1991. London's last private medical school. *Journal of the Royal Society of Medicine* 84: 682.

Myres, John L. 1944. A century of our work. *Man* 44: 2–9.

Napier, E. Elers. 1862. *The Life and Correspondence of Admiral Sir Charles Napier, K.C.B.* 2 vols. London: Hurst and Blackett.

Newman, Charles. 1957. *The Evolution of Medical Education in the Nineteenth Century*. London: Oxford University Press.

O'Malley, C.D. 1954. Andreas Vesalius' pilgrimage. *Isis* 45: 138–44.

Outram, Dorinda. 1984. *Georges Cuvier: Vocation, Science and Authority in Post-Revolutionary France*. Manchester: Manchester University Press.

Powell, Sally. 2004. Black markets and cadaverous pies: the corpse, urban trade and industrial corruption in the penny blood. In: Andrew Maunder and Grace Moore, eds. *Victorian Crime, Madness and Sensation*. Aldershot: Ashgate, pp. 45–58.

Prideaux, William Francis and L.S. Livingston, eds. 1917. *A Bibliography of the Works of Robert Louis Stevenson*. London: Frank Hollings.

Rae, Isobel. 1958. *The Strange Story of Dr James Barry: Army Surgeon, Inspector-General of Hospitals, Discovered on Death to be a Woman*. London: Longmans, Green.

Rae, Isobel. 1964. *Knox, The Anatomist*. Edinburgh: Oliver and Boyd.

Rehbock, Philip F. 1983. *The Philosophical Naturalists*. Madison: University of Wisconsin Press.

Rehbock, Philip F. 1990. Transcendental anatomy. In: Andrew Cunningham and Nicholas Jardine, eds. *Romanticism and the Sciences*. Cambridge: Cambridge University Press, pp. 144–60.

Richards, Evelleen. 1989. The "moral anatomy" of Robert Knox: the interplay between biological and social thought in Victorian scientific naturalism. *Journal of the History of Biology* 22: 373–436.

Richards, Evelleen. 1994. A political anatomy of monsters, hopeful and otherwise: teratogeny, transcendentalism, and evolutionary theorizing. *Isis* 85: 377–411.

Richardson, Ruth. 2000. A necessary inhumanity. *Journal of Medical Ethics* 26: 104–6.

Richardson, Ruth. 2001. *Death, Dissection and the Destitute*. 2nd ed. London: Phoenix Press.

Ritvo, Harriet. 1997. *The Platypus and the Mermaid and Other Figments of the Classifying Imagination*. Cambridge MA: Harvard University Press.

Rodgers, M.E. 2005. Human bodies, inhuman uses: public reactions and legislative responses to the scandals of bodysnatching. In: Austen Garwood-Gowers, John Tingle, and Kay Wheat, eds. *Contemporary Issues in Healthcare Law and Ethics*. Edinburgh: Elsevier, pp. 151–72.

Rosner, Lisa. 1991. *Medical Education in the Age of Improvement: Edinburgh Students and Apprentices 1760–1826*. Edinburgh: Edinburgh University Press.

Bibliography

Ross, James A. and Hugh Y.W. Taylor. 1955. Robert Knox's Catalogue. *Journal of the History of Medicine and Allied Sciences* 10: 269–76.

Roughead, William, ed. 1921. *Burke and Hare*. Edinburgh: William Hodge.

Roughead, William. 1929. *The Murderers Companion*. New York: Readers Club.

Rupke, Nicolaas A. 1994. *Richard Owen: Victorian Naturalist*. New Haven: Yale University Press.

Ruse, Michael. 1996. *Monad to Man: The Concept of Progress in Evolutionary Biology*. Cambridge MA: Harvard University Press.

Savulescu, J. 2006. Conscientious objection in medicine. *BMJ* 332: 294–7.

Secord, Anne. 2002. Botany on a plate: pleasure and the power of pictures in promoting early nineteenth-century scientific knowledge. *Isis* 93: 28–57.

Secord, James A. 2000. *Victorian Sensation . . .* Chicago: University of Chicago Press.

Shapin, Steven and Simon Schaffer. 1985. *Leviathan and the Air-Pump: Hobbes, Boyle, and the Experimental Life*. Princeton NJ: Princeton University Press.

Showalter, Elaine. 1992. *Sexual Anarchy: Gender and Culture at the Fin de Siècle*. London: Bloomsbury.

Stepan, Nancy. 1982. *The Idea of Race in Science: Great Britain 1800–1960*. London: Macmillan.

Stephen, Kathy. 1981. *Robert Knox M.D., F.R.S.E. (1791–1862)*. Edinburgh: Scotland's Cultural Heritage.

Stevenson, Robert Louis. 2002. *The Strange Case of Dr Jekyll and Mr Hyde and other Tales of Terror*. Ed. Robert Mighall. London: Penguin Books.

Stevenson, Robert Louis. 2006. *Strange Case of Dr Jekyll and Mr Hyde and Other Tales*. Ed. Roger Luckhurst. Oxford: Oxford University Press.

Stocking, George W. 1987. *Victorian Anthropology*. New York: The Free Press.

Summers, Montague. 1941. *Gothic Bibliography*. London: Fortune Press.

Taine, Hippolyte A. 1881. *The Ancient Regime*. London: Sampson Low, Marston, Searle and Rivington.

Tansey, Violet and D.E.C. Mekie. 1982. *The Museum of the Royal College of Surgeons of Edinburgh*. Edinburgh: Royal College of Surgeons of Edinburgh.

Thomas, Dylan. 1953. *The Doctor and the Devils*. London: J.M. Dent and Sons.

Turner, William, ed. 1868. *The Anatomical Memoirs of John Goodsir FRS Late Professor of Anatomy in the University of Edinburgh*. 2 vols. Edinburgh: A. and C. Black.

Urry, James. 1989. Headhunters and body-snatchers. *Anthropology Today* 5: 11–13.

Van Heyningen, Elizabeth. 2004. Medical practice in the Eastern Cape. In: Harriet Deacon, Howard Phillips and Elizabeth van Heyningen, eds. *The Cape Doctor in the Nineteenth Century: A Social History*. Amsterdam: Rodopi, pp. 169–94.

Waldby, Catherine and Robert Mitchell. 2006. *Tissue Economies: Blood, Organs, and Cell lines in Late Capitalism*. Durham: Duke University Press.

Walkowitz, Judith. 2004. Jack the Ripper. In: Chris Jenks, ed. *Urban Culture: Critical Concepts in Literary and Cultural Studies*. 4 vols. London: Routledge, IV, pp. 166–208.

Bibliography

Wallace, Mark Coleman. 2007. *Scottish Freemasonry 1725–1810: Progress, Power, and Politics.* PhD thesis, University of St Andrews.

Walls, E.W. 1964. John Bell, 1763–1820. *Medical History* 8: 63–9.

Watson, Robert Spence. 1897. *The History of the Literary and Philosophical Society of Newcastle Upon Tyne (1793–1896).* London: Walter Scott.

Wearing, J.P. 1990. *The London Stage 1930–1939: A Calendar of Plays and Players.* 3 vols. Metuchen NJ: The Scarecrow Press.

Wells, Thomas Spencer. 1873. *Diseases of the Ovaries.* London: D. Appleton.

Wilde, Oscar. 2005. *The Complete Works of Oscar Wilde. Volume 3: The Picture of Dorian Gray: the 1890 and 1891 Texts.* Ed. Joseph Bristow. Oxford: Oxford University Press.

Wilson, Jamie. 2001. Body snatching. *Student BMJ* 9: 29.

Wilson, John B. 1987. A surgeon's private practice in the nineteenth century: Sir William Fergusson's Edinburgh day books 1832–39, with some extracts from his London day books 1839–77. *Medical History* 31: 349–53.

Wise, Sarah. 2004. *The Italian Boy: Murder and Grave-Robbery in 1830s London.* London: Jonathan Cape.

Index

Abernethy, John: as a teacher, 29, 31, 51, 63; conservative opinions, 132; teaches Richard Owen, 136; teaches Alexander Walker, 148
Aborigines Protection Society, 49, 106
Academy of Sciences, Paris, 23, 44, 47
Adam, Alexander, 16–18
"Aesculapius", *see* Potts, Laurence Holker
Africa, *see* Cape Colony
Ainley, Henry Hinchcliffe, 169
Alcock, Rutherford, 111
Alder Hey Children's Hospital, 173
Alexander, Thomas, 65
Alfort Veterinary School, 54
Alison, W. P., 99, 187
Anatomical and Physiological Society, Edinburgh, 95
anatomical models, 4, 7, 42, 106, 117–18, 139
Anatomist, The (play), *see* Bridie, James
anatomy: as radical science, 4–6, 87, 89, 117–18, 137; and medical training, 10, 21, 55, 58, 60–3, 74–5, 89, 95, 105, 142; moral objections to, 21–2, 60, 63, 82, 106; and atheism, 21, 43; examinations, 25–6; public interest in, 116, 118, 139, 163; *see also* anatomy schools; artistic anatomy; comparative anatomy; transcendental anatomy
Anatomy Act (1832), 2, 6–7, 26, 89–91, 94, 97, 101, 104, 105, 111, 141, 164, 166
anatomy schools, 9, 27, 60–1; *see also under named teachers*
Andrews, Captain, 39
animal experimentation, *see* vivisection
Anthropological Review, 144, 145
Anthropological Society of London, 3, 129
Anthropological Society of Paris, 159
anthropology, 51–2, 122–9, 144, 159
anti-vivisectionism, 27, 29, 82–3, 172
apes, anatomy of, 123, 135–6, 137, 154–5
Apothecaries Act (1815), 30, 32, 61
archetype, ideal, 23, 113, 137, 151
Army Medical Department, 30, 42
arrested development, 63, 113, 133, 137, 143, 144, 154
artistic anatomy, 116–17, 139–40, 146–7, 149
Association of Teachers of Anatomy, 7, 92–4, 98, 103–4
atheism, 3, 21, 36, 43, 153, 161
Athenaeum Club, London, 116
Audubon, John James, 64–5
autopsy, 4, 10, 24, 83, 98, 158, 173
"Aztec" children, 143–5, 152, 155

Baartman, Saartjie, 36
Baird, George Husband, 20
Ballingall, Sir George, 27, 94, 99, 187
Barclay, John: early career, 27; denied university chair, 28, 42; museum, 51, 54; partnership with RK, 55; final illness, 56–7; obtains bodies for dissection, 59; as a teacher, 63, 136, 142, 148
Barnum and Bailey's circus, 144
Barry, James, 37–8
Beane, Sawney, 80
beauty, science of, 24, 140, 146–51
Béclard, Pierre, 49–50, 182
Bell, Sir Charles, 54, 82, 99
Bell, Sir John, 26
Bell, T., *see* Roberton, John
Belzoni, Giovanni Battista, 53, 183
Berlioz, Hector, 1
Bertram, James G., 164
Bichat, Xavier: RK's biography of, 4; inspires RK, 24–5; RK idolises, 49–50, 140
Birnie, Thomas (RK's nephew), 110, 142
Bishop, John, 76
Blackwood's Magazine, 73–4, 90
Blainville, Henri Marie Ducrotay de: RK attends lectures by, 46–7; RK

Index

translates works of, 102; paper on the orangutan, 106
Blake, C. Carter, 62, 160
Blandin, Philippe Frédéric, 64
Blumenbach, Johann Friedrich: on cranial morphology, 51, 123; on embryonic development 134
Body Snatcher, The (film), 83, 171
body-snatchers, 6, 26, 58–9, 105–6, 162–3, 165
Boers: in Cape Colony, 33–6; RK's opinion of, 37; ill feeling towards British, 41
Bonn, Andreas, 52
Boyer, Alexis, 49
Braxfield, Robert Macqueen, Lord, 14
Breadalbane, John Campbell, 2nd Marquis of, 65, 102, 118
Brewster, David, 57
Bridgewater treatises, 113–14
Bridie, James: *The Anatomist*, 169–70
Bristol Royal Infirmary, 173
British Association for the Advancement of Science, 108, 117, 200
British Medical Association, 158
Brookes, Joshua, 62
Brotherhood of the Friends of the Truth, *see* Oineromathic Society
Brotherhood of the Magi, *see* Oineromathic Society
Brussels, 31
Buchanan, George, 28, 52
Buckton, Oliver S., 168
Buffon, Georges-Louis Leclerc, Comte de, 43, 132
Burke, Edmund, 3, 148
Burke, William: sells body to RK, 66; domestic circumstances, 67; West Port murders, 67–8; trial, 68–9; link with David Paterson, 70; execution, 71; confession, 71–2; in fiction, 164–5, 167, 170–1
burking, 78, 84, 171
Burnett, Bishop, 40
Burns, Robert, 15
Bushmen, *see* San

Caledonian Mercury, 70, 73
Callanan, Laura, 126
Calvinism, 128
Campbell, John, 128
Campbell, William, 107
Camper, Pieter, 123, 134
Cancer Hospital, London, 158, 160
cannibalism, 1, 76, 78–84, 89, 90, 129, 159, 164
Cape Colony, South Africa, 32, 33–41, 49, 51–2, 58, 79, 105, 110–11, 114–15, 124–5, 127
Cape Corps, 33, 38–9, 41
Capel, Georgina, 31
Carlile, Richard, 83
Carlyle, Thomas, 80, 83
Carpenter, W.B., 109
chain of being, 47, 123, 135
Chambers, Robert, 138; *see also Vestiges of the Natural History of Creation*
Chaplin, Simon, 21
Cheselden, William, 147
cholera, 88–9, 101, 142
Chomel, Auguste-Francois, 49
Christian Examiner, 90, 127
Christison, Robert: investigates West Port murders 69; professional opposition to RK, 99, 101
Cloquet, Hippolyte, 64
Clydesdale, Matthew, 27
Cobbett, William, 14
Coigny, Comtesse de, 43
Coleridge, Samuel Taylor, 21
Collège de France, 43
commando raids, 37–8, 58
comparative anatomy, 5, 23, 24, 27, 44–5, 54, 63, 87, 105, 106, 136–7
Constable, Michael, 81
Cooper, Sir Astley, 75
Cory, G. E., 33
Court of Cacus, *see* Leighton, Alexander
Cox, Robert, 65
Craigie, David: inspector of anatomy, 91–4; relations with anatomists, 97; recommended for professorship, 110
Cruikshank, Andrew, 170
Crystal Palace, 139
Curse of Frankenstein, The (film), 167
Curtin, Philip D., 125
Cuvier, Frédéric, 85
Cuvier, Georges, Baron: RK on, 8, 43, 46, 48, 50, 139, 140, 145; career, 44; personal appearance, 45; museum, 45, 54, 117; relations with Geoffroy, 46, 87; opinions on Blainville and Lamarck, 47; RK's last meeting with, 54; Plinian Society proposes to honour, 57; scientific theories, 63, 87, 123, 136, 148; meeting with Owen, 136

Daft Jamie, *see* Wilson, James
Darwin, Charles: on unity of type, 23; on Monro *tertius*, 25; and RK, 64, 157; *Descent of Man*, 148; *The Origin of Species*, 152, 156–7
Darwinism, *see* natural selection

Index

Davies, Alan T., 128, 129
Day, Horatio Grosvenor, 119
Deseret, Phineas, 124
Desmond, Adrian, 5
Dick, William, 27, 61
Dickens, Charles, 122
Disraeli, Benjamin, 126, 161
dissection, anatomical: distasteful, 1, 3, 21–2, 60, 74, 80–2, 104, 142, 149–51, 173–4; in medical training, 6–8, 10, 26, 58–63, 89–90, 97, 101–2; as punishment, 26, 69, 71, 82–3; of animals, 32, 51, 52, 85, 93, 102; in Paris, 42–3, 48–9; compulsory, 61; dangers of, 74, 106, 142; in fiction, 162–4
Doctor and the Devils, The (play and film), 172
Douglas, Hugh, 10
Dr. Jekyll and Sister Hyde (film), 167
Dugong, 85
Duméril, Andre, 23
Dumfries, 89
Dundas, Henry, 13, 14
Dupuytren, Guillaume, 93

Ecole de médecine, Paris, 48, 90–1
Edinburgh: slums, 6, 16, 66–7, 80, 167; town council, 13, 15, 95–6, 99, 100, 109–10; Surgeons' Square, 14, 19, 27, 58, 59, 64, 66, 67, 68, 72, 88, 91, 92, 101, 109, 112; Nicolson Square, 51; Argyle Square, 63, 101, 102, 105, 112, 119–20; West Port district, 66–7; Burkomania, 78–9; Nicolson Street, 86, 112; cholera threat, 88; Clarke Street, 119
Edinburgh Courant, 72
Edinburgh Medical and Surgical Journal, 28, 91
Edinburgh Philosophical Journal, 41, 51
Edinburgh Royal Dispensary, 97
Edinburgh University: new buildings opened, 15; medical students in, 19–20, 29, 61, 97; MD degree, 19, 29, 30, 95; museum, 42, 51, 52, 55, 85, 87, 95; compulsory lectures, 55, 94; criticism of, 95, 102; supply of bodies to, 97, 101, 103, 107; chair in pathology, 99–100; chair in physiology, 109
Edwards, Owen Dudley, 10, 71
Edwards, W. F., 53, 183
Egypt, Napoleon I's expedition to, 43, 44
Egyptian Hall, Piccadilly, 122
Elephant Theatre, 171
embryology, 5, 11, 43, 47, 63, 113–14, 132–4, 137, 144, 145, 153–4, 156

epigenesis, 43
ethics, medical, 10, 170, 172–4
Ethnological Journal, 131
Ethnological Society, London, 49, 114, 115, 130, 144–5, 159
eugenics, 170
evolution, 2, 5, 11, 46, 47–8, 130, 134–8, 145, 152–4, 156–7, 196; see also natural selection

Fau, Julien, 146
Fergusson, William: assistant to RK, 65, 88, 92; meeting with Burke and Hare, 66, 68; acquaintance with Mary Paterson, 67; career as a surgeon, 94, 97, 109, 143; meets RK in London, 159; in fiction, 168
Fisherrow, East Lothian, 88–9
Fleeson, James, 39, 41
Flesh and the Fiends, The (film), 172
Fletcher, John, 112
Fonblanque, Albany, 79
Forbes, Edward, 65, 95–6
formalism, 87
Forster, B. M., 90
Fosbrooke, John Edward, 119–20
Foucault, Michel, 11
Frankenstein (novel, film), 166
Frankenstein Meets the Wolf Man (film), 338
Fraser, G. S., 33, 39
freemasonry, 15, 49
French Revolution, 3, 13, 14, 42–4, 52, 79, 83, 87
Friends of the People, Society of, 13–14
functionalism, 45, 87
funeratories, 103–4, 107, 112

Galton, Francis, 154, 196
Gant, Frederick James, 140, 141
General Medical Council, 8, 118, 169
Genga, Bernardino, 147
Gentleman's Magazine, 126
Geoffroy Saint Hilaire, Etienne: RK's opinion of, 8, 43, 46, 139; early career, 44, 45; relations with Cuvier, 46, 87; transmutation theory, 47–8, 63; theory of arrested development, 63, 113, 134, 154
Geoffroy Saint Hilaire, Isidore, 158
George Heriot's School, Edinburgh, 13, 14
Glenorchy, Lord, *see* Breadalbane
Goethe, Johann Wolfgang von, 23–4, 44, 46, 47, 113, 146, 148
Goldschmidt, Richard, 11
Goodsir, Harry, 65, 96

223

Index

Goodsir, John, 9, 95, 96, 103, 109, 140, 168
Goodsir, Robert, 96
Gould, Steven Jay, 137
Graaf Reinet, 34, 37, 39, 40
Graham's Town, 37, 39, 40
Grainger, Richard Dugard, 81
Grant, Robert, 56, 57, 136, 156, 197
Gray, James, 17
Great Exhibition (1851), 118, 139
Great Fish River, 33, 37
Greed of William Hart, The (film), 171
Greenhill, William, 106
Grégoire, Henri, 52
Greville, Robert Kaye, 57
Grey, Henry George, 3rd Earl, 118
Grey, Lady, 32
Greyfriars Kirk, 25, 103
Guy's Hospital, 55, 123

Hamilton, James, 99
Hammer Films, 167
Handyside, Peter, 9, 92, 94, 96, 98, 101, 112, 193
Hare, William: sells body to RK, 66; home life, 67; West Port murders, 67–8, 72; gives evidence for Crown, 69; relations with David Paterson, 70; reviled in press, 73; 76, 80; in fiction, 164–5, 167, 170
Hartley, Lucy, 148
Haslar Naval Hospital, Gosport, 31
Haydon, Benjamin, 116–17
hermaphrodites, 113
Hibbert-Ware, Samuel, 57
Hilsea Hospital, Portsmouth, 32
Hodgkin, Thomas; student life, 47, 48–9; friendship with RK, 53, 57, 61, 86, 88, 114; museum curator, 55, 123; interest in aboriginal peoples, 57–8, 114; on West Port murders, 78; recommends Craigie for chair, 110
Hogarth, William, 82–3
Holmes, Oliver Wendell, 1, 128
Home, Everard, 53
Hope, James, 103
Hope, Thomas Charles, 99
Hôpital de la gendarmerie, Brussels, 31–2
Hôpital de la Pitié, 1, 48–9
Hospital Pupil's Guide, see Potts, Laurence Holker
Hottentot, see Khoi
House of Frankenstein (film), 166
Howe, James, 99
Hunt, James, 129
Hunter, John, 123
Hunter, William (anatomist), 82, 147
Hunter, William (RK's lodger), 110

Hunterian museum, London, 53–4, 136
Institut de France, 44, 118
"Italian boy" murders, 76, 90, 163

Jack the Ripper, see Whitechapel murders
Jacyna, L. S., 5
Jameson, Robert, 42, 45, 51, 55
Jardin des Plantes, 43, 44, 117
Jardin du Roi, see Jardin des Plantes
Jenner, Edward, 16
Johnson, Samuel, 79
Jones, John Paul, 15
Jones, Thomas Wharton, 65, 66

Kahn, Joseph, 118, 139
Kant, Immanuel, 132
Kaufman, M. H., 9
Khoi, 33–4, 35–8, 52–3, 79, 105, 114, 125, 127, 131, 132, 137, 155
King's College, London, 62, 109
Kirkcudbright, 14
Knox, Archibald (RK's brother), 14, 176
Knox, Edward (RK's son), 158, 160, 201
Knox, Elouisa (RK's sister), 14
Knox, Frederick John (RK's brother): birth, 14; correspondence with RK, 35, 41; works at RK's school, 86, 93; zoological studies, 86–7, 96–7, 102; cholera epidemic, 88–9; emigration, 102–3, 106; life in New Zealand, 106–7, 192
Knox, Isabella (RK's daughter), 110, 117
Knox, Janet (RK's sister), 14, 110, 176
Knox, John (protestant leader), 3
Knox, John (RK's brother), 14, 176
Knox, John (RK's son), 110, 111
Knox, Mary (RK's daughter), 53, 110, 158, 183
Knox, Mary (RK's sister), 14, 110, 117, 119, 142, 176
Knox, Paxton (RK's brother), 176
Knox, Robert
LIFE: birth, 13, 14; smallpox, 16; attends High School, 16–18; *dux* of school, 18; matriculates at Edinburgh University, 20; studies transcendental anatomy, 23–5; president of Royal Physical Society, 24; fails anatomy examination, 25–6; joins Barclay's class, 27; graduates MD, 28; highland holidays, 29; studies under Abernethy, 29; commissioned Hospital Assistant, 31; treats wounded from Waterloo, 31–2; physician at Hilsea, 32; sails to Cape Colony, 32–3; army surgeon in the Cape, 33–40; quarrel with

Index

Stockenstöm, 38–41; duel, 40; returns to Edinburgh, 41; joins Wernerian society, 42; studies in Paris, 42–50; freemasonry, 49; visits London, 53; marriage, 53; fellow of Royal Society of Edinburgh, 54; curator of College of Surgeons museum, 54–5; partnership with Barclay, 55–6; fellow of Edinburgh College of Surgeons, 56; private teacher, 57–8, 61–3; meets Audubon, 64–5; West Port murders, 66–8; questioned by Christison, 69; threats made against, 71–2; writes to *Mercury*, 73–4; censured by committee, 75; cetology, 85–6; resigns museum conservatorship and army commission, 86; on philosophical anatomy, 87–8; success as a teacher, 88; on cholera epidemic, 88–9; Association of Teachers, 92–3; founds Anatomical Society, 95; shortage of cadavers, 97–8; applies for chair in pathology, 99–100; visits Holland, 102; Argyle Square school, 105; partnership with Lonsdale, 107; alleged plagiarism, 108–9; fails to obtain salaried post, 109; wife and children, 110; Edinburgh school fails, 112; proposed African expedition, 114–15, 118–19; Glasgow school fails, 115; lectures on race, 116; manages Thibert's museum, 117–18; signs false certificate, 119–20; expelled from Royal Society, 120; moves to London, 121; ethnological shows, 122, 130–6; transcendental theories, 130–8; Royal Free school, 140–1; on "Aztec" children, 143–4; blackballed by Ethnological Society, 145; theories of beauty, 146–50; on species change, 154–6; reaction to *Origin of Species*, 157; pathologist at Cancer Hospital, 158–9; lodgings in Hackney, 158–9; honorary fellow of Ethnological Society, 159; death and burial, 160; posthumous reputation, 2, 12; biographies of, *see under* Lonsdale *and* Rae
ATTITUDES AND OPINIONS: dislike of dissection, 3, 142, 150–1; radical views, 3, 16, 25, 42–3; contempt for authority, 3, 7, 25, 68, 89, 102, 109; religion, 3, 110; "atheism", 3, 153; enthusiasm for science, 8, 32, 140, 160; showmanship, 11, 62, 96, 110–11; outspokeness, 25, 101, 107, 139; abstemious habits, 28; dislike of Celts, 32, 48, 126, 143; interest in race, 35–6, 51–3, 64, 109, 124–31, 159; anticolonialism, 37, 38, 53, 124–5, 128, 131, 159; antivivisectionism, 82; wit, 93, 101, 105; transcendentalism, 112–13, 146, 151, 152–6; alleged "racism", 125, 128
PERSONAL APPEARANCE: 16, 28, 61–2, 110
IN FICTION: 1, 10, 161, 164–72, 174
PUBLISHED WORKS: *The Edinburgh Dissector*, 105; journal articles, 106, 112, 116, 144, 152; *Great Artists and Great Anatomists*, 139; *Manual of Artistic Anatomy*, 140, 146; *Manual of Human Anatomy*, 140; *Fish and Fishing*, 142; *The Races of Men*, 1, 124–31
Knox, Robert (RK's father), 13–15, 25
Knox, Robert (RK's son), 110, 142–3
Knox, Susan (RK's daughter), 110, 142
Knox, Susan (RK's wife), 53, 110, 111
Knox, Thomas, Earl of Ranfurly, 16
Knox, William (RK's brother), 14

l'Herminier, F. J., 49
Lacroix, Jules, 164
Lafayette, (General) Marie-Joseph Paul Yves Roch Gilbert du Motier, Marquis de, 4
Laird, Margaret, 67, 71
Lamarck, Jean-Baptiste: theories, 8, 47, 136, 138, 140; career in Paris, 44; Cuvier's opinion of, 47; RK's opinion of, 47
Lamarckian inheritance, 132
Lancet, The: on RK, 9, 97; RK's obituary, 53, 128; on anatomy, 62, 76, 82, 84, 87, 120, 136, 166; writings by RK in, 100, 102, 106, 107, 142, 144, 152, 153, 158; reviews, 130, 140, 169; on Royal Free School, 140–1
Larrey, Dominique Jean, Baron, 160
Lasteyrie, Charles-Philbert, Comte de, 49
Lawrence, Sir William, 59, 132, 135
Le Vaillant, Francois, 34, 49
Leighton, Alexander: *The Court of Cacus*, 59, 67, 76, 164–5
Lightfoot, Robert, 1
Lincoln, Lord, 119
Lind, Jenny, 119
Lindqvist, Sven, 125
Linnaean Society, London, 152, 156
Linnaeus, Carl, 134, 200
Liston, Robert, 27, 55, 61, 64, 63, 91, 116
Lizars, Alexander, 63, 92, 94, 96, 98, 101, 102, 103, 109
Lizars, John, 59–60, 61, 63, 94, 102, 109
London: anatomy schools, 19, 29, 58,

59–60, 62, 75, 76, 87, 90, 101, 102, 105; RK on, 34, 42, 121, 139; exhibitions in, 52, 53, 118, 122, 143–4; museums, 54, 55, 117, 118, 136; Hyde Park, 59; bodies obtained from, 61, 76, 92; Clapton, 143; *see also* Crystal Palace; Royal College of Surgeons; Royal Institution; University College
London Medical Gazette, 82, 89, 90, 108, 112, 113, 114
London University, *see* University College London
Lonsdale, Henry: *Life of Robert Knox*, 8–9, 15, 18, 34, 53, 56, 61, 65, 68, 72, 73, 74, 82, 100, 101–2, 110; career, 67, 109, 112; RK's pupil, 95, 96; RK's friend and partner, 107, 111, 135
Lothian, Marquis of, 89
Lovett, William, 118
Lucae, Johann, 151
Lyceum Theatre, Edinburgh, 169
Lyndhurst, Lord, 126

Macbeth (play), 121
Mackay, John, 10
Mackenzie, William, 91, 92, 95
Mackintosh, Sir James, 89
Macnee, John, 10, 69, 76, 78
Macnish, Robert, 75
Macready, William Charles, 121
macroevolution, 11, 153
Maga Club, Edinburgh, 95
Magubane, Zine, 52
Makanda, *see* Nxele
Malcolm, Sir Charles, 130, 145
Marsden, William, 140, 158
Marshall, Tim, 166
Mavor, Osbourne Henry, *see* Bridie, James
McDougal, Helen, 67, 69, 71
McGrigor, Sir James, 42, 65, 86, 119
Meckel, Johann Friedrich, 107
Meckel-Serres law, 133
Medical Act (1858), 8, 158
Medical Circular, 141, 142
medical regulation, 6–7, 61, 89, 90–1, 92, 118, 120, 158, 169–70
Medical Times, ii, 105, 106, 107, 111, 116, 120, 122, 124, 128, 129, 140
Melbourne, William Lamb, 2nd Viscount, 91–3
Mercey, Frederic de, 164
microscopy, 96–7
Miller, Alexander, 65, 66
Miller, James, 109
Milne, David, 119

"missing link", 144, 145, 155
Mitchell, Mary, *see* Paterson, Mary
monogenism, 52–3, 129, 131–2
Monro, Alexander, *primus*, 25, 55
Monro, Alexander, *secundus*, 25, 27, 55
Monro, Alexander, *tertius*: lectures, 7, 25, 26, 62–3, 94, 95, 111, 112; writings, 25, 81; museum, 42, 51; career, 54, 55, 92, 99, 179; dissecting room, 66, 71, 91, 98; obtains bodies, 76, 97, 103, 107, 112
monsters, hopeful, 11, 153
Monthly Journal of Medical Science, 139
Murray, Lord, 114
Muséum d'Histoire naturelle, Paris, 44, 45
museums, anatomical, 2, 3, 4, 11, 36, 42, 48, 51–6, 64, 65, 69, 78, 85–6, 95, 102, 106, 115, 117–18, 136, 139, 141, 159, *see also named museums*

Napier, Edward Delaval Hungerford Elers, 161
Napier, Francis, 8th Lord, 15
Napoleon I of France, 3, 4, 15, 16, 30, 32, 43, 128, 164
Napoleonic wars, 14, 19, 27; *see also* Waterloo, battle of
natural selection, 5, 8, 148, 152, 153, 156–7, 200
Naturphilosophie, 23, 44, 47, 113, 132, 157
North, Christopher, *see* Wilson, John
Nxele, 37, 38

Oineromathic Society, 96
Oken, Lorenz, 23–4, 128, 137, 178
Old Surgeons' Hall, Edinburgh, 19, 61, 91, 93, 101, 102, 105
Oliphant, John, 149
orangutan, 106, 134, 135, 137, 155
Ord, John Walker, 65
organ transplantation, 172–4
Osborne, John Henry, 119–20, 141
Ostend, 31
Outram, Dorinda, 45
Owen, Richard: early career, 56, 136; anatomical studies, 80, 106; transcendental views, 136–8; on the Aztec children, 143–4; anti-evolutionist views, 155–6

Pae, David, 165
Paine, Thomas, 16
Paley, William, 22, 43
Paleyism (argument from design), 138
Paré, Ambroise, 74
Paris: anatomical training in, 1, 7, 25,

Index

42–50, 59, 61, 90–1; RK visits, 54, 56, 117; bodies obtained from, 107; Owen visits, 136
Partridge, Richard, 62, 76
Paterson, David, 67–71, 165
Paterson, Mary, 67–8, 72, 149–50, 162, 165, 168, 169, 172
Pattison, Granville Sharp, 87
penny dreadfuls, 161, 163
Phrenological Society, Edinburgh, 124
Pillans, James, 18
Pinkerton, John, 129
Pitt, William, the younger, 14
Plinian Society, Edinburgh, 57
Polygenism, 123, 131
Portland Street School of Medicine, Glasgow, 115
Potts, Laurence Holker, 21
Powell, Baden, 152
Powell, Sally, 163
preformation, 43, 154
Punch, 80, 134

Quain, Jones, 97, 101
Queen's College, Edinburgh, 107, 119–20
Queensberry, 6th Marquess of, 75
Quetelet, Adolphe, 124

radicalism, 3, 6, 13–16, 25, 29, 79, 87, 89, 117–18, 128, 137, 138, 157
Rae, Isobel, 9
Ranger (ship), 15
Redfield, James W., 143
Reform Bill, 88, 89
Rehbock, Philip F., 5
Reid, Francis, 119
Reid, John: RK's pupil, 57; RK's assistant, 93; career, 95, 97; accuses RK of plagiarism, 108, 109
Renshaw, Henry, 159, 160
Reynolds, George W. M., 79, 161–2
Richards, Evelleen, 2, 5, 128, 134, 137, 152, 153
Richardson, Sir Benjamin Ward, 159
Richardson, Ruth, 6, 71, 89
Richardson, William, 112
Roberton, John, 147, 149
Robertson, A., 92, 94, 101
Robinson, Sir John, 75
Robson, Dame Flora, 169
Roux, Joseph-Philibert, 49
Royal Academy, London, 123, 147
Royal College of Physicians, Edinburgh, 30
Royal College of Surgeons, Edinburgh, 2, 3, 22, 53–6, 61, 85, 91, 117, 120

Royal College of Surgeons, England, 27, 140–1
Royal Free Hospital, London, 140–1
Royal High School, Edinburgh, 16–18, 19
Royal Infirmary, Edinburgh, 19, 59, 91, 101, 103, 107, 108, 185
Royal Institution, Edinburgh, 87
Royal Institution, London, 72, 116
Royal Medical Society, Edinburgh, 95, 131
Royal Society of Edinburgh, 28, 54, 75, 85, 86, 100–1, 120–1
Ruskin, John, 146
Russell, Lord John, 97, 118
Russell, Margaret, 192

St Bartholomew's Hospital, 29, 142, 144
saltatory evolution, 8, 311, 319
San, 2, 36, 37, 38, 122, 155
Scherer, Archibald (RK's father-in-law), 14
Scherer, Mary (RK's mother), 14
Scott, Sir Walter, 71, 75
Scottish Academy, 109, 116, 146
Selkirk, Helen, Countess of, 15
sexual selection, 148
Sharpey, William, 92, 93, 94, 109
Shaw, George Bernard, 170
Shelley, Mary, 166
Shelley, Percy, 161
Sherriffs, E. B., 94
Sim, Alastair, 170
Simpson, James Y., 65
Sinclair, Sir George, 61, 187
Skidmore, Thomas, 117–18
Slater, George M., 170
Slaughter, Tod, 170, 171
slavery, 2–3, 37, 125, 127, 128–9, 180
smallpox, 14, 16, 106
Smyth, Thomas, 131
snakes, 36, 64
Society of Apothecaries, 61, 119–20
Somerset, Lord Charles Henry, 39–40
Somerset, Lord Fitzroy, 86
Somerset, Captain Henry, 40, 41
Somerville, James: on supply of bodies, 69, 76, 91–2; Inspector of Anatomy, 98, 101, 103–4, 107, 111
Son of Frankenstein (film), 166
species change, *see* evolution
Speer, Thomas Charlton, 19
Spence, James, 65
Spineto, Marquis, 72
Stanley, Lord, 114
Stark, John, 101
Stephen, Kathy, 9

Index

Stevenson, Robert Louis: *The Body Snatcher*, 150, 161, 167–9; *Dr Jekyll and Mr Hyde*, 167
Stockenström, Andries: Landrost of Graaf Reinet, 37–8; quarrel with Knox, 38–40, 52
Stockenström, O. G., 38–41
Struthers, Sir John, 9, 112, 115
Syme, James: 27, 55, 61, 85–6, 99, 100, 101, 116
syphilis, 32

Taylor, Donald, 172
The Times, 1, 36, 76, 143, 170, 173
Thibert, Felix: museum, 117–18, 139
Thomas, Dylan, 172
Thomson, Allen, 96, 109
Thomson, John, 99–100, 109
Thomson, William, 100
"tiger arm", 112–13, 133, 145
Todd, Sweeney, 80, 170
Town Yetholm, 64
Traill, T. S., 85, 99, 101
transcendental anatomy, 4–5, 7, 8, 10, 23–4, 25, 44, 46, 63, 65, 102, 105, 112–13, 126, 130, 132, 136, 137, 139–40, 145–6, 148, 151, 152–4, 156–7, 159
Tyrell, Frederick, 58

Unity of plan, 4–5, 23–4, 46, 87, 133–5, 156
Université de France, 44
University College London, 65, 97, 101

Venus, 147–9, 151
Vesalius, Andreas, 74
Vestiges of the Natural History of Creation, 138, 140, 153
Victoria, Queen, 158
vivisection, 3, 27, 29, 82–3, 169, 172
Voltaire (François-Marie Arouet), 21
Voyer, Marquise de, 43

Wakley, Thomas, 119–20
Wakley, Thomas Henry, 140–1
Walker, Alexander, 148
Wallace, Alfred Russel, 129, 152, 156
Warburton, Henry, 89–90
Ward, Alexander, 105
Warren, James L., 119
Waterloo, battle of, 30–1, 160
Watson, Alexander, 54
waxworks, anatomical, 8, 117, 149; see also anatomical models
Weber, Ernest Henry, 108
Wells, Thomas Spencer, 158
Werner, Abraham, 42
Wernerian Natural History Society, 42, 51, 53, 65, 136
West Port murders: 7, 9, 10, 65, 66–77, 78, 80, 81, 82, 83, 86, 88, 89, 100, 141; in fiction, 163–9, 171
whales, anatomy of, 51, 85, 86–7, 114
Whelpdale, Andrew, 96
White, Charles, 123, 195
White, Frederick John, 119–20
Whitechapel murders, 168
Williams, Thomas, 76
Willshire, Thomas, 37
Wilson, James, 68
Wilson, John, 73–4
Wilsone, W. Syme (RK's son-in-law), 53, 116
Wishart, John Henry, 56
Wolves of Tanner's Close, The (play), 170
Wood, Alexander, 13
workhouses, 59, 89, 103–4
Wright, Thomas Giordani, 57, 74, 75
Wright, William, 142

Xhosa, 33, 36–8, 49, 59

Zoological Society, London, 136
Zoologist, The, 152, 156
Zulu, 36

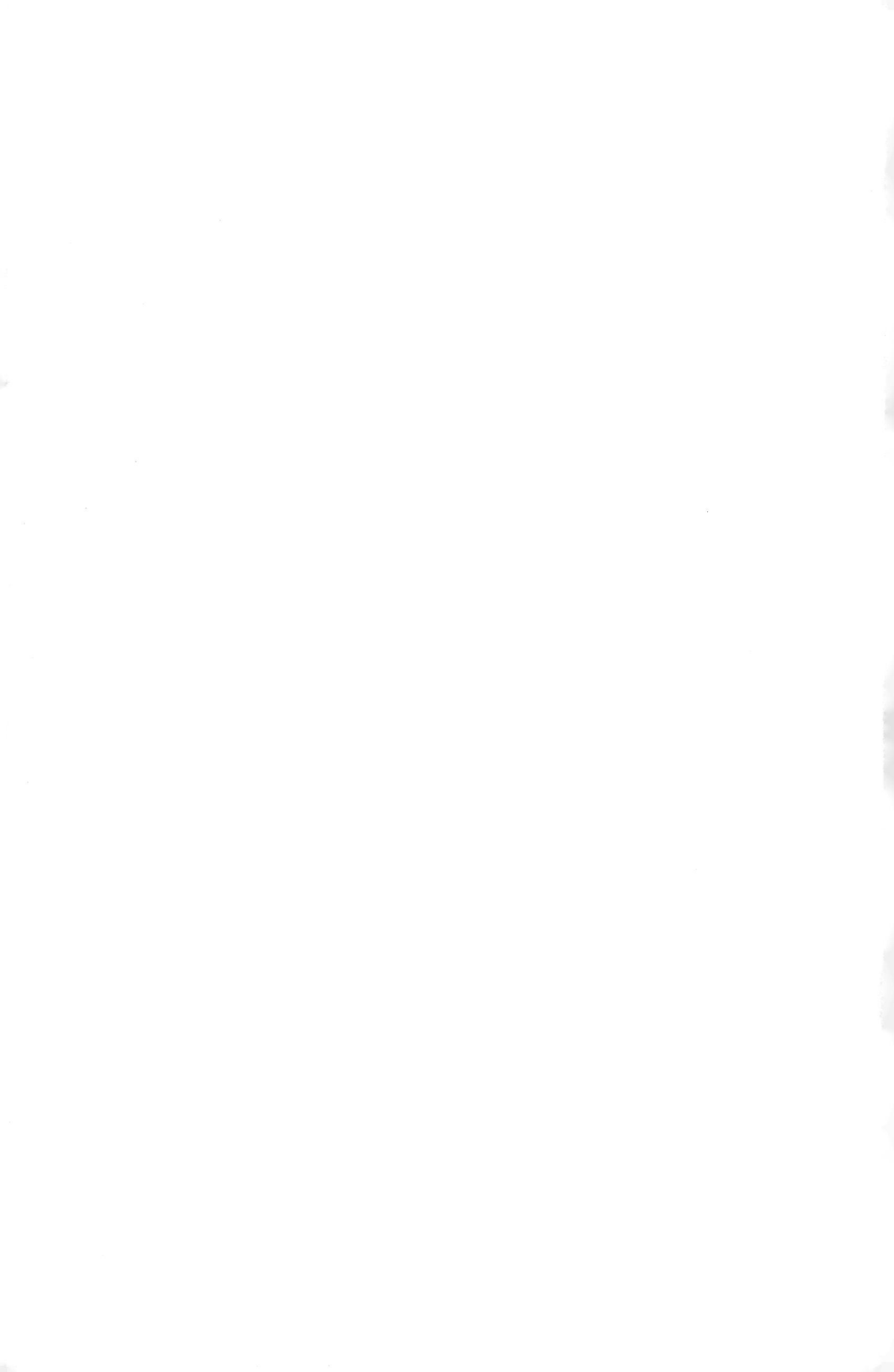